THE SENILE BRAIN

A Clinical Study

BY

R. S. ALLISON
V.R.D., M.D., F.R.C.P., D.P.M.

Senior Physician, Neurological Department
Royal Victoria Hospital, Belfast

LONDON
EDWARD ARNOLD (PUBLISHERS) LTD

First published 1962

Printed in Great Britain at the Villafield Press
Bishopbriggs, Glasgow

PREFACE

THIS work is principally a record of personal experience. It was begun 20 years ago and since then has been greatly stimulated by realization of the possibilities there are for extension of purely clinical methods of investigation in the field of organic brain disease, especially in later life.

The poet Robert Browning encouraged the youth of his day not to fear growing old because, as he said, the best was yet to be. This may well be true in the psychological sense but in the physiological it is probable, as the seventeenth century Bishop Hough is claimed to have remarked:[3] " Whatever may be said in favour of it, old age is a losing game ". Part of the purpose of the book is to focus attention upon ways and means of ensuring that points in the game are not given away unnecessarily.

Theoretical aspects of the subject have probably not been given the attention that is their due and there are many omissions, the lack of which will be apparent to the informed reader. But the relationship existing between the cortex, diencephalon and upper brain stem is still undecided, and in the cortical realm of function the views held by protagonists of the old schools are being criticized by the experimental psychologist, who seeks to delineate some factor or factors in brain injured persons which may influence and determine the varied disturbances of intellectual function shown by them. It is for these reasons that the aim has been to make the book primarily descriptive and to concentrate on details of clinical observations made in individual cases.

I have had much help and encouragement from Dr. Macdonald Critchley, through whose kindness I had the privilege of working at the National Hospital, Queen Square, and Institute of Neurology in 1953. I am deeply indebted also to Dr. J. H. D. Millar, Dr. G. F. Adams, Dr. G. J. C. Dawson, and Dr. L. J. Hurwitz for their helpful criticism. Also to Dr. H. H. Stewart, Mr. A. R. Taylor, Mr. C. A. Gleadhill, and Mr. D. S. Gordon for allowing access to some patients under their care and for permitting details of their cases to be included in the text.

Grateful acknowledgments are also due to Surgeon Captain J. G. Danson, (R.N., Retired), and to the late Dr. K. Sax for their assistance in translation of some references in the German literature, and to

Dr. G. Johnston, S. H. O. in the Neurological Department, for his help in assisting with proof reading and other details. It is a pleasure also to acknowledge the invaluable assistance given by my wife and Mrs. E. O. Russell, Secretary, in helping to compile records and in the typing of the manuscript.

GREENWOOD,
  MARINO,
  CO. DOWN.

CONTENTS

Introduction   I

Chapter   I   Case-taking in organic mental states   7

   II   General physical examination   27

   III   Neurological examination   42

   IV   Organic mental testing   66

   V   Acute disturbances of consciousness   93

   VI   Chronic amnesic syndromes   111

   VII   Disorders of speech and language   132

   VIII   Disorders of speech and language   156

   IX   Disorientation   173

   X   Agnosia and apraxia   202

   XI   Differential diagnosis: psychoneurosis and affective disorders; focal from diffuse cerebral lesions.   221

   XII   Treatment   261

   Index   283

Introduction

HUMAN life expectancy has materially improved in the past fifty years. The population of Great Britain " is today larger by ten millions, and of the fifty millions in this country now no fewer than seven millions are over 60 years of age ". So wrote Thomson[1] in 1949, and as Medawar[2] suggests, it may be that the shift in the age spectrum of the population towards senescence will lead in time to " at least a numerical tyranny of greybeards ". The discovery of antibiotics has taken away the deadly risk attached to pneumonia, once described by Charcot as " that great enemy of old people ", and in another sense by Osler as " the friend of the aged ".[3] But other dangers beset persons in later life and not the least of these is premature intellectual decline, which it has been forecasted may be the chief source of admissions to mental hospitals in the future.[4] In middle-aged and elderly people its approach is often signalled by impairment of memory, loss of initiative or drive or apparently inexplicable behaviour. It is undesirable, however, that these symptoms should invariably be construed as indicative of " presenile dementia ", for such has been the change in attitude to the subject in recent years that, without proper investigation, the label is no more justified than would be a diagnosis of " chronic bronchitis ", made solely on the presence of cough and sputum. Not only may focal cerebral lesions due to vascular accidents or tumours mimic the diffuse cerebral cortical atrophy of true presenile dementia in giving rise to superficially alike clinical pictures, but the brain may not primarily be affected, the symptoms of intellectual decline being secondary to toxic or metabolic disturbances arising as the result of disease in other organs. The possibility, too, of apparent decline being related purely to an affective disorder has also to be taken into account.

The concept of presenile dementia is attributed to Binswanger (1898), " presenile " (used in the temporal sense) referring to the tendency of symptoms to develop between the ages of 40–60 and " dementia " simply implying impairment of memory and intellect.[5] Between 1892–

1

1908 Arnold Pick[6] contributed several papers to the literature on the curious form of presenile cerebral cortical atrophy, which now bears his name. This affects grey and white matter of both hemispheres and often has a focal and clear-cut distribution, frontal or temporal lobes or both being most commonly involved. Although accepted as a cause of presenile dementia this disease is rare and considerably more so than its counterpart, which was first described by Alois Alzheimer[7] and is characterized by diffuse cortical atrophy, the presence of senile plaques and changes in the intracellular neurofibrils. The rôle of atheroma and arteriosclerosis in the genesis of dementia in old people was recognized principally by Marcé (1863), but Claude and Lhermitte[8] state that Campbell in England also emphasized the connection. However, although it was known that intellectual deterioration occurred in other brain diseases, including general paralysis of the insane and Huntington's chorea, until thrity years ago interest centred chiefly around clinical means of differentiating between Alzheimer's and Pick's diseases. The publication of Macdonald Critchley's lectures on " The Neurology of Old Age "[9] stimulated renewed interest in the presenile dementias, and since then the concept has been broadened and endowed more with generic than specific status. Points of similarity have been recognized between conditions once thought to be separate entities, as, for example, between so-called " carbon monoxide poisoning " and hypoxia or anoxia, and attention has been focused more on aetiology. This work has been helped by advances in neurosurgery and modern methods of investigation by contrast radiography, electroencephalography and biochemistry. It has been recognized for some time that both Pick's and Alzheimer's diseases, although probably less rare than is sometimes thought, account for only a small proportion of cases of presenile intellectual deterioration: in a recent series of cases in women the proportion was 6%.[10] Much more common are cerebral vascular disease, post-anoxic effects, cerebral tumour and trauma, which together with neurosyphilis, Alzheimer's and Pick's diseases comprise the etiology of the great majority of cases.

Indeed, the time may have come when the term " dementia ", so closely identified as it is on the clinical side with irreversible and progressive cerebral changes, may be discarded except in such instances as investigations have shown its use to be justified. In its place and certainly more appropriate for yet undiagnosed cases is the term " organic mental state ", which if less euphonic is not so sinister in its connotation and appears to be coming into more general use. It emphasizes a principle which is often overlooked, namely that as a rule memory impairment and disturbances in behaviour in later life have an organic basis, and that in some cases at least, if the cause can be promptly recognized and treated, symptoms may be reversible. In favour, too, of an alternative designation it may be said that in some cases, e.g. post-traumatic, post-anoxic, there may be no progressive deterioration, or treatment may lead to its arrest, as in general paralysis and certain cases of chronic subdural haematoma or tumour. Even when no treatment is available and deterioration is progressive, provided care is taken to avoid acute confusional episodes, only a proportion develop delusions, hallucinations and other frank expressions of psychosis, many remaining in a more or less static condition for years until their lives are mercifully ended by a stroke or sudden heart failure from coronary occlusion.

The purpose of this work is to review the early symptoms and signs of intellectual decline, especially as they occur in later life, to describe appropriate methods of clinical examination and to discuss causes in relation to their differential diagnosis and treatment. It is unfortunate that the subject should lie in a sort of no man's land between psychiatry and neurology because the psychiatrist may not be asked to see patients until they have reached an advanced state of deterioration. On the other hand, the neurologist and neurosurgeon in dealing with focal cerebral lesions, usually pay more regard to physical than to mental aspects of their cases. This does not apply, of course, to speech and language disorders or to certain other aspects of agnosia and apraxia. But their approach is influenced by the traditional mosaic theory of cerebral function so that with focal circumscribed lesions they expect only selective intellectual defects, the characteristics and extent of which have not always been correlated with more general aspects of intellectual function and behaviour. In the absence of gross evidence to the contrary it has been tacitly accepted that intellectual function in general is undisturbed. *Per contra*, when signs of intellectual deterioration have appeared to be disproportionately great it has been assumed that the results of mental testing must of necessity be discounted.

Recent monographs on the organic mental states to which we have referred include those of Bini,[11] Klein[12] and Mayer Gross, Dewan and Spaulding.[13] The subject is of great potential interest, as it opens up possibilities for extension of orthodox medical casetaking procedures into a field as yet little disturbed by the modern clinician, although bearing in its soil the footprints made by Arnold Pick and other early observers.

The clinical material forming the basis of this review consists of 198 patients practically all of whom were seen initially in neurological outpatients or in consultation with colleagues at the Royal Victoria and Claremont Street Hospitals, Belfast, between the years 1946–1959.* The figure represents an average of about one case per month over the thirteen years' period. In accepting cases for particular study two principal criteria were used:

1. The chief, presenting features should point to impairment of memory and intellect. Disturbances of mood and behaviour were often seen in conjunction, but it was not considered necessary that there should be physical signs of organic neurological disease; many patients indeed had no such signs.

2. Patients recovering from cerebral vascular accidents, cerebral trauma or anoxia, or suspected of having a space-occupying intracranial lesions, were accepted, but it was essential for their inclusion that they should exhibit persistent signs of mental disorder, the latter in many instances being more difficult to manage than the physical aspects of their disability.

All patients, if not already in hospital, were admitted with a view to further observation and investigation, the duration of their stay extending over several weeks and many being brought back subsequently for review at intervals over a period of some years. In several instances, either through the results of surgical operation or autopsy, it was possible to correlate the pathological findings with the clinical features, and in those cases in which more immediate confirmation was denied the outcome was often rendered apparent by follow-up procedures.

Table 1 shows the age and sex distribution of these cases. Although

TABLE 1.—*Age and Sex Distribution of Patients with Organic Mental States*

Age when first seen	Males	Females	Total
under 40	10	3	13
41–45	7	6	13
46–50	14	17	31
51–55	19	15	34
56–60	24	14	38
61–65	26	8	34
66–70	13	11	24
over 70	7	4	11

* The exceptions were 5 pensioners seen originally during the second world war and 16 other patients examined in the National Hospital, Queen Square, during a period of study leave in 1953.

the prevalence is seen to rise steadily until the age of 60 and thereafter to dwindle, significance should not be attributed to this as geriatric services in Belfast are well organized and it is probable we were dealing only with a fraction of the total material available, many patients over the age of 60 being referred to the other centres directly. There were 120 men and 78 women, the proportion of the former being greater in all age groups except 46–50. Table 2 shows the pathogenesis. For various reasons in only a proportion of the cases was a firm diagnosis

TABLE 2.—*Pathogenesis in 198 Organic Mental Cases*

Cerebral tumour (44)

Cerebral vascular accidents or " Strokes " (43)

Chronic presenile dementia due to arteriosclerosis, atherosclerosis, Alzheimer's, Pick's diseases or unknown causes (38)

Post-anoxic encephalopathies and chronic amnesic states (17)

General paralysis of the insane (13)

Affective disorders with minimal evidence of organic mental changes (13)

Chronic subdural haematoma (8)

Post-traumatic encephalopathies (8)

Huntington's chorea (5)

Parkinsonism and chronic arteriosclerotic dementia (? Jakob Creutzfeld disease) (4)

Hepatic encephalopathy (3)

Subacute encephalitis of unknown causation (1)

Chronic insulin hypoglycaemia in a diabetic (1)

reached during life or confirmed after death. In a substantial number the cause eluded recognition. Further, it would not be fair to suggest that the known causes in this particular series of cases are representative of the etiological pattern of organic mental disease states as a whole. The number of cases attributed to cerebral anoxia, for example, may appear to be an overestimate and the high proportion of patients with cerebral tumour is probably only an expression of the fact that the neurosurgical and neurological departments at our hospital occupy the same building and that there is close liaison between them. It is readily conceded, too, that the low proportion of affective disorders and psychoneurosis is quite unrepresentative of the extent to which these conditions may be responsible for mental illness in old people. Thus, O'Connell[14] who investigated a number of mental patients aged 65 or over, found a depressive syndrome in more than one-quarter, delusions of guilt and unworthiness, paranoid and hypochondriacal complaints colouring their depression and there being no evidence of intellectual deterioration. Their comparative absence in this series is intentional because only " mental diseases which have a cerebral pathology " Bleuler,[15] were considered. The few cases referred to have been included because of the difficulty there was in ruling out an organic mental state.

BIBLIOGRAPHY

1   THOMSON, A. P. (1949). Problems of ageing and chronic sickness. *Brit. Med. J.*, **2**, 243.
2   MEDAWAR, P. B. (1958). Old age and natural death. In " The Uniqueness of the Individual ". Methuen, London. Quoted by Zuckerman, Sir Solly in *Radio Times*, Nov. 13, 1959.
3   ROLLESTON, Sir Humphry (1932). " Medical Aspects of Old Age." Macmillan, London.
4   LEWIS, A. (1946). Ageing and senility. A major problem of psychiatry. *J. ment. Sci.*, **92**, 150.
5   MAYER-GROSS, W. (1938). Discussion on the presenile dementias. *Proc. Roy. Soc. Med.*, **31**, 1443.
6   PICK, A. (1901). Hirnatrophie als Grundlage von Herderscheinungen. *Wien. klin. Wsch.*, **17**.
7   ALZHEIMER, A. (1907). Über eine eigenartige Erkrankung der Hirnrinde. *Zbl. ges. Neurol. Psychiat.*, **18**, 177.
8   CLAUDE, H. and LHERMITTE, J. (1910). De certains états psychopathiques des veillards liés à la sclerose et à l'atrophie du cortex cérébral. *Encéphale*, **5**, 177.
9   CRITCHLEY, M. (1931). The neurology of old age. *Lancet*, **1**, 1333.
10 ROBERTSON, E. E. and MASON BROWN, N. L. (1953). Review of mental illness in the older age group. *Brit. Med. J.*, **2**, 1076.
11 BINI, L. (1953). " Le Demenze Presenile ". Rome.
12 KLEIN, R. and MAYER-GROSS, W. (1957). " The Clinical Examination of Patients with Organic Cerebral Disease." London.
13 DEWAN, J. G. and SPAULDING, W. B. (1958). " The Organic Psychosis." University Press, Toronto.
14 O'CONNELL, B. A. (1954). Psychiatric illness in the elderly. A follow-up study. *Brit. Med. J.*, **2**, 1206.
15 BLEULER, M. (1951). Psychiatry of cerebral diseases. *Brit. Med. J.*, **2**, 1233.

CHAPTER I

Case-taking in Organic Mental States

BASICALLY the same clinical methods are used in the examination of organic mental states as in other conditions but a different kind of approach is required because of the difficulty in getting these patients to give an adequate account of their symptoms. This difficulty may be due to a number of causes: inability to express themselves; impairment of memory; genuine loss of insight; desire to conceal the fact that they are unwell; the presence of accompanying severe emotional disturbances. In most cases two or more of these causes are acting in concert. Some examples may be given.

The first occurred some years ago on a ward round with students. The patient, a farmer aged 56, with a left fronto-temporal chronic subdural haematoma, had been admitted the day before with a three-week history of "behaving peculiarly and neglecting his work" and of increasing weakness of the right arm. He lay propped-up in bed with pillows, his left arm behind his head, his right lying immobile on the counterpane. Despite the fact that the bedclothes were freshly soaked with urine he appeared to be unaware of the fact or if aware in no discomfort. Occasionally he would yawn or rub his nose and at times his gaze might be distracted by someone passing through the ward, but, otherwise, he said nothing and stared at his visitors with indifference. A student was invited to question him and the following dialogue ensued:

Student: " What do you feel wrong, Mr. M.?"

Patient: " Eh?"

Student (speaking with more emphasis): " What do you feel is wrong with you? What are you complaining of?"

Patient (rubs his nose again and passes the palm of his hand over his face): ". . . eh?"

Student: " Can you hear me?"

Patient: " Ay, I can hear you all right!"

Student: " Have you any pain?"

Patient (with apparent interest): ". . . yes . . . yes . . . pain in the appendix " (fumbles with the bedclothes, pulling them down and points to the left lower abdomen) ". . . here!"

Student (putting a hand on the abdomen at the site indicated): " Is this where you have the pain?"

Patient: " No . . . further up." (Points now to his right breast and yawns disinterestedly.)

Notable points in this case were the patient's unconcern, the urinary incontinence, yawning, rubbing the nose and his suggestibility which was brought out by the question about pain, this apparently determining the form taken by his confabulation. There was, of course, no question of his having any abdominal lesion.

A second case was that of a retired soldier, aged 62, whose mental state in the three years following the first interview slowly progressed to one of global dementia. However, when first seen neither his appearance nor his behaviour suggested anything very unusual and it was only on questioning him that memory and speech difficulties became apparent. Neatly dressed and preserving much of his military bearing, he exchanged greetings very naturally and engaged readily in " small talk " about the weather. But instead of accepting a chair as his wife had done he remained standing, looking about him uncertainly. Then he asked if he might remove his overcoat and having done so proceeded to fold it carefully and place it on a nearby vacant chair.

The doctor's letter had mentioned headaches, failing memory and difficulty in finding the way out of doors, so the interview proceeded:

Examiner: " Tell me about yourself, Colonel . . . I understand you have not been well?"

Patient (leans forward, knitting his brows): ". . . well doctor . . . eh . . . ah . . . yes, that's it . . . I've . . . I have no desire to do the things I used to do . . . you know . . . no pep . . . if I try . . . I . . . I . . . ah . . . get irritated."

Examiner: " Yes, I understand . . . tell me more about it!"

Patient (looks embarrassed and turns to his wife. She prompts him to mention the headache): ". . . oh, yes . . . over the left eye . . . here (pointing) and it goes down into the left shoulder."

Examiner: " Yes . . . tell me what else bothers you?"

Patient (more embarrassed, clasps his hands): ". . . I . . . I . . . well . . . no (laughs shortly) . . . well I suppose it's just the lack of interest!"

Later the subject was changed to fishing in which sport the patient had previously been expert and much interested:

Examiner: " Where did you fish in the old days?"

Patient: " Well, I did a lot of ground . . . so . . . what I mean is . . . in the County Antrim . . . whenever I go anywhere I fish wherever I can . . . I was up in North Russia fishing . . . when was that? . . . I . . . I'm afraid I can't remember . . . some time ago."

In this case " small talk " was well-preserved as were also the niceties of behaviour, but there was unexpected orderliness in the care taken to fold the coat. His wife said she had noticed this characteristic

T.S.B.

in recent years although previously he had not been a " fussy " person. His talk was disjointed and ungrammatical and despite his obvious efforts to concentrate he had great difficulty in expressing himself. However, it was noticeable that he did better when discussing fishing.

In these two instances there was either incongruous behaviour or expressive speech defects with memory impairment, but in many other organic mental patients not showing these features, one might have been tempted into thinking relatives' stories were exaggerated on account of the patient's air of self-possession, facile talk and ready answers. If the mistake was made of expressing doubt as to the plausability of their answers some patients became truculent so that the interview was only prevented with difficulty from ending stormily through one or both parties losing their tempers. This was one kind of difficulty encountered; another was that if an attempt were made to take the history systematically by asking a series of questions about shortness of breath, dyspepsia, headache, etc., the patient might follow these leads and recite a whole train of symptoms, the inconsistence of which would create the false impression that one was dealing with a neurotic. Such behaviour might have been related to loss of insight but was more often the expression of a desire to divert attention from the real difficulties, or to pretend that they did not exist.

Another problem arose in patients showing pronounced emotional disturbances from whom it was impossible often to get any satisfactory statement. Some wore an air of unconcern although at the same time adopting a watchful or wary attitude as would a witness in court. Questions were answered as briefly as possible, the patient never proffering information and conveying the impression that he was suspicious or fearful of being trapped into making some unguarded admission. At the opposite extreme was the patient who was most willing to co-operate but whose obvious anxiety and emotional tension was so great as to lead one to suspect the possibility of an underlying depressive state. An example of the last kind was a business manager, aged 55, in whom neurological examination subsequently revealed papilloedema and a right-sided visual field defect. At operation a left temporo-parietal astrocytoma was found. His main complaint was of headache, which had been steadily increasing in intensity over the preceding three years.

Its chief effect, he said, had been to make him feel depressed and his tense, worried expression and repeated tendency to sigh throughout the interview bore out his words. He pointed to his head to indicate the site of the pain and imitated its crushing, severe character by gesticulation, at the same time re-iterating that he wished to be truthful and not make it out to be worse than it

actually was. Then he burst into tears and wept uncontrollably, trembling
with emotion. When he had recovered from this outburst he admitted a fear
that his power of concentration might become so bad that he could no longer
continue at his work. His memory had been failing; he was not eating and
had lost weight, and at night he could not sleep for the pain. He denied any
other worries, had no ideas of reference, of personal unworthiness or suicidal
intent. His son said that his father had always been a most conscientious type
of man and that there had not been any previous nervous breakdowns.

Kurt Goldstein,[16] whose pioneer studies into the behaviour of brain-
injured subjects has done much to unravel the tangle that formerly
surrounded this subject, notes that " the characteristic difference
between the older and more recent orientation in psychopathology is
that the former regarded the observable symptoms simply as manifestations of changes in different functions or structures, whereas in the
new approach many symptoms are seen as expressions of the change
which the patient's personality as a whole undergoes as a result of
disease, and also as expressions of the struggle of the changed personality to cope with the defect and with demands it can no longer meet ".
Among these symptoms are changes in mood; curious reactions on the
part of the patient to what Goldstein refers to as " catastrophic situations "; variability in performance, and evasions of different kinds.
In his view variations in performance are not simply due to disturbance
in the patient's capacity for sustained attention or interest " becaue it
has never been possible to demonstrate the independent existence of
these supposed disturbances. Painstaking observation, as a matter of
fact, discloses that attention, interest, memory, fatigue, etc., vary quite
as the performances vary. They are sometimes good, sometimes bad.
. . . The clue can be found through careful observation of the patient's
behaviour as a whole, in the light of tasks which he performs and those
in which he fails ".

Some of these symptoms have already been referred to in the case
illustrations given but they may now be considered in more detail.

Changes in mood.

The mood or prevailing emotional state displayed by a patient with
disturbed brain function depends on three principal factors: the extent
of clouding of consciousness, if any is present; his previous personality
and temperament; and the kind of situation with which he is faced.
In clouding of consciousness, delirium is associated with angry, aggressive or hostile moods or expansiveness and elation. In disorientation
the mood is usually placid and unconcerned. Until " full " consciousness is regained it is often uninhibited and usually not altogether
appropriate to the situation (see chapter V). Previous personality and

temperament also colour the mood, lively and sociable characters often retaining these qualities despite considerable intellectual impairment and memory loss. Organic brain disease may have the effect of throwing into greater prominence former hysterical or obsessional characteristics, over-conscientiousness, undue sensitiveness, tendencies to worry or to paranoid thinking. These contribute towards one patient's casual air of unconcern so that his mood resembles " la belle indifférence " of the hysteric, and to another's exaggerated sense of distress at his condition or the length to which he will go to conceal it. Next in importance to previous personality and temperament is the extent of intellectual impairment. This influences mood and behaviour very considerably, accounting for the many swings in one direction or another that may be observed in the course of a single day. Thus, as a rule, when faced with a task of peculiar difficulty, many of our patients responded either by over-reacting, when they might become anxious or aggressive, by under-reacting when they became sullen or made facile excuses for their failure, or by pretending that the problem presented no difficulty and brazening-out their mistakes. The same patients, however, were animated, pleased and interested in what they were doing when the activity upon which they were engaged presented no especial difficulty.

Catastrophic reactions.

These may appear suddenly without warning although more often indications of their near approach are signalled by increasing anxiety or tension. The catastrophic reaction occurs when the patient becomes acutely aware of his inability to perform a task, and it is the very antithesis of hysterical indifference or benign acceptance of disease.[16] In the reaction as described by Goldstein[17], the patient " looks dazed, changes colour, becomes agitated, anxious, starts to fumble; a moment before amiable, he is now sullen, evasive, exhibits temper, or even becomes aggressive. It takes some time before it is possible to continue the examination ". Afterwards the patient may express concern for having behaved in this way although he will usually have no clear idea why he did so.

Variability in performance.

This is as characteristic of organic mental states as are catastrophic reactions and mood changes. Thus, in one of our patients, a man who was subsequently found to have a right parietal astrocytoma, there was evidence of cortical sensory loss in the contralateral hand so that the nature of objects placed therein could not be recognized by touch alone.

When he was admitted to hospital and tests were repeated variable responses were obtained, on some days the patient exhibiting absolute astereognosis and on other days not. His suggestibility also seemed to be increased and as an electroencephalogram and lumbar encephalography had yielded negative results, for a time he was thought to be hysteric. Even in every-day activities, as the nurses' records show, the performance of patients with organic brain disease varies greatly. One day they may exhibit a dressing dyspraxia which cannot be demonstrated on the next or urinary incontinence on one day and not on another. Undoubtedly performance is influenced to some extent by psychological factors, objects in the environment owing their significance to a large extent to the setting in which they are placed,[18] and the attitude of the doctor, nurses and others in attendance do much to determine its character. It also varies in respect to the type of activity in which the patient is engaged, affective influences playing a considerable part. As has been seen, the retired soldier illustrated this point for he did better when talking about his fishing than when trying to describe his disabilities.

Stratagems and evasions.

In contrast to the psychoneurotic, who tries to impress the examiner with the severity of his ailments, the brain-injured patient is usually at pains to conceal his disabilities and this attitude leads to the elaboration of characteristic stratagems, denials and evasions. Thus, if one asks a patient whose memory is affected to give the names of reigning monarchs or prime ministers in recent years he will declare that he had never been interested in such matters or paid any attention to them. If given a sum to do, he may point out that it is a long time since he was at school. Shown a picture, he may plead that he cannot find his glasses, or, if these are produced, that for some time he had been considering having them changed. One man, whose difficulty in registering a name and address had been demonstrated some days previously, must have made a point of learning it by heart because at each subsequent ward round he would repeat it triumphantly to the embarrassment of some of us who had forgotten the details. Other patients were observed practising tests surreptitiously in the performance of which they had failed previously and those with unilateral astereognosis would often make use of their good hand to identify objects. Patients with defective memories or defects in spatial orientation often became excessively orderly in the manner in which they arranged their personal belongings and were greatly perturbed when anyone upset these arrangements by moving objects out of their fixed place. The retired soldier's concern over his overcoat illustrated this tendency, the object of which was to enable him to find it promptly and to put it on when the time came for departure. When these patients deteriorated still further so that they forgot where they had put things, their tendency was to excuse themselves by suggesting that someone must have stolen the object in question or deliberately hidden it. One could multiply such examples almost indefinitely. Dysphasic difficulties were usually found to be responsible for the habitual silence of many organic mental patients. But they attempted to conceal their defects by " sitting-in " on conversations between other patients, nodding their heads and expressing other signs of would-be appreciation of what was being said. Filibustering tactics, by which they attempted to dominate a discussion and so prevent awkward personal questions being asked, were much less commonly seen.

PROCEDURE ON EXAMINATION

Different methods of case-taking were tried over the years to meet the difficulties in patients with organic mental states and the one adopted, as will be seen, is a combination of the neurological and psychiatric approach, certain points of the latter discipline having been introduced to supplement the former. Whatever method is adopted in case-taking, however, *the cardinal principle is to ensure that the notes provide as much detail of the patient's appearance and behaviour during the interview as they do of the symptoms of which he complains.* Examination may be divided into four stages:

1. Patient's statement, appearance and behaviour.
2. Statements of relatives and friends.
3. Physical examination.
4. Mental testing (usually conducted at subsequent interviews).

Patient's statement, appearance and behaviour.

First impressions being important the medical student should be taught to study his patient objectively, attention being paid especially to the following points:

Dress.

Is this neat or untidy? Is there evidence of carelessness in fastening neckties or buttons? What is the state of personal cleanliness, i.e., is this in keeping with the patient's situation? Has he any difficulty in dressing or undressing himself? In shaving does he tend to neglect one half of the face?

Appearance.

Is his appearance unremarkable or unusual in the sense that he looks anxious, depressed,* apathetic, unconcerned, sullen, suspicious or over-confident.

Behaviour.

Is this appropriate to the occasion or not? Does he show increased emotional lability and, if so, whether towards laughter or tears? Does he tend to joke or make " wise-cracks "? Can his interest be held or is it readily diverted by chance stimuli? Does he appear to be indifferent to his surroundings, cautious or wary, liable to take offence, or anxious to create a good impression?

Talk.

Is he capable of " small talk " about the weather, etc.? Does he remain silent unless spoken to? Are questions referred to the person accompanying him or does he quote from notes made on pieces of paper? Is gesture much used? Does he show any tendency to perseveration? (See p. 100.) Are statements made hesitatingly or does he break off in the middle of a sentence? Does he have difficulty in finding the right word or tend to be prolix, irrelevant or circumstantial in his talk?

Thought content.

Does he recognize that he is not well or deny illness and protest against being examined? Does he take a serious or light-hearted view of his case? What explanations does he offer for his symptoms: does he blame himself, other people or some circumstance in his environment?

Needless to say the above list is incomplete and, indeed, it is neither possible nor desirable to draw up a series of questions that would cover all eventualities and enable an examiner to record the results of his examination in the form of ticks and crosses. After trying to put the patient at ease by some preliminary remarks about where he lives, mutual acquaintances or his journey to town, one should ask: " What do you feel wrong?" or " I understand you have not been well—perhaps you would like to tell me about it?" and then allow him to proceed on his own, prompting him to continue only when necessary and avoiding leading questions. If one can conduct the interview

---

* Charles Darwin's[19] illustration will be recalled, " A party of natives in Tierra del Fuego endeavoured to explain to us that their friend, the captain of a sailing vessel, was out of spirits, by pulling down their cheeks with both hands, so as to make their faces as long as possible."

without making notes so much the better, but it is often desirable to jot down fragments of conversation, although such notes must be made as inconspicuously as possible. Later, if necessary, they can be elaborated, significant points relating to appearance and behaviour inserted in parenthesis and actual statements quoted verbatim.

Statement of relatives and friends.

This part of the examination should be conducted separately and, if possible, two or more persons who have known the patient well should be interviewed. Surprising as it may seem, relatives sometimes appear to be unaware that there is anything seriously wrong with the patient's intellectual functions or memory, being more inclined to attribute any unusual behaviour to worry or to assume that failing memory is something that may be expected to occur naturally between the ages of 50–60. Not infrequently, relatives would claim that the patient had " never had a good memory ", and however plausible their reasoning might be to explain aberrations of behaviour one had the impression that their reaction was determined through a misplaced sense of loyalty, or through a desire to defend themselves against any possible criticism of neglect. However, as is well known, persons who live together often fail to note changes in each other that would at once be apparent to a stranger and too much need not be made of the point except to indicate how important it is to gain the relatives' confidence first, if any worth-while information is to be obtained by talking to them.

In this connection the observations of Wolff and Chapman[20] are of interest. They reviewed the mental states in a series of patients who had been operated upon for circumscribed brain tumours or arterio-venous anomalies and found that, although the site of damage in the cerebral hemisphere was important as regards its effect on sensory and motor function and speech, the form and extent of impairment of highest integrative functions were independent of the site or nature of the lesion. When the amounts of brain tissue removed at operation (30–150 g.) were compared with the extent of deterioration, a curve plotted from the data suggested that there was a logarithmic relationship between them. For example, the excision of 30–60 g. of cerebral hemisphere tissue led only to slight departures from the normal (reduction in the patient's versatility and his capacity to maintain function under stress, loss of spontaneity or " sparkle " and diminished drive or initiative). Such patients complained of feeling tired and found learning new skills too fatiguing. They talked less and were " slow on the uptake ". They were less interested in social activities and more easily frustrated and made angry. They tried to do one thing at a time and preferred familiar activities, shunning anything that was strange or novel and limiting their actions to a routine that was well within their capacities. The removal of greater amounts of brain substance led to more apparent defects, but it was only after the removal of 90–120 g. that other members of the patient's family, friends or fellow employees recognized that something was " radically wrong ".

These points should be taken into consideration therefore, in trying to establish from relatives the probable duration of symptoms of intellectual decline. Once they understand how they can help they may be able to recall episodes that occurred some years before the onset of more definite and overt symptoms. Thus, in the case of a woman aged 54 with arteriosclerotic dementia in whom it was alleged symptoms had only been of six months' duration, her son was able to recall an incident some four years previously that probably had a bearing on her subsequent state. On this occasion he and his wife had been invited to dinner at his mother's, but when they sat down to table it was discovered she had forgotten to cook the meat although she had prepared a special sauce to which he was very partial and had all the other accessories ready. This incident, which is similar in many respects to that described by Penfield and Evans[21] in a woman after unilateral frontal lobectomy, had apparently been the first of a series which when pieced together indicated that the duration of symptoms had been much longer than at first had been supposed. Commenting on the behaviour of patients who had sustained extensive brain damage, as after frontal leucotomy, Goldstein[22] points out that they have usually little difficulty in dealing with concrete situations but " if the situation confronts him with a problem which can be solved only after having given account to himself what to do before acting, then he may show deviations and failure ". Brickner[23] also reported on the sequelae of frontal lobectomy. He mentions a business executive who when confronted with a complicated deal found it impossible to hold all the relevant facts together in his mind.

SYMPTOMS

In about one-third of the cases in this series the onset had been sudden, symptoms making their appearance within a few minutes, hours or days and thereafter the patient's condition slowly improving, remaining more or less static or slowly deteriorating. Cases of cerebral anoxia, trauma and cerebral vascular accidents accounted for the majority of these and it was noted among the last-named that apoplectic coma was less common than were transitory attacks of " confusion ", which either preceded or followed the appearance of hemiplegia and aphasia. In several instances this confusion was sufficiently bizarre as to cause concern about the patient's sanity. Thus a man aged 77, who was still sufficiently active mentally as to take a keen interest in his business, was resting in bed one day on account of troublesome sciatica when his son visited him to get him to sign some cheques. He signed the first two correctly, but on coming to the third, after writing his name, began making figures for the amount all over the cheque until the paper was nearly covered. When his son asked him what he was doing he replied inconsequently, demanded his clothes and when an attempt was made to reason with him became noisy and aggressive. Later he became incontinent of urine and the next day was found to have a left-sided visual defect. In another case, a woman of 70, in whom a similar vascular accident occurred, this was only discovered after she became acutely hallucinated, declaring that she could see a choir standing on a balcony, and on two other occasions respectively, a man dressed in red, and the ceiling of the room festooned with roses. At the same time she was restless, refusing to stay in bed, resented interference and was noisy and disorientated in time and place.

Another interesting feature seen on a number of occasions following the onset of hemiplegia was the occurrence of disturbance of the body image. Thus, one man denied that his paralysed left arm was his own and declared that " someone has put the arm in my bed so that I can do exercises with it ". This symptom is considered together with other aspects of body disorientation in Chapter IX.

Among patients with gradual modes of onset, *headache* was some-times one of the first symptoms to be complained of, but it was rarely possible to get much detail as to its character because either the patient had forgotten or the relatives could not supply the necessary infor-mation. In only four cases did it reach the kind of severity described on p. 9, and this was the only instance in which an acute depressive reaction had been precipitated by headache. In the others behaviour was more neurotic and had it not been for the presence of accompanying physical signs its true cause might have been overlooked. Two of these patients had astrocytomata (left temporo-parietal and parietal respectively), a third a right frontal meningioma and the fourth a right frontal metastasis from a squamous cell carcinoma of the bronchus. Especially severe headache was noted also in 2 of the 8 cases of chronic subdural haematoma in this series.

However, it should not be thought that headache was a common presenting symptom in middle-aged and elderly patients with space-occupying lesions for when the histories of 40 proved cases of tumour were reviewed it was found that in 15, or 37·5%, there had been neither headache nor papilloedema. These 15 cases comprised:

> 5 meningiomata:
>> 2 right frontal
>> 1 falx cerebri
>> 2 left temporal
>
> 5 infiltrating gliomata:
>> 2 left temp. astrocytoma
>> 2 left fronto-temp. astrocytoma
>> 1 left temp. pariet. glioblastoma multiforme
>
> 1 Acoustic neurinoma (left)
> 1 Suprasellar epidermoid cyst
> 1 Ependymoma of 4th ventricle
> 2 Multiple metastases from primary mammary or bronchial
>> carcinoma

Further, in 8 other cases, not included in the above, headache and papilloedema had only occurred late in the history, i.e. 3–4 weeks before the patient was seen, other symptoms having preceded them for months or years as the case might be. These findings support Moersch *et al.* in their contention as to the relative infrequency of these symptoms and signs in elderly patients with tumours, a fact which presumably may be due to physiological cerebral atrophy permitting of greater accumulation of cerebrospinal fluid.[25] Cushing and Eisenhardt[26] in their account of meningiomas refer to disturbances of memory and other signs of mental impairment in some cases, especially those with frontally-sited tumours, but in discussing convexity meningiomas they remarked that mental symptoms were notable by their absence. Sachs,[27] however, described 8 cases of meningiomata, some frontal, some parietal, others temporal, in all of which the earliest symptoms were those of dementia. In 3 headache was not complained of and in only one case was it a prominent feature. Only 3 showed papilloedema. The following case is a further example of how this type of tumour may simulate dementia due to global cerebral cortical atrophy.

The patient was a widow, aged 63, when seen in 1950, and had always been strongly left-handed. The relatives said that she had had a severe emotional shock some 3 years previously, the effect of which had been to deprive her of energy so that she would lie in bed all day and take no interest in her home or friends. Her gait had been unsteady over the same period and on several occasions she had been incontinent both of urine and faeces. But when asked to describe her symptoms all she would say was: " I have had a lot of worry and one thing and another . . . indeed I can hardly tell."
On examination she showed fatuous unconcern and increased emotional lability, laughing and crying readily. There was great difficulty in getting her

to register a name and an address, memory for past events was vague, her defects in this respect being global and not affecting recent events more than distant. She was completely disorientated in time and place but not for persons. Neurologically there were no unequivocal signs, but when the arms were outstretched the left tended to deviate or " float " slowly upwards. Further, although she could recognize objects placed in the right hand, it was impossible to get her to do so with the left hand. How much this was indicative of a true astereognosis it was difficult at the time to say because she was so unco-operative. Tendon reflexes were equally brisk, and although there was some increase of tone in both lower limbs there was no suggestion of voluntary muscular weakness. At times the right plantar was extensor, the left always being flexor.

At first opinion was inclined towards the diagnosis of a global dementia but fluctuations in the level of consciousness were observed, at times the patient passing into a drowsy stupor and at others exhibiting some expressive dysphasia. The possibility of a chronic subdural haematoma was considered but at operation a large right fronto-temporal meningioma was found. This was successfully removed and six months later her mental state had enormously improved; she was able to register well and was fully orientated, memory for past events having also recovered.

In patients found later to have diffuse cortical atrophy headache was seldom mentioned spontaneously although varying answers were given when they were prompted to think about it. It was then described as " a dull heaviness " or as a feeling " as if the head was lifting off ". One case, a woman of 60 with early dementia illustrated in her history the tendency for migraine to decrease in intensity and frequency with the onset of cerebral arteriosclerotic changes. Although a victim of migraine since adolescence, headaches had been materially less in the 3 years preceding examination, over which period gradual deterioration in her intellect and behaviour had been observed.

Epileptiform fits were observed by relatives in a fair proportion of patients with failing memory and intellectual decline but not noticeably more often in those with global dementia than with space-occupying lesions. However, the character of the fits differed. Leaving out of account the few patients who had had epilepsy since childhood, major seizures with convulsions were much less common in global dementias than were temporary " lapses " or minor fits. Describing these, the wife of one patient said: " when he is talking he may suddenly break off in the middle of a sentence, stare vacantly, turn his head from side to side and appear as if he were thinking deeply before resuming what he was saying . . . but he usually loses the thread and has to be prompted and if it happens at table he has to be reminded to go on with his meal." Of the 40 patients with tumour there was a history of epileptiform seizures in 11 or 27·5%, in 6 the fits being Jacksonian in type and in 5 generalized with convulsions. In one instance (right frontal oligodendroglioma) recurring major fits had been noted for some 20 years and in another (left temporal meningioma) for 15 years. But, although there were 12 cases of meningioma in the series in only 3 of these were fits reported.

Disturbances of gait.

" The most characteristic type of gait seen in old age is the *marche à petits pas*," Critchley.[9] In our series this was often seen as were also motor disabilities taking the form of gradually increasing weakness of one side or affecting both lower limbs and associated with exaggeration of tendon reflexes, extensor plantar responses and spasticity. But even more striking and certainly more difficult to appraise were cases in which there were no definite pyramidal, extrapyramidal, cerebellar or sensory signs but in which unsteadiness in walking was the principal complaint. This was the presenting complaint in 15 of our cases. Some appeared to be unaware or unwilling to admit any disability and had to be restrained from attempting to walk unaided, but in the majority the frequency of falls, or their own sense of insecurity had induced anxiety so that they were reluctant to venture unaided. Typical of the descriptions given by relatives and patients were the following: " he walks as if drunk "; " she will suddenly fall backwards or forwards "; " he walks as if he were feeling his way cautiously on a slippery surface "; " he takes peculiar short steps ".

In the elderly, unsteadiness of gait, momentary giddiness or actual loss of balance leading to falling is most commonly related to basilar insufficiency, from carotico-vertebral atheroma (p. 35). In such cases ischaemic infarcts may be found in the cerebellum. A classical example was the centenarian Dr. Holyoke, mentioned by Critchley,[9] who wrote: " in walking I was apt to lose my equilibrium and sometimes to stagger like one intoxicated, particularly if I looked up to see the town clock or how the wind blew ". At post-mortem examination atrophy of the cerebellum was the most striking abnormality. In such instances the absence of signs of ataxia on formal testing may lead to the suspicion of hysteria, but we have yet to meet a case in an elderly subject in which this was so and recall that on one occasion this false assumption led to a patient falling and sustaining an impacted fracture of the neck of the femur. In their recent paper, Meyer and Barron[28] quote Bruns (1892) as having been the first to describe ataxia of gait in patients with frontal lobe tumours and these authors discuss three mechanisms by which a frontal lesion may affect gait:

1. An expanding lesion may cause displacement of intracranial contents, leading to cerebellar and medullary compression.

2. A similar train of events may lead to stretching of the eighth nerve and vertigo of labyrinthine origin (Clovis Vincent).

3. Localized frontal disease, especially mesially-placed lesions, may cause an actual apraxia of gait (Gerstmann and Schilder, Van Bogaert and Purdon Martin).

In retrospect we think it likely that in the majority of our cases the disturbances of gait were either of cerebellar origin and due to carotico-vertebral atheroma or apraxic in nature and related to diffuse cerebral cortical atrophy. Feeling their way as a person would on a slippery surface, or when crossing a badly-lit and strange room aptly describes the mode of progression adopted by most of these cases. Petrén,[29] quoted by Critchley, noted that after a few steps the patient might feel he could go no further, and Denny-Brown[30] has applied the epithet " magnetic ataxia " to the curious way in which the feet may seem to be glued to the floor. In many of our cases the gait was more sugges-tive of apraxia than of ataxia. As one patient, a man of 75 said: " I think, doctor, I have lost my *mental* balance . . . I do not connect up things properly. . . ." Methods used in the clinical examination are described in Chapter III.

Sudden falls or *drop-attacks* are also not uncommon in elderly people, the usual complaint being that without any preliminary warning the patient has fallen precipitously to the ground. Serious injuries may result, the nose and face being badly bruised, or fractures and dislocations being sustained. More often, however, the victims escape with superficial bruises but are usually badly shaken and emotionally upset by the experience. Although an epileptic origin may be suspected this is usually not the case, there being no evidence of any clouding of consciousness. In Sheldon's[31] series unexplained falls were sometimes related to vertigo (7%), in such cases deafness and tinnitus being commonly associated symptoms. Sudden throwing the head back was another exciting cause but few instances could be attributed to postural hypotension. Sheldon emphasizes the loss of postural tone in muscle after these attacks, which is a fairly constant feature.

Apart from a few cases in which the first abnormality to be noted was *incontinence of urine*, and others with disturbances of *sleep rhythm* (one patient finding that he could not sleep at nights, others being excessively drowsy by day), the earliest disabilities noted concerned mind or intellect.

Tiredness or lack of energy was often complained of and could be more appropriately described as loss of initiative or drive. It was probably the great alteration in this respect noticed by relatives that caused them so often to declare that a patient was " not the man he used to be ". Thus one man, formerly a witty raconteur and a social asset at any party became changed in these respects, being content to remain silent and to follow the lead of others. A woman, who had been a school mistress and highly efficient in her work until 4 years before, gave up her post because she said she was " worn out " and had no energy, and it was reported that she had either lain in bed or sat idle about the house all day. Another with Huntington's chorea, for 8 years before the true nature of her disability was discovered, had been temperamental, " sulking after trivial disagreements, complaining of loss of energy, and being irritable, unreliable and difficult to live with ". A third, a woman of 65, for a year had changed from her former pleasant, affable self into an extremely rude and offensive person, quarreling frequently with her neighbours and spreading discreditable and false rumours about the private lives of her son and daughter-in-law.

Of intellectual symptoms, *impairment of memory* for past events headed the list and as will be seen, it was particularly difficult to assess, because some patients who were reported to have no difficulty in remembering were found on examination to be grossly disturbed in this respect, whilst in others amnesic disorders were more apparent than real. These disabilities are considered in Chapter VI.

Disturbances of speech and language.

These were also commonly reported, very typical of the statements of relatives being the following: " she cannot get the right word and uses the wrong name for things ", or " he often breaks off in the middle of a sentence and leaves it unfinished ". Difficulties in recalling familiar names were common, such being often referred to simply as a tendency to " stammer ", the inference being that they were simply due to emotional upset connected with worry. In one case, that of a journalist aged 52, it was possible to obtain a very complete history from his wife and his employers. Long before the appearance of more definite signs of deterioration in his spoken and written speech (possibly some 7–10 years before), a gradual falling-off in his literary style and ability had been apparent and was undoubtedly the first symptom of his subsequent dementia. In another case, a woman of 46, the first and only indication of the approach of dementia was difficulty in reading. During this period changes of glasses were prescribed without benefit and routine ophthalmological and neurological examinations were negative. The patient stated that when she looked at print she had difficulty in recognizing the letters by their shape and, further, that with long words she could only see part of the word, the part to her right being blurred or indistinct. As she said " I can't see the end of long words so I have to go through them and spell them letter by letter ". In other patients print was described as appearing to be " jumbled ".

Disturbances of behaviour.

These were remarked by relatives in a number of patients in whom the onset of symptoms had been gradual. Some of these were clearly related to absent-mindedness, e.g. forgetting to put on a waistcoat, or when given a set of fresh underwear putting these on over the old, but others by reason of their bizarre character suggested the existence of some underlying form of agnosia or apraxia, e.g. attempting to take soup with a knife; stirring a cup of tea with a fork; when offered a cup of tea, dipping the fingers in it and then rubbing them in the hair. Such symptoms usually indicated either rapidly advancing deterioration or that the patient had already reached an advanced state by the time he was first seen. As a rule such learned activities as using a knife and fork at table, shaving and combing the hair were retained. However, the histories showed that these patients often had difficulties in constructional tasks, e.g. rehanging curtains after " spring-cleaning ". One woman had to await her husband's return each evening before she could prepare the meal because she could not manipulate the dials on her electric stove. Some workmen were reported to have forgotten how to use tools or to be unable to assemble parts. In yet other patients eccentricities of behaviour appeared to be related to the presence of disturbances of temporal and spatial orientation.

Tendencies towards *delusional thinking* were only occasionally reported and when delusions occurred they were never organized or well-integrated and were invariably connected with the particular difficulties a patient might be experiencing at the time, e.g. forgetting where he had put things and accusing other people of stealing them; forgetting that he had been told something and maintaining that his relatives and work-mates had deliberately withheld information for some reason or other. One man, who was employed in the shipyard, failed one evening to notice that the whistle to cease work had sounded and became panic-stricken when approached by a body of men hurrying to get home. He admitted afterwards that he had been under the mistaken impression that they were about to attack him.

Organized hallucinatory experiences were equally uncommon. Allen[32] reported the case of a man in whom spontaneous stereognostic sensations occurred following the removal of a large meningioma from the posterior Rolandic area of the left cortex. The patient was convinced that he was holding an object in his right hand. Sometimes this felt smooth and round like a ball, at other times it had jagged edges like a piece of granite, or was flat and smooth like a lady's small mirror. When an actual object was placed in his left hand he felt another similar object spontaneously in the right hand. These stereognostic sensations disappeared a week after the operation. No similar cases were encountered, but a curious proprioceptive hallucination occurred in a man of 52, a chartered accountant, who was suffering from ulcerative colitis and hepatic insufficiency. Following the prescription of an opiate to control severe diarrhoea, he became restless, excited and declared that he was wearing two pairs of pyjama trousers. Later, he insisted that he had four arms and four legs, two on either side, and when he went to defaecate he could not be got back into bed because, as he said, he had to wait " to empty the other bowel ". After some days he recovered and was able in retrospect to confirm the intensity and vivid character of his recent experiences. In this case the hallucinations were clearly related to toxaemia but the nature of the occupation may have played some part in determining their character. In some cases of global dementia, and others with space-occupying lesions giving rise to hemianopic defects, visual after-images were mentioned. Thus, a patient with general paralysis disturbed the hospital one night because he saw " the night nurse approaching and carrying five rifles to attack me ". Bartlett[33] believes that deprivation of part of the brain responsible for receiving conscious impressions of the customary appearance of objects may be an important factor in inducing hallucinations. He mentioned the case of an old man of 84 who was partially blind and had hallucinations very similar to those of the patient described on p. 17. Deafness may have the same effect in inducing auditory hallucinations.

Possible Etiological Factors

One of the principal difficulties of case-taking in organic mental states is to assess how much importance should be attached to psychogenic factors, which as a rule friends and relatives are usually only too ready to offer in explanation of the changes observed in the patient. Genuine examples of misfortune such as unavoidable loss of employment, death of a close friend are often cited as causes and it is likely that these may have been responsible to some extent for precipitating overt signs of intellectual failure in predisposed subjects. However, in the presence of symptoms of the kind which have been described, psychogenic factors rarely play any important part in causation and one must be careful not to be misled into investing them with any etiological significance.

Of much more importance it is to gain the relatives' and friends' mpression of the patient's previous personality and temperament and his intellectual level. Obsessional and perfectionist qualities, the occurrence of previous mood swings or hysterical tendencies should be noted and the primary educational level ascertained. The last-named can often be estimated by the standard reached by the patient on leaving his primary or elementary school, or the naïve disclosure that " he was never a great scholar ". Previous nervous breakdowns should be noted together with his former interest in and capacity for work, his hobbies or sparetime pursuits, degree of sociability. One should also try and obtain an accurate family history, especially as regards other members of the family having been similarly affected in the later years of life.

Enquiry should also be made into some of the known aetiological causes of organic mental states. When symptoms are of relatively short duration the possibility of the patient having sustained a minor head injury should always be considered, although it must be admitted that in most of our cases of chronic subdural haematoma neither the patient nor his relatives were able to supply a history of such injury. Cardiac decompensation leading to cerebral circulatory failure is a common cause of organic mental symptoms and enquiry should be made as to attacks of breathlessness on exertion, substernal pain or swelling of the ankles. When the patient is known to have been a chronic dyspeptic, enquiry should be made for previous haematemesis or melaena, the extent of blood loss at the time and whether or not the patient was transfused. Any surgical operations in the previous 5 years should also be noted, especially as regards the type of anaesthesia used and recovery therefrom, extent of shock and duration of bed rest after operation. The patient's previous habits as regards diet and alcohol should be taken into account and, where there has been excess drinking, the pattern ascertained. If the patient is a known diabetic, enquiry should be made as to the frequency of hypoglycaemic reactions, the dosage of insulin and the attention paid to dietetic restrictions.

BIBLIOGRAPHY

16 REINHOLD M. (1953). Human behaviour reactions to organic cerebral disease. *J. ment. Sci.*, **99**, 130.

17 GOLDSTEIN, K. (1942). " After Effects of Brain Injuries in War," p. 69. Heinemann, London.

18 PATERSON, A. (1942). Emotional and cognitive changes in the post-traumatic confusional state. *Lancet*, **2**, 717.

19   DARWIN, C. " Expressions of the Emotions in Man and Animals." John Murray, London.

20   WOLFF, H. and CHAPMAN, L. (1957). Studies in human cerebral hemisphere function: adaptive capacity after loss of hemisphere tissue. *Med. Clin. N. Amer.*, p. 175–8.

21   PENFIELD, W. and EVANS, J. P (1935). The frontal lobe in man: a clinical study of maximum removals. *Brain*, **58**, 115. Quoted by Brickner, R. M. (1939).

22   GOLDSTEIN, K. (1944). The mental changes due to frontal lobe disease. *J. Psychiat.*, **17**, 187.

23   BRICKNER, R. M. (1939). Conscious inability to synthetize thoughts in a case of right frontal lobe tumour. *Arch. Neurol. Psychiat.*, **41**, 1166.

24   MOERSCH, F. P., CRAIG, W. McK. and KERNOHAN, J. W. (1941). Tumours of the brain in aged persons. *Arch. Neurol. Psychiat.*, **45**, 235.

25   SPILLANE, J. D. (1952). Discussion on the differential diagnosis of early dementia. *Proc. Roy. Soc, Med. Joint Meeting No.* 4, p. 374.

26   CUSHING, H. and EISENHARDT, L. (1938). " Meningiomas, Their Classification, Regional Behaviour, Life History and Surgical End Results." Thomas, Springfield, Illinois.

27   SACHS, E. (1950). Meningiomas with dementia as the first and presenting symptom. *J. ment. Sci.*, **96**, 998.

28   MEYER, J. S. and BARRON, D. W. (1960). Ataxia of gait: a clinicophysiological study. *Brain*, **83**, 261.

29   PETRÉN, K. (1900). Über den Zusammenhang zwischen anatomisch bedingter u. funktioneller Gangstörung im Greisanalter. *Arch. Psych.* **33**, 818; *ibid.* (1901), **34**, 444. Quoted by Critchley, M. (9).

30   DENNY-BROWN, D. J. Nerv. and Ment. Dis., **216**, 9. Quoted by MEYER and BARRON (1960).

31   SHELDON, J. H. (1960). On the natural history of falls in old age. *Brit. Med. J.*, **2**, 1685.

32   ALLEN, I. M. (1928). Unusual sensory phenomena following removal of a tumour of the sensory cortex. *J. Neurol. Psychopath.*, **9**, 133.

33   BARTLETT, J. E. A. (1951). A case of organized hallucinations in an old man with cataract. *Brain*, **74**, 3, 363.

CHAPTER II

General Physical Examination

AN organic mental state may often be recognized simply by talking to a patient and observing his behaviour, in this way the condition being distinguishable from a psychoneurosis or affective disorder. But physical examination is essential for determination of its underlying cause and as these are diverse it must be as detailed and comprehensive as possible.

A catalogue of personal experience relating to some of the principal causes of organic mental disease in later life already has been given. This makes no pretence at being complete, but it is doubtful if any useful purpose would be served by trying to devise a classification that would meet all eventualities because in a number of cases the cause defies recognition or at the best is only imperfectly understood. An alternative plan would be to focus attention on the cerebral neurone and enumerate the many potentially noxious agents that may affect its natural functioning—e.g. hypoxia, vitamin deficiency, metabolic disturbances, water and electrolyte imbalance. But symptoms may not be entirely dependent on disturbance of *cerebral cortical* function and, often, more than one of these causes is responsible. So, the discovery or exclusion of such possibilities, although of value, is not so much the objective in examination as to *decide whether symptoms are due to primary dysfunction of the brain or to disturbances arising in other organs. This is one of the principal aims of physical examination. The other is to help in deciding, when the signs point to primary disease of the brain,* whether they *are expressive of a diffuse or focal cerebral affection.*

Two types of patient have to be considered. First, those presenting with symptoms of acute clouding of consciousness. These are discussed in Chapter XI. Second, cases in which symptoms have been of gradual onset and are related chiefly to impairment of memory, intellect, speech, visual, motor or sensory function. The examination outlined in this chapter refers to the latter group of patients.

Physical appearance.

Some time should be allowed for general inspection of the patient before proceeding to systematic examination of the heart, lungs and other organs as otherwise certain important conditions which are often

27

associated with mental symptoms may be overlooked. One of the best examples of these is myxoedema, a disease which Asher[34] avers is " one of the most important, one of the least known, and one of the most frequently missed causes of organic psychosis ". Wayne[35] suggests that the term myxoedema should be reserved for cases in which skin changes are present and hypothyroidism preferred for general use, as skin changes need not be present in hypothyroidism. The most typical physical signs are consistent slowing of the pulse rate, subnormal body temperature; decreased sweating; periorbital puffiness, dryness and yellowness of the skin; intractable constipation; hoarseness, dysarthria; deafness and paraesthesiae. Defective eyebrows in their outer-thirds is often quoted as a sign but is unreliable. Supraclavicular padding may be observed but this is usually less pronounced than the obesity and " puffy " appearance of the face. Characteristic of myxoedematous subjects is their extreme sensitivity to cold: they like to sit by the fire; in bed they require plenty of blankets. They are also very susceptible to morphine, insulin and barbiturates, acute mental confusion and coma being readily precipitated by incautious use of these drugs. The yellowish discolouration of the skin may simulate Addisonian anaemia but it is not due to rise in bilirubin but to excess of serum carotene. Deafness is not conductive but of perceptive type. Clinical diagnosis is readily confirmed by estimation of the basal metabolic rate, or, as are now used more often, radio-active iodine tests to measure thyroid uptake of ^{131}I, and estimation of the serum cholesterol. The latter is over 300 mg. per 100 ml. in a high proportion of cases of myxoedema. In some instances myxoedematous symptoms are secondary to primary pituitary disease and there is danger in giving thyroid of precipitating acute adrenal insufficiency or severe hypoglycaemia, if adequate cortisone replacement is not undertaken first.[36] Dementing-like symptoms may also occur in alcoholics under treatment by disulfiram or Antabuse, owing to the effect of the drug in depressing the metabolic rate, but they are reversible and disappear on its withdrawal. Sometimes, however, even with such aids, diagnosis may be difficult. Thus, in one of our cases, a woman aged 50, whose physical appearance and dullness of wits suggested myxoedema, pulse rate and temperature were normal. The serum cholesterol was slightly elevated but the uptake of iodine was within normal limits. Thyroid extract was cautiously administered, $\frac{1}{2}$ gr. daily at first and the dose then gradually increased until she was taking 2 gr. daily. However, at this stage she complained of palpitation and as the heart sounds were rapid and irregular the drug was stopped. Subsequently she was found to have a primary squamous-celled carcinoma of the vagina, which was too advanced for radical surgical treatment. Some improvement in her mental state, however, followed deep irradiation.

The case just referred to is, indeed, a reminder that physical examination in all patients suspected of having organic mental disease must include careful palpation of the breasts, neck, axillae as well as making a rectal and vaginal examination. It is as well to remember also that organic mental symptoms may be the presenting features in cases of malignant disease in which no secondary cerebral deposits are found. Examples of such have been reported by Charatan and Brierley[37] in which subsequent examination of the brain has been found to show no macroscopic or microscopic evidence of cancerous infiltration or actual tumour. In all three of their cases, however, secondary deposits were found in the liver. There was also evidence of cerebral oedema as shown by increase in weight of the brain and by honeycombing of the cerebral white matter. They conclude that in such cases liver damage from metastases may be a contributory factor in causing mental symptoms. The precise nature of the metabolic disorder associated with bronchogenic carcinoma is still unknown, although Denny-Brown[38] has suggested that some metabolite may be present in carcinomatous cases which interferes with the metabolism of pantothenic acid. McGovern, Miller and Robertson[39] recently reported two similar cases of bronchogenic carcinoma with mental symptoms, in neither of which the liver was affected. In both instances, too, mental symptoms preceded diagnosis of the growth in the chest. The fluctuation and varying character of the mental symptoms were thought to be indicative of an underlying biochemical disorder and it was noted that a raised blood ammonium level was found in one instance. The value of ammonia estimations in such cases, however, is doubtful. In addition to the primary vaginal carcinoma already referred to, there were two instances in this series of primary breast cancer giving rise to organic mental pictures and a fourth case in which the primary seat of new growth was in the lung. In the last-named secondary deposits were found in the liver, adrenals and brain.

This was a woman of 70 in whom previous history was irrelevant until July 1955, when she began to lose interest in her home and friends and to complain of loss of appetite and abdominal discomfort. Her mood was melancholy and she was preoccupied with the idea that she had cancer. By the end of the year she was spending the greater part of the day in bed and seemed to be unusually somnolent. In February 1956, by which time she had lost much weight and developed some pigmentation of the skin and of the buccal mucosa, Addison's disease was suspected, but cortisone treatment led to no improvement and her condition became more and more lethargic.

When first seen in March 1956, she was cachectic and lay motionless in bed with the eyes closed and apparently sleeping. But when one raised the eyelids, instead of being turned upwards, the eyeballs were found to be staring straight at the observer much in the same way as was described by Cairns *et al.* in their case of " akinetic mutism " (see p. 94). It was virtually impossible to get her to co-operate in mental testing and negativistic behaviour was very pronounced, food being refused. However physical examination in detail was negative. Plantars were flexor and there was no papilloedema or evidence of cranial nerve palsies. An E.E.G. showed diffuse slow activity. X-rays of the skull, chest and lumbar encephalography gave normal results.

Death occurred in coma a month later. At necropsy both lungs were studded with tiny firm nodules (1–4 mm. in diameter) which were best appreciated on palpation. In the left lower lung there was a small tumour, which was lying in relation to a peripheral bronchus and to the wall of a large pulmonary vessel. In the liver a similar tumour was found measuring some 3 cm. and situated on the posterior surface of the right lobe. Tumour nodules were also found in the adrenal cortices, and in the brain there were four small tumours (each of about 2 cm. diameter), two in the frontal regions and two in the occipital. Histological examination showed the lung tumour to be an adenocarcinoma, which was well differentiated in some parts, where it consisted of acini lined by irregular columnar cells. Other parts were more anaplastic. The hepatic, adrenal and cerebral nodules showed a similar structure.

Early signs of *Parkinsonism* may be misconstrued when the presenting symptoms are mental, the immobility and dejected appearance being mistaken for depression or attributed to side-effects of drugs being used in treatment, such as Rauwolfia Serpentina or phenothiazine derivatives. Examination should be repeated after withdrawal of the drugs. Increased postural tone in the neck and shoulder girdle muscles can readily be demonstrated by standing behind the patient, grasping his head between the two hands and making to and fro passive lateral movements of the head upon the neck. Similarly, it can be shown in the shoulder girdles by suddenly pushing forward the arm from behind. Absence of associated swinging movements of the arm on one or both sides in walking is another important sign and dissociation of head and ocular movements upon the patient's turning his gaze to the side may be noted. The complex tremor of Parkinsonism is quite unlike that due to emotional causes although its intensification under the stress of emotion is well-recognized. Tremor is often inconspicuous in the arteriosclerotic form of the disease, Critchley.[40] Mental changes, however, are common and early in their appearance, the occurrence of symptoms after an apoplectiform attack or of emotional instability with facile laughter and tears being suggestive of a vascular basis. Another suggestive feature is the occurrence of extensor plantar responses. The combination of dementing symptoms with bilateral pyramidal features and signs of Parkinsonism was seen in four cases and, although no pathological confirmation was obtained, these were thought possibly to be instances of Jakob Creutzfeld's disease.

There may be some hesitancy in attributing obscure mental symptoms to *hepatic insufficiency* in the absence of jaundice, spleno-megaly, ascites and other gross signs. Yet, as experience has shown, mental symptoms are often the first indicators and may be apparent at a time when even liver function tests reveal no abnormality. They occur in about 20% of patients after portacaval anastomotic operations, performed for the relief of severe and recurrent haematemeses,[41] and in one of our cases the Cruveilhier-Baumgarten syndrome[42] was demonstrable clinically and confirmed at autopsy. In these cases symptoms are due probably to nitrogenous substances absorbed from the intestine by-passing the liver and reaching the brain. Phillips *et al.*[43] obtained symptoms identical with those seen in hepatic coma by giving cirrhotic patients ammonium-containing cation exchange resins. But although the blood ammonium was often elevated they found no corre-lation between the extent of this and the clinical signs of hepatic coma. However, despite negative laboratory tests, careful inspection often provides valuable guides to incipient liver failure and chief among these are involuntary movements, hepatic foetor, reddening of the palms of the hands, " spider " naevi on the skin of the face, trunk and extremities, and an " earthy " pallid complexion, without clinical signs of anaemia. The involuntary movements have been discussed by Foley and Adams,[44] Sherlock *et al.*[45] and are best demonstrated by getting the patient to extend his arms horizontally, with the fingers spread. Foley and Adams note: " a peculiar intermittency of sustained muscle contraction that presents as an irregular flapping movement when the arms and legs are held outstretched, a fluctuating rigidity of the limbs, grimacing, sucking. . . ." The actual movements are said to occur at irregular intervals of a fraction of a second to several seconds and to consist of " lateral deviations of the fingers, flexion-extension of the fingers at the metacarpophalangeal joint, and flexion-extension at the wrist ". When the arms are outstretched in a pronated position the flexion phase is always more rapid than the other and movements tend to occur in bursts, at a rate of one every second or two. In the more severe cases flexion-extension movements may be observed at the elbow and at the shoulder. In most cases there is in addition a fine 6–9 per second tremor of the outstretched fingers. This sign is not pathognomonic of hepatic failure and has been observed in other conditions, e.g. uraemia, polycythaemia vera, steatorrhoea, severe malnutrition, lupus erythematosis,[46] but when seen in association with fluctuating and recent impairment of memory, peculiar conduct and general lethargy, it should always arouse suspicion of impending liver failure. The " meaty " foetor of the breath is also characteristic. It may be so strong and compelling as to be recognizable at a distance, but often it is necessary to get the patient to exhale forcibly in order to detect it. Of liver function tests probably one of the most sensitive is the serum albumin level, figures below 3 g. per 100 ml. being indicative of liver failure. Other methods of confirming the diagnosis are by prescribing a high protein diet for 7–10 days and observing the patient for signs of deterioration in his mental state or the appearance of slow wave forms on repeated electroencephalography. Until recently one would have hesitated to diagnose hepatic encephalopathy in the absence of signs of liver failure, yet in one case, a man of 55, the first and (at the time) only symptoms of the multilobular cirrhosis from which he died 3 years later were changes in behaviour, chronic amnesia, periodic mental confusion and typical " flapping " tremor. The manner in which these symptoms waxed and waned at first gave rise to the suspicion that they were hysterical. Liver function tests were carried out and he was given a week's trial on a protein diet of 150 g. daily but the results were negative and it was not until a year and a half later, when he was readmitted to hospital in hepatic coma and found to have ascites and an enlarged spleen, that the diagnosis was finally confirmed. Probably in cases where diagnosis is in doubt it may be more rewarding to see what beneficial effect results from a short 10 day oral course of neomycin, combined with a low protein (10 g. daily) diet.

The presence of *anaemia* may be difficult to detect in old people because of epiphora and inflammatory redness of the conjunctiva of the lower eyelids but undue pallor of the buccal mucosa and of the palms of the hands is suggestive. Mental symptoms are common in subacute combined degeneration and sometimes occur early, constituting the presenting features. Their occurrence in patients with pernicious anaemia was noted by Addison in his original description of the disease and there is no correlation betweeen the severity of the spinal cord signs and the mental state.[47] Before the onset of overt anaemia the only clues to diagnosis may be complaints of numbness and "pins and needles " in the hands and feet, and slight lemon-yellow tinting of the skin and sclerotics. In such cases, where the peripheral blood picture is normal, estimations of the serum vitamin B_{12} level and sternal marrow puncture are required and assay of the reticulocyte response to vitamin B_{12}. But probably the most satisfactory manner of demonstrating failure of absorption is to label the cobalt content of the vitamin with its radio-isotope ^{60}Co and then estimate the 24 hour urinary excretion after an oral dose of labelled vitamin B_{12}. Normal subjects excrete 7–22% of the injected dose; in cases of subacute combined degeneration the range is between 0·3–1·0%.[48] Chronic blood loss from hiatus hernia, haemorrhoids, diverticula may also lead to the development of severe hypochromic microcytic anaemia. In their survey of old people living at home Hobson and Pemberton[49] found malnutrition and signs of scurvy fairly common among those who tended to live on a diet of tinned meat, biscuits, jam, tea and condensed mild. Signs of vitamin C deficiency must, however, not be confused with senile purpura.

Cardiovascular System.

Cerebral function is maintained by the pumping action of the heart conveying blood through the carotid and vertebral arteries and the vessels comprising the circle of Willis to the brain. Fluctuation in the rate of utilization of oxygen and glucose, which are the chief food-stuffs contained in the blood substrate, are met by corresponding changes in the cerebral blood flow rate and in health this mechanism is sufficiently elastic to meet the varying demands put upon it. The concept of " cerebral circulatory insufficiency " implies that, either through cardiac or arterial disease, the supply of blood to the brain is not being adequately maintained and, although it has only been introduced in recent years, there are signs that its application may revolutionize orthodox thinking in respect to the interpretation put upon the neurological and mental symptoms, which may be associated with cerebral vascular disease.

In examination of the cardiovascular system, therefore, the principal objective is to find out if there is any abnormality that could give rise to cerebral circulatory insufficiency, because of all causes of organic mental disorder in middle and later life this is probably the most common. Congestive heart failure, which in elderly persons especially is often accompanied by acute mental symptoms of confusional type, is a good example in which the connection between cause and effect is easily recognized. The reduction in cerebral blood flow, which is found in this condition, is proportionate to the fall in cardiac output and related also to peripheral resistance, brought about by cerebral vasoconstriction. The mental symptoms are due to hypoxia, the cerebral neurones being unable to extract enough oxygen for their needs.[50]

In other cases the connection may not be so obvious. The radial, femoral, dorsalis pedis and posterior tibial vessels should be palpated and the adequacy of the blood supply to the limbs estimated by the skin temperature and the presence or absence of trophic changes. In two of our patients with cerebral vascular disease there was a previous history of intermittent claudication. Similarly, in relation to the state of the myocardium, enquiry should be made for a previous history of substernal pain on effort. In a number of cases this was forthcoming and in others the electrocardiograms showed evidence of ischaemic heart disease, with or without signs of previous coronary occlusive episodes.

The discovery of arterial hypertension with persistent elevation of systolic and diastolic pressures may tempt one to attribute any co-existent mental or neurological symptoms to hypertensive encephalopathy, but before doing so three points at least should be taken into account. First, moderate degrees of hypertension are not uncommon in the elderly and in many cases have no significance. Second, the hypertension may be secondary or compensatory to increase of intracranial pressure caused by a cerebral tumour or cerebral vascular accident; and third, it may be secondary to renal or adrenal disease, or superimposed upon a background of cerebral arteriosclerosis.

Symptoms in hypertensive encephalopathy differ from those seen in other forms of cerebrovascular disease: they have a more fluctuating course, progressive dementing features being rare, whereas epileptiform and acute confusional symptoms are more common. On histological examination of brains from patients dying of this condition Foley[51] found miliary infarctions, increased vascular permeability with transudation of blood elements into the surrounding tissues, petechial haemorrhages and oedema. In life malignant hypertension is recognized by the marked rise in diastolic and high systolic pressure, rise of blood urea and the occurrence of papilloedema with multiple retinal haemorrhages and exudates. Good results attend treatment with ganglion-blocking drugs, the chances of prolonged survival being increased by the absence of any signs of gross impairment of renal function, but accompanying atherosclerosis is a limiting factor in the success of treatment, especially in old patients.[52]

Indeed, mention of this is a reminder of the dangers attendant upon lowering the blood pressure in old persons. In 3 of our patients, whose previous symptoms had included headache, dizziness and recurring dyspepsia, the reason for their referral was because, following the incautious prescription of hypotensive drugs, they had developed symptoms of incipient dementia. Bedford[54] has described how the same effects may be brought about as a result of hypotensive surgery or inadequate precautions being taken to maintain pressure levels during and after operations.

Formerly in cerebral vascular disease attention was focused chiefly on the intracranial vessels derived from the circle of Willis: the anterior, middle and posterior cerebral arteries. As Beevor [53] showed, the branches of these vessels, which penetrate and supply the cortex, are end arteries and do not anastamose with the contiguous branches, although there is some anastomosis between the three chief arterial systems: the anterior, middle and posterior cerebral arteries, " at the confines of their areas ". Apoplexy was thought to be due to haemorrhage, thrombosis or embolism involving one of these vessels and occurring in the first two named as the result of atheroma.

In recent years it has been recognized that in many cases the intracranial vessels may be unaffected by atheroma, the seat of this being on the proximal side of the circle of Willis in one or more of the great vessels in the neck, before their entry into the skull. The diffuse cerebral atrophic changes or focal infarctions that may result from obstruction of such vessels are not thrombotic but ischaemic in origin and caused by hypoxia due to cerebral circulatory insufficiency. Sometimes indeed, the vessel supplying the region of the ischaemic infarct is patent. In the field supplied by the carotid system, ischaemic infarcts are found chiefly in the frontal, temporal and parietal lobes, and with vertebral stenosis in the occipital lobes, cerebellar foliae and caudal half of the pons.[55] Hutchinson and Yates describe chronic amnesic syndromes resembling early dementia in patients in whom post-morten examination revealed bilateral internal carotid stenosis, and their experience has been borne out by others.[56,57] However, as atheromatous obstruction of one internal carotid artery alone had not led to ischaemic cerebral infraction in any of the ten cases examined, they concluded that when signs of infarction are present this usually indicates inadequacy of the circle of Willis and atheromatous changes causing narrowing of other main vessels. For this reason the title " caroticovertebral stenosis " is preferred to " internal carotid stenosis ".

There are several clinical methods of testing the patency of the carotid arteries. The simplest is by direct palpation of the vessel in the neck at a point opposite the thyroid cartilage and above the bifurcation of the main vessel into internal and external branches. If there is no pulsation on one side after repeated palpation, stenosis or obstruction due to thrombosis may be inferred. When a pulse is felt it cannot be assumed that the internal carotid is patent because its pulsation may be transmitted from the external carotid artery, which lies adjacent. The superficial temporal artery should also be palpated as pulsation in the latter would suggest that the obstruction was distal to the bifurcation and in the internal carotid.[58, 59] A second method is by auscultation; in a fair proportion of cases of internal carotid stenosis, a systolic bruit can be heard on listening over the vessel or its parent trunk. Indeed, auscultation should never be omitted when stenosis is suspected as often bruits are heard over the skull or over the eyeball. Angiography usually shows that, although the internal carotid is obstructed, the external carotid is patent and often of greater diameter than its fellow, a collateral circulation having been opened up between the angular branches of the external maxillary and the infraorbital branches of the internal maxillary arteries and branches of the ophthalmic artery. In this way blood meeting with obstruction in the internal carotid artery (the site is usually just distal to the bifurcation) is diverted into the external carotid and by collateral channels reaches the internal carotid as it emerges from the cavernous sinus within the skull. In one of our cases in which the internal carotid was obstructed on the left side and in which there was angiographic evidence of anastomotic channels having been opened up, a bruit was heard over the right eyeball. In this case the right internal carotid was patent.

A third method of testing the patency of the internal carotid artery is to try and feel it at a higher level as it passes lateral to and just behind the tonsil, deep in the neck and before entering the carotid canal. Unfortunately, successful palpation at this site is not always reliable as pulsation may still be transmitted from the external carotid [59] and as the vessel is crossed here by the stylopharyngeus muscle, clonic contractions of which may simulate pulsation. Further, it is often not possible to get patients to relax sufficiently to enable one to insert the finger into the required position. Preliminary cocainization is usually necessary to abolish the gag reflex. The gloved forefinger is then inserted through the side of the mouth to behind the tonsil and gentle pressure exerted in a lateral direction.

Another method of investigation in suspected cases of internal carotid stenosis or thrombosis is by ophthalmodynamometry. Using the Baillairt ophthalmodynamometer, Weitzman and Spalter [60] found a significant lowering of retinal artery pressure on the ipsilateral side in 9 out of 11 cases of internal carotid occlusion. In a number of cases with other neurological conditions the average pressure difference between the retinal arteries was 3% systolic and 4% diastolic. In cases of carotid occlusion the ipsilateral pressure was lower by an average of 43% systolic and 50% diastolic. The least reduction was 22% and the greatest 84%. Preliminary cocainization of the eyball is necessary. The retinal vessels are then focused by an ophthalmoscope and the dynamometer applied via the outer canthus to the surface of the eyeball. Gentle increasing pressure is exerted and the moment at which the retinal arteries are seen to collapse marks the systolic pressure, the diastolic being coincident with the moment when pulsation re-appears in the vessels, as pressure is reduced. This method has been in use for over two years and we have seen no untoward effects. Considerable practice is necessary, however, and allowance must be made for the fact that in many cases initial differences in pressure may disappear in time with establishment of a good collateral circulation, thus making results equivocal.

The use of carotid compression in association with electroencephalo-graph and angiographic methods of investigation in these cases is discussed in Chapter XI.

Respiratory system.

Examination of the chest in organic mental states is important because of the frequency of bronchogenic carcinoma in the older age groups and the tendency of these tumours to metastazise in the brain. In their recognition, little reliance can be placed on clinical methods and as cerebral symptoms may predominate, there being no signs referable to the chest, there is much to be said for the routine practice of having radiograms in all patients over the age of forty presenting with mental or neurological symptoms of recent origin. Bronchoscopy has also a recognized place in diagnosis where a tumour is suspected on clinical or radiographic grounds. Thus, Somner *et al.* [61] report that in 276 patients with bronchogenic carcinoma a visible abnormality on bronchoscopy was found in 189 (68%) and histological evidence of the disease was obtained by bronchial biopsy in 168 (61%). They emphasize the value of " blind " biopsy in obtaining histological proof of carcinoma in cases where bronchoscopic appearances have been normal.

Alimentary system.

Gastro-intestinal haemorrhage, when sudden and sufficiently severe as to cause cerebral circulatory failure may lead to such anoxic damage to the cerebral cortical neurones that dementia ensues. This unfortunate sequence was seen in only one of our cases but in some others transient acute confusional symptoms were prominent, the origin of which was not apparent until after thorough physical examination had been made. In such cases enquiry of the relatives will usually reveal a previous history of dyspepsia, due to gastric or duodenal ulceration, but the possibility of cirrhosis of the liver should also be borne in mind. In cirrhotic patients indeed, gastro-intestinal haemorrhage may act as a precipitating cause of hepatic coma.

Acute confusional symptoms may also be precipitated in chronic alcoholism, gastric carcinoma and in patients existing on an inadequate diet by persistent vomiting and diarrhoea. In such instances the combination of symptoms of clouding of consciousness with oculomotor palsies, ataxia of the limbs and blurring of the margins of the optic discs may suggest a diagnosis of Wernicke's encephalopathy. This nutritional disease, which is amenable to intensive treatment by vitamin B_1 (thiamin) has to be differentiated from intracranial meningeal metastases and carcinomatosis of the meninges,[62] which may give rise to similar clinical pictures. However, in Wernicke's disease the cerebrospinal fluid shows no increase of cells or protein and the blood pyruvate level is raised.[63]

Vomiting has other noxious effects in leading to loss of electrolytes and dehydration. Formerly the clouding of consciousness seen in *dehydration* was attributed to increased permeability of the blood-cerebrospinal fluid barrier permitting toxins from the gut to reach the brain, but it is now recognized that it is due simply to the diminished cerebral blood flow creating stagnant hypoxic conditions. Patients with chronic duodenal or gastric ulcers are subject to these complications especially when there is co-existent pyloric obstruction or renal damage and alkaline powders have been taken to excess for the relief of pain. In the latter event, as pointed out originally in this country by Cooke[64] a state of *alkalosis* may arise. Although less potent than dehydration, alkalosis induces cerebral hypoxia by the high blood pH levels interfering with the dissociation of oxyhaemoglobin. I am indebted to Professor G. M. Bull for notes on the following case, which is an example of the harmful effects that may be induced.[65]

The patient was a man of 39 who had been in the habit of taking alkaline stomach powders several times daily over a period of years for relief of pain, due to chronic duodenal ulceration. Although there was no radiological evidence of obstruction, he had been vomiting and on admission to hospital was in a drowsy, confused mental state and resisted examination.

The results of blood investigation were as follows (normal values in brackets).

Packed cell volume	32·5%	(48%)
Plasma volume	1·33 l.	(3 l.)
Total blood volume	1·97 l.	(6 l.)
Blood urea	622 mg.%	(20–40 mg.%)
Chlorides	450 mg.%	(365 mg.%)
Na	309 mg.%	(330 mg.%)
CO_2 combining power	100 vol.%	(55–70 vol.%)
Blood pH	8·0	(7·25)
Effective renal flow	15 ml.	
Glomerular filtration rate	5 ml./min.	
Urine flow	2·5 ml./min.	

Samples of blood were taken from the internal jugular vein and oxygen saturation was found to be 33 and 38% in two samples. Allowing for the pH of the blood at the time, and reading from Barcroft's curves for oxyhaemoglobin dissociation at different pH, oxygen saturation in the cerebral tissues must have been about 8–10 mm. Hg., in comparison with the normal figure of 35 mm. Hg.

Reference has already been made to hepatic encephalopathy. It is rare in such cases to find the liver enlarged but the spleen is often palpable and, occasionally, as in the Cruveilhier-Baumgarten syndrome, where anastomotic connections are established through the inferior mammary arteries, a bruit can be heard on auscultation over the lower end of the sternum or over the liver.

Finally, the urine must, of course, be tested routinely for albumin, sugar and specific gravity. In addition, when liver disease is suspected, a search is made for amino-acids. We had no instance of porphyria in our series but in obscure cases it is advisable to test for the presence of porphyrobilinogens. Mental symptoms in this condition may remit or persist for many years after an attack; or again underlying mental instability may be rendered apparent by an attack, Gibson and Goldberg,[66] Hierons.[67]

BIBLIOGRAPHY

34 ASHER, R. (1949). Myxoedematous madness. *Brit. Med. J.*, **2**, 555.

35 WAYNE, E. J. (1960). *Brit. Med. J.*, **1**, 115.

36 MONTGOMERY, D. A. D. (1957). Myxoedema. In "Whitla's Dictionary of Medical Treatment", 9th Edn. Ed. Allison R. S. and Crozier T. H. Baillière, Tindall and Cox, London.

37 CHARATAN, F. B. and BRIERLEY, J. B. (1956). Mental disorder associated with primary lung carcinoma. *Brit. Med. J.*, **1**, 765.

38 DENNY-BROWN, D. (1948). Primary sensory neuropathy with muscular changes associated with carcinoma. *J. Neurol. Psychiat.*, **11**, 73.

39 McGOVERN, G. P., MILLER, D. H. and ROBERTSON, E. E. (1959). A mental syndrome associated with lung carcinoma. *Arch. Neurol. Psychiat.*, **81**, 341.

40 CRITCHLEY, M. (1929). Arteriosclerotic parkinsonism. *Brain*, **52**, 23.

41 WALKER, R. M. (1957). Portacaval anastomosis. *Lancet*, **1**, 56.

42 CRUVEILHIER (1829–35) "Anatomie Pathologique du corps humain." Vol. 1, xvi. livr. pl. vi—Maladies du veines. Paris, Baillière. Baumgarten von P. (1907): Über völlstandiges Offenbleiben der Vena umbilicalis: zugleich ein Beitrag zur Frage des Morbus Bantii. *Arb. path. Anat. Inst.*, **6**, 93.

43 PHILLIPS, G. B., SCHWARTZ, R., GABUZDA, G. J. JNR. and DAVIDSON, C. S. (1952). The Syndrome of impending hepatic coma in patients with cirrhosis of the liver given certain nitrogenous substances. *New. Engl. J. Med.*, **247**, 239.

44 ADAMS, R. D. and FOLEY, T. M. (1953). The neurological disorder associated with liver disease. *Res. Publ. Ass. Res. Nerv. Ment. Dis.*, **32**, 198.

45 SHERLOCK, S., SUMMERSKILL, W. H. J., WHITE, L. P. and PHEAR, E. A. (1954). Portal-systemic encephalopathy: neurological complications of liver disease. *Lancet*, **2**, 453.

46 SMYTH, C. and McCAW, N. B. (1957). Hepatic-type " flapping tremor " occurring in patients without hepatic disease. *J. Amer. Med. Ass.*, **165**, 31.

47 HERMAN, M., MOST, H. and JOLLIFFE, N. (1937). Psychosis associated with pernicious Anaemia. *Arch. Neurol. Psychiat.*, **38**, 348.

48 BERLYNE, G. M., LIVERSEDGE, L. A. and EMERY, E. W. (1957). Radioactive vitamin B_{12} in the diagnosis of neurological disorders. *Lancet*, **1**, 294.

49 HOBSON, W. and PEMBERTON, J. (1956). The health of the elderly at home. *Brit. Med. J.*, **1**, 4967.

50 SCHEINBERG, P. (1950). Cerebral circulation in heart failure. *Amer. J. Med.*, **8**, 148.

51 FOLEY, J. M. (1956). Hypertensive and arteriosclerotic vascular disease of the brain in the elderly. *Proc, Ass. Res. Nerv. Ment. Dis.*, **35**, 171.

52 HARINGTON, M., KINCAID-SMITH, P. and McMICHAEL, J. (1959). Results of treatment in malignant hypertension. *Brit. Med. J.*, **2**, 5158.

53 BEEVOR, C. E. (1907). The cerebral arterial supply. *Brain*, **30**, 29.

54 BEDFORD, P. D. (1955). Adverse cerebral effects of anaesthesia in old people. *Lancet*, **2**, 259.

55 HUTCHINSON, E. C. and YATES, P. O. (1957). Carotico-vertebral stenosis. *Lancet*, **1**, 2.

56 FISHER, M. (1954). Occlusion of the carotid arteries: further experiences. *Arch. Neurol. Psychiat.*, **72**, 187.

57 HURWITZ, L. J., GROCH, S. N., WRIGHT, I. S. and McDOWELL, F. H. (1959). Carotid artery occlusive syndrome. *Arch. Neurol. Psychiat.* **1**, 491.

58 GURDJIAN, E. S. and WEBSTER, J. E. (1949). " Spontaneous Thrombosis of The Carotid Arteries in the Neck." *Trans. Amer. Neurol. Ass.*, 50.

59 Ibid. (1955). The place of the carotid bifurcation in the production of the stroke syndrome. *Trans. Amer, Neurol. Ass.*, 198.

60 WEITZMAN, E. D. and SPALTER, H. (1959). Use of retinal arterial pressure as a diagnostic tool in internal carotid disease. *Arch. Neurol. Psychiat.* **81**, 708.

61 SOMNER, A. R., DOUGLAS, A. C., HILLIS, B. R., MARKS, B. L. and GRANT, I. W. B. (1958). Value of Bronchoscopy in clinical practice. *Brit. Med. J.* **1**, 5079.

62 FISCHER-WILLIAMS, M., BOSANQUET, F. D. and DANIEL, P. M. (1955). Carcinomatosis of the meningea. *Brain*, **78**, 42.

63 SPILLANE, J. D. (1947). " Nutritional Disorders of the Nervous System." Livingstone, Edinburgh.

64 COOKE, A. M. (1932). Alkalosis occurring in the alkaline treatment of peptic ulcers. *Quart. J. Med.*, **1**, 527.

65 ALLISON, R. S. (1956). Clinical consequences of cerebral anoxia. *Proc. Roy. Soc. Med.*, **49**, 609.

66 GIBSON, J. B. and GOLDBERG, A. (1956). The neuropathology of acute porphyria. *J. Path. Bact.*, **71**, 495.

67 HIERONS, R. (1957). Changes in the nervous system in acute porphyria. *Brain*, **82**, 176.

CHAPTER III

Neurological Examination

PATIENTS with organic mental symptoms may have no neurological signs, but this assumption should not be made until examination has been conducted in detail and any equivocal features have been carefully evaluated. The rule is applicable especially when no general metabolic or other cause can be found to account for the patient's disturbed mental state. Conversely, when neurological signs are present, the chief object is to determine whether these are indicative of a focal, circumscribed lesion or of diffuse changes affecting both hemispheres. Bilaterally more or less symmetrical signs are fairly common in diffuse cerebral atrophy, but signs confined to one side are usually convincing proof of the presence of a focal cerebral lesion.

It is not proposed to enter into details of clinical methods except where some modification from standard procedure is required to compensate for the patient's altered mental state.

SPECIAL SENSES

Patients were tested routinely for their ability to recognize peppermint, cloves, etc., but no appreciable differences in response from the normal were noted. An olfactory hallucination was the presenting symptom in one case, the patient, a woman of 55, complaining of a recurring strong smell of coal gas. This would persist for about 10–15 minutes and sometimes it occurred twice or thrice in the day, although she might be free for some weeks at a time. So real was it that she was continually urging her husband to search for possible leaks and to complain to the Gas Company. When these appeals were ignored or treated as imaginary she became depressed and neglected her household duties. Her first admission to hospital was determined by an attempt at suicide through taking an overdose of barbiturate. Electric convulsion treatment was given and there was some improvement in her mental state, but shortly after she returned home hallucinations recurred and, following an intense headache, she had an epileptiform fit. Angiography revealed a large aneurysm situated at the junction of the middle cerebral and internal carotid arteries, which at operation was found to be pressing on the left temporal pole.

Ophthalmoscopy. Two questions arose over the interpretation to be put on the findings on ophthalmoscopy. First, when an intracranial tumour was suspected, what significance was to be attached to normal appearances of the discs? As already mentioned, in a number of patients later proved to have tumours or subdural haematomata there was no evidence of papilloedema at any stage in their illnesses. Further, in some others papilloedema appeared too late to be of any assistance in early diagnosis. Some of the patients referred to us, indeed, had had lumbar punctures in the belief that the absence of papilloedema removed any possible contra-indication to the procedure. In fact, lumbar puncture was often responsible for accelerating their decline and creating a state of surgical emergency. The other difficulty lay in the significance to be attached to blurring of the disc margins, increased tortuosity of retinal vessels, variations in calibre and constriction of veins at arterio-venous crossings in patients in whom systemic blood pressure was elevated. Raised blood pressure levels were to be expected in many of these older patients and it is known that such may occur in response to increase in intracranial pressure as from a tumour. Whilst recognizing that distinct swelling of the discs may be seen in arteriospastic retinitis without any accompanying haemorrhagic exudates and degenerative retinal changes,[68] our attitude was not to give too much weight to such findings unless the diastolic pressure was much elevated (125–160 mm. Hg) and haemorrhages and cotton wool patches were widely distributed over the retina.

Visual fields. It is often difficult to get patients with organic mental disease to co-operate sufficiently to enable perimetric tests to be made and the same may apply to confrontation tests. But as *hemianopia* may be the only neurological sign of a focal lesion it is important to try and confirm or exclude its presence by other means. Sometimes the response to menace may be taken as a guide or a hemianopic defect may be suggested by the absence of optokinetic nystagmus to one side on rotating a drum with figures on it before the patient in clockwise and anti-clockwise directions. Another way is for the examiner to seat himself in front of the patient and engage him in talk. Meanwhile, an assistant standing behind him projects into each of his half-fields in turn a brightly-coloured object such as an orange or better, a flower held by its stalk. The presence of hemianopia or visual inattention on one side is then confirmed by the patient ignoring the stimulus on that side and at once turning his gaze towards it when it is presented on the other. The patient should not be told to look at the examiner; he does this unconsciously but if specifically directed to do so may disregard stimuli on both sides under the impression that this is what he is required to do.

Colour vision. Lack of appreciation of colour may be limited to one homonymous half-field in which case it can be detected by the confrontation method, each eye being tested separately and a brightly coloured object being displayed in each half field in turn. But, before doing so one should determine whether the patient can recognize the colours of objects set before him and pick out different shades from among Holmgren's wools. Inability to do so would indicate colour imperception.

Homonymous hemianopia was present in a number of our cases, either alone or in association (more commonly) with ipsilateral motor and sensory defects. The right halves of the visual fields were affected more often than the left. In lesions affecting the temporo-parietal rather than the occipital region hemianopia is often incongruous, there being no accurate bisection of the visual field into two regions, according to whether visual acuity is intact, or not.[69] In most of our cases with posterially-placed lesions, however, gross incongruity of the fields could seldom be demonstrated, although macular sparing was obvious in many of those who were able to co-operate sufficiently in perimetry. Occasionally there was no such sparing, the blind halves being sharply defined right up to the fixation point, and one of these was a man of 55, whose chief complaints had been inability to see to the right and " numbness " in the corresponding half of his body. At post-mortem a tumour was found replacing the left thalamus and involving the internal capsule and left cerebral peduncle.

Of interest in connection with hemianopia is the extent to which subjects are aware of their visual defects. Some of our patients complained that their " sight " was not good, or that the right or left eye was defective, this being their way of interpreting the loss of vision to one side. Others, however, although seemingly unaware of any visual impairment, when asked to draw a house or some other object neglected details on their hemianopic side and when shown a map sited well-know places not as they should be, some on one side, some on the other, but all on their non-hemianopic side. Various explanations have been suggested to explain this phenomenon, some of the factors thought to determine awareness being: anteriorly-placed lesions involving the chiasma or optic tract; incongruity of homonymous defects; sudden onset of hemianopia, absence of macular sparing. And those determining unawareness: posteriorly-placed lesions affecting the optic radiations; congruous field defects; hemianopia of gradual onset, and the presence of macular sparing. But the matter is far from being so simple as to be capable of such ready explanation.[70] The lack of awareness in some cases may indeed be an example of

" organic repression " and analagous to other attitudes adopted by patients with brain disease, some of which have already been referred to in a previous chapter. Further, the normal tendency to perceive whole objects when presented only with parts of the whole may play some part in determining unawareness, for hemianopic patients when shown half of a square or circle, so placed as to project into their blind field, declare that they see a whole square or circle, as the case may be.[71] There are some grounds for thinking, too, that the phenomenon of unawareness is related to development of a pseudo-fovea or new macula, the patient learning to shift his gaze so as to bring to bear a point on the retina slightly to the side of the former fixation point.

Visual inattention for one side was often the first evidence of a developing hemianopia or the sole indication of a posteriorially-placed lesion affecting the visual pathway. It could readily be detected by confrontation. The patient was instructed to keep both eyes open and to fix his gaze on the examiner, who extended his arms to either side and made discreet finger movements, first on one side, then on the other. When the patient could recognize these movements individually, movements on both sides were then made simultaneously. Ability to detect single stimuli in either half-field, but failure to recognize simultaneous stimuli, the patient invariably selecting the one on the unaffected side, is typical of visual inattention. Another recognized method is to prepare a blackboard or card upon which are inscribed a series of digits and/or letters arranged in form of a square, each quadrant of which contains the same letters or digits. The patient is then seated in front of the board, given a pointer and directed to point to a " 7 ", " 9 ", " B ", or " G " etc. Patients with unilateral visual inattention make selections exclusively or predominantly from the digits or letters on the opposite side of the board.

The occurrence of *sudden blindness* or transient episodes of impaired vision in patients over the age of 50 should raise suspicion at once either of cranial (temporal) arteritis or of internal carotid stenosis (p. 35). The former is recognized by the association of visual symptoms with severe headache and tenderness over the scalp, where the affected vessels may be felt as swollen tender cords. Pain is often complained of also in the face and jaws, especially on chewing, and the erythrocyte sedimentation rate is raised. But when the short ciliary arteries forming the arterial circle of Zinn around the optic nerve head (Meadows[72]), or the retinal blood vessels are first affected, these signs may be absent and blindness the only symptom. Both eyes may be affected simultaneously, or first one and then, in the course of a few days, the other. Diplopia may occur from involvement of the oculo-motor mechanism with third or sixth nerve palsy. Parsons-Smith[73] points out that eye complications occur in half the cases and that not infrequently these are the presenting features. On ophthalmoscopy there may be little to be seen or the appearances may be those of papilloedema, thrombosis of the central artery of the retina or macular haemorrhages and exudates. Early recognition is important as vision may be saved through the adoption of prompt treatment (see p. 272). *Cortical blindness.* In cortical blindness, due to bilateral destruction of the occipital cortex, the patient is not as a rule aware of being blind. As Duke Elder [74] says " he is not plunged into darkness, but so far as he himself is concerned has nothing in front of him to see ". The pupils respond to light. Voluntary ocular convergence and accommodation are still possible, but reflex ocular movements of convergence and accommodation are lost. In *visual agnosia* by contrast, there is no absolute blindness; particular aspects of an object with which the patient is familiar may be seen. But he still cannot recognize the object for what it is, although able to do so promptly when allowed to employ his other sense, i.e. those of touch or hearing. Psycho-visual reflexes connected with the responses to convergence and accommodation are unaffected.

Visual acuity. Impairment of previously good reading ability may be one of the first signs of organic mental disease and was indeed the presenting symptom of such in four of our cases. Errors of refraction, cataract, opacities in the vitreous, optic atrophy or retrobulbar neuritis, and retinal degenerative changes have to be considered, but if these can be excluded the possibility of a dyslexia must always be taken into account. Particularly suggestive is the finding that the patient has no difficulty in seeing small dots on a sheet of paper and is yet unable to read even the largest test type. The testing of such patients is considered in Chapter VIII.

Hearing. Acuity of hearing was tested by the distance from one ear a patient could hear whispered voice sounds when the other ear was occluded. When necessary, this simple test was supplemented by audiometry. In otosclerosis there is depression of hearing throughout the different range of frequencies and especially for higher frequencies, the latter effect being typical of pure nerve deafness. In doubtful cases Hallpike's fractional method of caloric stimulation of the labrinth was used, in favour of a tumour compressing the eighth nerve being loss of hearing for high frequencies, combined with much diminished or absent caloric response. Frequently in otosclerotic cases there is no response to stimulation with water at 44° C and only a poor response to stimulation at 30° C. Defective hearing, as might be expected in older patients, was fairly common and occasionally tinnitus was the presenting symptom of a depressive disorder, the patient blaming the noise for his inability to concentrate and loss of interest. In one case the combination of nerve deafness, tinnitus and ipsilateral cerebellar ataxia, in a middle-aged woman showing signs of impairment of memory and intellect, led to a correct diagnosis of acoustic neuroma, but this was the only instance in the series. Radiological evidence of erosion of bone or widening of the internal acoustic meatus is to be expected only in about one half of such cases. Of other neurological signs, probably of most value in determining the likelihood of an acoustic neuroma is impairment or absence of the corneal reflex on the affected side, a sign which was present in 51 out of 53 cases investigated by Parker.[75] This author also drew attention to the infrequency of facial pain or neuralgia in cases of tumour of the acoustic nerve.

Recurring attacks of acute vertigo simulating Ménière's disease were reported in two patients who were later found to have tumours involving the middle part of the temporal lobe. In one of these the subjective sense of movement was in the vertical plane, the patient when driving his car, suddenly experiencing the impression that it was reversing or falling over backwards, and only with difficulty maintaining his position at the steering wheel. It was not until he had had nine such attacks (in three of which, following the aura, consciousness was lost) that a contralateral quadrantic field defect was detected and the true nature of his condition revealed.

In addition to hearing tests, patients with organic mental states were also required to demonstrate their capacity for recognizing the nature of familiar sounds, e.g. running water from a tap, jingling keys and money, tearing or crushing paper. Auditory agnosia was more rare than visual agnosia but these aspects are considered further in Chapter X.

CRANIAL NERVES

Contracted and sluggishly reacting pupils were not uncommon in these older patients but *Argyll Robertson pupils* were only seen once (in the absence of other evidence of neurosyphilis), and this was in a man with diffuse cerebral atherosclerosis causing mild dementia. However, in view of the importance of this sign in neurosyphilis it is of interest that in some of the cases of general paralysis it was absent. Thus, in two patients presenting with mental symptoms, positive blood and cerebrospinal fluid Wassermann reactions, paretic Lange curves, and increase of cells and protein, the pupils were normal, both in their appearance and responses, and in three other cases the only abnormality was diminished response to light. Unequal, contracted pupils occurred in two cases and in two others, one of whom had a unilateral partial external ophthalmoplegia, there was *ptosis* of the upper lid. *Tremor of the face*, often present only on talking, very fine and confined to the angles of the mouth and nasolabial folds was seen in about half of the cases and in about an equal proportion there was coarse ataxic tremor of the tongue and some *slurring dysarthria*.

Unilateral *facial weakness* was often an important localizing sign of a contralateral intracranial space-occupying lesion, but being slight, was easily overlooked if reliance were placed on getting the patient to bare his teeth and shut the eyes tightly. A better way was to get him to talk and watch his face carefully for any signs of asymmetry of movement in the nasolabial folds. Early facial weakness could often be detected in this way when it was not apparent by any other test. It is also important in patients with expressive speech defects to test for signs of facial or tongue apraxia. This was done by asking the patient to purse his lips or to whistle, and by getting him to put out his tongue and lick his lips. In the absence of paralysis failure to perform such skilled movements was usually accepted as evidence of oral apraxia, a condition which, as will be seen by reference to Chapter VII, was often found in association with severe expressive speech disorders. In patients with dysarthria attention was especially directed to movements of the soft palate and tongue. In spastic conditions the tongue cannot as a rule be protruded beyond the teeth; in ataxic dysarthrias there is no difficulty in protrusion but voluntary movement is impaired by coarse tremors of trombone type and rapid to and fro movements or protruding and withdrawing movements of the tongue cannot be performed.

Motor Functions

Determination of the *handedness* of patients with organic mental disease is important owing to the relationship that exist between this and cerebral dominance, a conception which drew its inspiration originally from Dax's observation of the frequency with which right-sided hemiplegia is associated with disturbances of speech and language and Broca's demonstration of the association of left-sided frontal lesions with aphasia. The dominant hemisphere, it has been thought, not only governs the preferred hand but is the seat of the faculties concerned with speech and language. Determination of handedness is the most widely recognized method of deciding which hemisphere is dominant, but eye and foot preference, although having less significance, must also be taken into account. Handedness is genetically determined and acquired sometime before the fifth or sixth year of life, but it may be modified by other post-natal factors. Thus, although most individuals are predominantly or exclusively right-handed and only a small proportion truly left-handed, many show mixed laterality, the right hand being preferred for some actions and the left for others.

Blau [76] gives a list of some 40 tests by which handedness or " preferred lateralism " may be determined. It is unnecessary to apply such detailed testing when the right hand is clearly preferred, but in others in which there is evidence of crossed lateralism careful tests should be made and we have used especially the following:

Hand:

which hand is preferred in writing, drawing,* striking a match, hammering, dialling the telephone, cutting with scissors, holding a knife, throwing a ball, combing the hair, brushing the teeth, blowing the nose, turning a tap or unscrewing a cork.

Eye:

which eye remains open when the patient looks through a small hole in a piece of paper?

Foot:

which foot is used for kicking a ball?
on which foot is the weight put in hopping?

This subject is considered further in Chapter VIII.

The demonstration of slight unilateral *motor weakness* or alteration of tone is, of course, a valuable sign of a contralateral focal cerebral lesion, but unless searched for carefully may readily be overlooked. A few minutes should be allowed for observing what happens when the patient extends his arms in front, with the backs of the hands uppermost and the fingers extended. He does this first with the eyes open and then with them closed. In the former event slight weakness or decrease in tone may bring out some irregular coarse tremor, limited to the affected side, or compensating movements may be seen to correct the tendency of one or other arm to droop. With the eyes closed, however, the tendency for the limb to fall away or lose height becomes more apparent, or it may drift outwards or upwards. In many confirmed cases of tumour this was the earliest and sometimes the only indication of motor deficit. In other patients, with the arms out-

---

* Evidence of handedness is also provided by the way in which persons represent smoke issuing from a chimney, right-handed persons usually representing it as blowing to the right, left-handed persons to the left. Similarly, left-handed persons represent objects as moving towards the left, right-handed persons towards the right.

stretched and the palms held uppermost, it was possible to demonstrate Babinski's pronator sign. Another useful test was to observe whether " mirror " movements occurred on the affected side when the patient was made to grasp an object with the sound hand.

Equally important for the detection of unilateral parietal lesions was the demonstration of diminished postural tone and slight ataxia in the contralateral limbs. No instance of parietal wasting of muscle was encountered, but this may affect the small muscles of the hand and have an " ulnar " or " median " distribution. It is said to occur especially with long-standing tumours such as meningiomata. However, the most constant sign in our patients was the way in which they neglected to make use of one hand in skilled activities which required the use of both hands, working together. This *motor neglect* could be demonstrated by spilling a box of matches and inviting them to pick them up as quickly as possible. With parietal lesions, and especiallly those affecting the subordinate hemisphere, the absence of any attempt to make use of the contralateral hand was very apparent, one hand only being employed in completing the task. In one patient, a woman with a primary carcinoma of the vagina (p. 28) and a chronic amnesic syndrome but no neurological signs, a curious feature was observed. When a number of objects were placed before her and she was asked to demonstrate their use, she picked up with her right hand objects situated on that side and with her left hand objects on the left side. One of these was a toothbrush and when the order of objects was re-arranged so that the toothbrush was then on the left side, she persisted (or perseverated) in picking it up and demonstrating its use with her left hand. Enquiry showed that she had always been right-handed.

Motor weakness confined to the lower limbs was seen in only two patients with tumours. The first gave a 6 months' history of slowly progressive hemiparesis, first affecting the left leg and later spreading to the arm (right fronto-temporal astrocytoma). The second was a sailor with a right frontal meningioma. In his case the only evidence of motor weakness had been a tendency to catch the toes of the (ipsilateral) right foot on the deck so that he had fallen many times. On testing him lying in the prone position, with the knees half-flexed, there was some tendency for the right leg to fall away, but the plantar reflexes were flexor, and it was difficult to detect any appreciable difference in the knee and ankle jerks, both of which, however, were unduly brisk.

In cerebral vascular accidents the sudden onset and hemiplegic character of the resulting paralysis were reliable clues. Only occasionally was an apoplectic type of onset observed in patients subsequently found to have cerebral tumours and these exceptions created no great difficulties in differential diagnosis. The chief problem rather was to decide whether the *hemiplegia* had been caused by (1) capsular haemorrhage, thrombosis or embolism, (2) internal carotid occlusion, or (3) intracerebral haemorrhage. Ten years ago the last two possibilities were rarely considered but on looking over old case notes it is obvious that in many patients the more or less sudden onset of paralytic symptoms may well have been due to one or other of these causes. For instance, some of them were found to have hemiplegia and an homonymous field defect but little evidence of sensory loss, pinprick and touch being felt over the trunk and being only slightly impaired over the extremities on the affected side, whereas loss of postural joint sensibility was pronounced in the fingers and often at the wrists. This selective and restricted sensory impairment with pronounced hemiplegia and hemianopia is difficult to reconcile with a capsular lesion, and in the light of more recent experience more suggestive of ischaemic cerebral infarction. A further point of differentiation concerns the initial state of consciousness in these patients rendered suddenly hemiplegic. In two recently proved instances of intracerebral haemorrhage, leading to haematoma formation, headache was associated with the sudden development of hemiplegia, but there was no initial loss of consciousness, the patient appearing perfectly lucid. In such cases it is recognized that clouding of consciousness may supervene later owing to expansion of the haematoma from further bleeding. In capsular lesions, it is our impression that impairment of consciousness is likely to be present from the onset of symptoms (of hemiplegia) or to supervene within a few hours, and that this may be due to the proximity of the internal capsule to the diencephalic centre regulating consciousness (see p. 96). In retrospect, it was noticeable in many of our atherosclerotic patients with acute cerebral vascular lesions that there had been little initial impairment of consciousness, although signs of such became apparent as a rule within the succeeding week and often persisted for some time before showing signs of resolving. This sequence of events is more in keeping with haemorrhage into the substance of one hemisphere or of occlusion of a vessel on the carotico-vertebral system, the hemiplegia and prolonged clouding of consciousness being due to ischaemic infarction. However, it is not suggested that this rule is absolute; in practice there were many inexplicable exceptions. Reviewing clinical aspects of carotid thrombosis, Elkington [77] discusses the wide varieties that may occur. The condition affects the left carotid more often than the right and is three times as common in men as in women. Comparatively rare are cases in which occlusion of the vessel in the neck gives rise to rapidly-developing massive contralateral hemiplegia with depression or loss of consciousness. Equally rare are cases in which sudden contralateral hemiplegia is associated with ipsilateral blindness, narrowing of the retinal vessels and subsequent optic atrophy. At the other extreme are cases in which carotid occlusion occurs without causing any symptoms. More common manifestations are transient episodes of unilateral disturbance, recurring at irregular intervals over many months or years. These often consist of weakness or numbness in one arm, blurring of vision in one eye or dysphasia. As such symptoms are usually associated with headache, which follows them, they may be mistaken for migraine. In other cases the chief complaint may be of recurring " dizziness ", " by which they mean, a feeling of confusion and impairment of consciousness rather than of vertigo ". Fits, although they may occur, are rare harbingers of carotid occlusion, the only indication of which is more often gradually developing contralateral hemiplegia and dysphasia, the arm and face being more affected than the leg. In all such cases in which carotid thrombosis is susupecte angiography is required to make an absolute diagnosis, but frtherd indirect information may be obtained by ophthalmodynamometry and the other procedures outlined in the section dealing with examination of the cardiovascular system. Symonds[78] has suggested that in certain instances it may not be necessary to employ angiography and better to make a direct surgical exploration of the vessel with the object of removing clot, and if possible, excising the diseased portion. This is most commonly situated just distal to the bifurcation of the carotid artery into its external and internal branches.

INVOLUNTARY MOVEMENTS

Tremor, although often considered as an integral feature of the process of ageing, actually is uncommon in old age. [79] Senile tremor has many points of similarity to " idiopathic " or " familial " tremor and typically affects either the head, jaw, face or hands. When it involves the head, fine rhythmical nodding movements result, these taking place either in an anteroposterior direction (affirmative gesture) or from side to side (gesture of negation). Tremor of the mandible may take the form of rhythmical chewing or champing movements, and in some cases where the lower part of the face is involved the movements may resemble those displayed by a rabbit nibbling grass. In the hands the involuntary movements are slow and coarse, resembling Parkinson's disease, fine and quick as in hyperthyroidism or they may be exaggerated by action, as is seen in cerebellar disease. The development of senile tremor is not usually a herald of impending mental dissolution, and is often seen in patients who live to a great age. Its chief importance lies in its distinction from other more serious varieties of tremor, e.g. Parkinsonism, hepatic encephalopathy. Although the typical involuntary movements of Huntington's chorea may be absent, [80] choreiform movements are usually found in association with the gradual dementing process, which is characteristic of the disease, and in about half of our cases they were the most conspicuous feature. Profusion of involuntary facial grimaces, shrugging movements of the shoulders and undue fidgetyness with frequent changes of posture, one leg being crossed over the other and then the positions reversed, are all suggestive. In some of our cases the presenting symptom was difficulty in walking and unless one has had previous experience of cases it is easy to fall into the error of assuming that the gait is hysterical. The patient advances the lower limbs in a hesitant and jerky fashion, the natural timing of movements being lost and the pattern interrupted irregularly by what appears at first sight to be purposeful and unrelated movements. These almost, but not quite, throw the patient off balance and the way in which he succeeds in retrieving this, taken into account with the frequent associated choreiform movements of the upper limbs, neck and face, convey a bizarre effect that is unmistakable. The electroencephalogram may show a flat record (low amplitude) but this is not pathognomonic and confirmation of the diagnosis is usually obtained through the family history indicating that other members of the family have been affected.

Apraxia of Gait. Reference has already been made to the peculiar disturbances of gait sometimes seen in elderly subjects with organic mental states. Meyer and Barron[26] describe a number of clinical tests which may be useful in distinguishing apraxia from ataxia. Some of the most useful we have found to be as follows:

(1) In ataxia of cerebellar origin the patient has no difficulty in lifting his feet off the ground and shows no tendency to shuffle, but walks drunkenly, his steps being irregularly-placed and usually widely separated. By contrast the apraxic patient's feet often appear to be rooted to the ground and progression is by short, irregularly-timed and hesitant steps.

(2) Apraxic patients often have difficulty (in bed) in changing to the upright from the recumbent position, although once upright they can maintain this position. Similarly, when instructed to turn over in bed, to cross one leg over the other, to tap on the floor with the heel or kick a ball they are unaccountably inept in their performance. Often such ineptitude is taken for " stupidity " or " lack of co-operation ", as when during examination one instructs the patient to flex his knee and

he persists in keeping it extended, a result which may well be due to his tendency to perseverate.

(3) In apraxia, a grasp reflex may sometimes be obtained in stroking the soles of the feet. Purdon Martin [81] remarked on something very similar some years ago in two cases of frontal tumour: " the plantar reflexes were peculiar in that they were very briskly flexor: the slightest touch of the sole produced full and immediate flexion of the great toe, unaccompanied by any withdrawal of the foot ", and again: " briskly flexor to an extreme degree, the merest touch of the sole causing full and immediate flexion ". In one of his cases showing this phenomenon the gait was apraxic.

(4) Apraxic patients, although able to take a few paces forwards, when instructed to reverse their direction and step backwards may be unable to do so, the familiar quality of the feet remaining " rooted " or " glued " to the ground becoming at once apparent.

(5) " Star gait " test for ataxia.[82] In this test the patient's attention is directed to an object some paces distant and with his eyes closed he is told to take three or four steps forward in its direction and then to reverse his steps by an equal number and go forward again. Ataxic subjects tend each time to veer to one side of the target. This test is far from being devoid of risk and only suitable for mildy affected cases, in which the results may be equivocal.

SENSATION

It is often difficult in organic mental cases to test sensation adequately, but the demonstration of unilateral sensory impairment may have such diagnostic significance that efforts to do so must always be made, standard procedures being modified where necessary to make up for specific intellectual defects or other difficulties in co-operation.

When the level of consciousness is seriously depressed only the response to pinprick can be ascertained. Otherwise, in testing touch, vibration and postural sensibility it is advisable first to spend some time explaining the procedure to the patient. Thus, using the tip of his forefinger as a stimulus, the examiner should let the patient both see and feel him touching his skin, and make sure he understands that he is required to say " yes " or make some appropriate gesture in response to each stimulus. When he has proved his ability to do this, the tests are then repeated with the eyes covered or the parts to be tested concealed from view. Occasionally, we met patients who denied that they could feel any touch. Whether this was due to negativism or determined by one or other of the factors that govern behaviour in brain-injured subjects is not known. But when the stimulus was increased by brushing the skin lightly with the whole hand they invariably recognized it, and once they had done so it was usually possible, by gradually reducing the strength, to get them to recognize even the lightest touch.

Similarly, in testing *postural sensibility*, the examiner should first encourage the patient to watch him making passive movements of the fingers and get him to indicate the direction of movement by calling " up " or " down ". When he has shown he can do this the same tests are then applied with the eyes covered. The interphalangeal joints of the fingers and great toes are first selected, passive movements being made distinctly and abruptly and care being taken to immobilize other joints. If no sensation of movement is felt in the joints being tested one then proceeds to test passive movements at more proximal joints, i.e. the wrists, ankles, knee and elbow joints. Needless to say, postural sensory loss should only be deduced when passive movements are correctly interpreted with the eyes open but are consistently neglected or misinterpreted when the eyes are covered.

Vibration sense is often diminished in old age,[83] so that too much reliance was not placed on this type of sensory loss alone. But the demonstration of *pseudo-athetosis* was sometimes useful in confirming the presence of defective postural joint sense in the fingers. To do this the patient's eyes were covered and he was instructed to extend his arms in front of him with the palms of the hands uppermost, in this position the slow sinuous and exploratory flexor movements of the fingers being usually most apparent. Another method of confirming extensive proprioceptive loss, involving more proximal joints, such as the wrists and elbows, was to take hold of the affected arm and raise it to a position well within the patient's view, the latter then being told to grasp the thumb with his sound hand. When he had demonstrated his ability to do this his eyes were then covered and the tests repeated, each time the limb being moved into a different position. Almost invariably patients with severe sensory loss reached into space beyond the actual situation of the limb and groped about in an exploratory fashion until they finally made contact with it. Having found the arm by groping in the air they then proceeded to work their way down it until they came to the hand and finally to the thumb (Photograph facing p. 58). In some cases in which there were associated disturbances of the body image, the examiner's hand was mistaken for that of the patient but such gross errors were unusual (see Chapter IX).

When routine testing with a single stimulus fails to demonstrate any gross sensory loss, the method of double simultaneous stimulation should be tried. This was used by Oppenheim,[84] who showed that when certain patients with organic brain disease were submitted to tactile or painful stimuli on both sides of the body simultaneously they often failed to acknowledge the stimulus on one side. He called this sign *tactile inattention.*

In testing for it one should, as before, first allow the patient to watch what is being done. This time, not only has he to report when he feels the stimulus but he must indicate the side and place upon which it is felt, e.g. " on the right hand ", " on the left hand ", " on both sides ", " on the right side of the face ", " on the right side of the face and the right hand ". Patients in whom there is appreciable clouding of consciousness or who have difficulties in registration or self-expression, and others in whom catastrophic reactions readily occur are unsuitable, as they cannot be expected to follow what to them must appear complicated directions. But, assuming that a patient is capable of cooperation, once he has understood what is required the tests should be repeated with his eyes covered. When sensory inattention is present single stimuli to either side are reported, but when bilaterally symmetrical stimuli are used, the one on the affected side is ignored, and this curious phenomenon may be demonstrable both for light touch and pain. In a few of our cases, indeed, it was so pronounced that when a bulky wad of cotton wool was applied to the " bad " arm and a thin wisp of the same material to the sound one, only the latter was reported. On another occasion, in the same patient, when the test was repeated with a pin and cotton wool respectively, the pinprick was ignored and only the light touch of the wool acknowledged. When a patient ignored the stimulus on one side his eyes were uncovered and he was invited to look and see what was being done. The effect of this was often to surprise him greatly for, as he might say, he could see now that he was being touched on both sides, but could not recall previously having felt any sensation on the affected side. Even with the evidence before their eyes, patients were sometimes reluctant to acknowledge it and were apt to comment that the feeling was not so strong as it was on the sound side. Whether this was true or not it was difficult to decide, but in some cases there was substance in their remarks for, when tested with single pinpricks, the response was less on the affected side and tactile stimuli were not reported so consistently as they were on the sound side.

Other writers since Oppenheim, convinced that the phenomenon cannot be explained simply on the basis of inattention have renamed it " extinction " or preferred to use the expression " perceptual rivalry " in relation to it. Its explanation is certainly not fully understood. It is analogous to visual inattention in its dependence on double stimulation and its occurrence in patients with minimal sensory defects. It is also related to *allaesthesia*, in which condition a single stimulus applied to a point on one side is referred by the patient to a symmetrical point on the opposite of the body. Allaesthesia was observed in only two of our cases and is probably of much rarer occurrence than sensory inattention, but Bender and his associates [85] have given a detailed account of such a case in a man suffering from diffuse encephalopathy. Bender [86] interprets Oppenheim's inattention as being more a positive extinction of part of the body image, but Denny-Brown *et al.*[87, 88] discount the rôle of primary disturbances in the body image and regard it as being an expression of defective spatial summation and part of the disturbed perceptual capacity shown by brain-damaged subjects in general, many of whom have difficulty in competing with more than one stimulus at a time. Jaffe and Bender,[89] however, demonstrated that persons recovering consciousness after anaesthesia, when stimulated simultaneously on the face and hand, at first only acknowledge the stimulus to the face, and Cohn [90] believes this represents a reversion to a more primitive type of perceptual thinking in relation to the body image. This is of interest as similar reversions to more primitive patterns of performance may be seen in the house drawings of brain-damaged subjects,[91] and Cohn's view is supported by the character of normal childrens' drawings of the human figure between the ages of $3\frac{1}{2}$–5 years. These invariably depict the face as forming the centrepiece, the extremities receiving but scant notice and there being little or no attempt to delineate fingers and hands.

In our experience sensory inattention (or extinction) was usually seen in patients in whom (1) there was slight clouding of consciousness, and (2) minimal sensory impairment. It was often demonstrable on the contralateral side in focal vascular and neoplastic lesions affecting the parietal region. Usually, the patients had only recently been admitted to hospital and there was some clouding of consciousness, however slight. Critchley [92] notes that inattention may be present one moment and not the next, and this was our experience too. As the level of consciousness rose it tended to disappear. It was also seen in some patients with diffuse cerebral cortical disease, and in one case the only abnormal finding in the brain at autopsy was softening in the thalamus and internal capsule, the result of a former thrombotic lesion. This was a woman who had originally been rendered dysphasic, hemiplegic and hemianopic. There had been considerable improvement in the first two disabilities over the succeeding years, but some sensory impairment and right-sided visual inattention had persisted. Her unusual mental attitude to the affected right arm is described on p. 197. Perhaps the best example of sensory inattention being of assistance in diagnosis, however, was the following:

The patient, a shipyard worker aged 58, had been admitted to hospital in the belief that he might be suffering from syringomyelia. This was because he had a large, third degree, burn on the back of the left hand for which he was unable to account. His relatives were not so much concerned about this as the fact that a week previously he had appeared one evening in the street clad in his night attire and had acted in a confused manner. He was a healthy-looking man, and general and neurological examination were negative. When tested with pin-prick and touch he responded naturally, although perhaps not so promptly on the left arm as on the right. However, no dissociated sensory loss was demonstrable. When simultaneous stimuli were used he invariably ignored the stimulus on the left arm. Mentally, there was defective memory for recent events, slight difficulty in registration and disorientation in time, but this was correct for place and persons. He was not dysphasic and except for some constructional difficulties showed no apraxia or agnosia. Talk was free and rather uninhibited, like his behaviour, the mood being elated and euphoric. E.E.G. showed diffuse abnormalities with slower rhythms over the left side but there was no focus. Blood and C.S.F. were normal. Lumbar encephalography showed some symmetrical ventricular dilatation. Despite the evidence of dementia, it was felt that the persistence of unilateral sensory signs justified further action, and as the result of a ventriculogram a chronic subdural haematoma was discovered, lying over the right parietal cortex. This was evacuated and subsequently the sensory inattention disappeared, the patient being able to resume work, although still exhibiting signs of general cerebral deterioration.

Cortical sensory loss. The chief tests used in evaluating cortical sensory function were: ability to locate the site of tactile stimuli; two-point discrimination, and stereognostic sense. To test for the first-named, the patient placed his hands with palms down, resting on the bed or table. The examiner then touched him on the back of one hand or lower forearm with a blunt-pointed pencil and asked him to indicate with the forefinger of the other hand where he had felt the touch. After a few trials the patient then closed his eyes and the tests were repeated, this time the points touched and the points indicated by the patient being marked on the skin with dots and crosses respectively. Five tests were made and the process then repeated for the other limb. Fig. 1 illustrates the results obtained in a woman aged 55 with a glioblastoma multiforme, which was diffusely infiltrating the upper and posterior part of the left temporal lobe, bridging the Sylvian fissure and extending into the parietal lobe. In addition to her difficulty in locating the site of tactile stimuli applied to the right hand and forearm, there was variable sensory inattention for both light touch and pinprick, some evidence of defective postural sensibility in the fingers, defective two-point discrimination and dystereognosis.

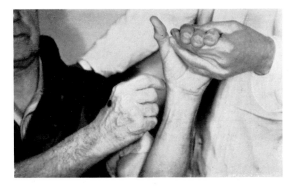

Patient experiencing difficulty in grasping his thumb on the affected side with the opposite or sound hand. He cannot find it with his eyes closed.

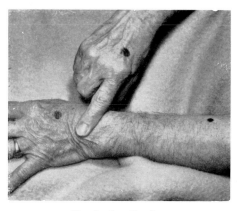

Tactile Localization

With his eyes closed the patient attempts to place his forefinger on the spot on the back of his hand just touched by the examiner. The other black spots represent points where he has previously been touched.

Two-point discrimination was tested over the finger pads by means of an aesthesiometer or two fine wooden orange sticks. Ten tests were made on each hand, the points being separated an inch or more at first and the distance then being gradually reduced. When the distance apart at which two points were felt as one had been determined, they were then gradually separated until two stimuli were received, the mean of these two readings being accepted as the critical distance. In making this test each application should be firm and abrupt, the points

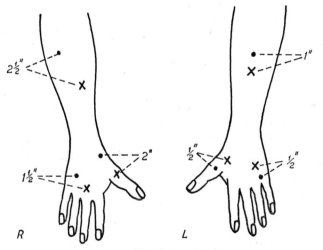

Fig. 1.—Tactile Localization

Case No. 106. The dots represent points at which the skin was touched firmly with a blunt pencil. The crosses indicate points where the patient located the touches with his other forefinger. Figures represent approximate distances between these points.

being left in contact with the skin for a second or two before being withdrawn. Normally, over the finger pads two points can be recognized as such when they are not closer together than 0·3 cm.; over the palm of the hand the distance they must be apart becomes greater: 1·5–2 cm.[69] More important, however, than actual distance between points is the subsequent comparison of results on the two sides. Thus in one case, (No. 117, in Table 3) the critical distance on the forefinger of the affected side was 1 cm. and at times 2 cm., whilst at symmetrical points on the opposite side the distance was only 0·25 cm.

In testing for *stereognosis* it is advisable to have a good assortment of objects, both large and small, common and uncommon, identical and otherwise. One may begin by testing recognition by touch in each

TABLE 3.—*Sensory impairment in 15 cases with cerebral lesions,*

Case No.	Lesion	Associated signs
70	L. temp. parietal (astrocytoma)	R. hemiparesis, dysphasia
91	R. parietal (meningioma)	Ataxic weak. L. arm
117	L. parietal (astrocytoma)	Ataxic weak. R. arm
48	R. fronto-parietal (meningioma)	L. hemiplegia, visual in-attention L.
39	L. thalamus, int. capsule, cereb. peduncle (thrombotic infarct)	R. hemiplegia, hemianopia, dysphasia.
41	L. thalamus and int. capsule (thrombotic infarct)	R. hemiplegia, hemianopia, dysphasia
142	R. parietal, deep-seated, (cystic astrocyt. invad. corp. callos.)	L. hemiplegia, hemianopia
177	L. int. carotid stenosis at bifurcation. No filling of ant. and mid. cereb. arts.	R. hemiparesis, hemianopia, dysphasia
86	R. parietal (meningioma)	Slight ataxic weak. L. arm, hemianopia
148	R. pariet. occipital (oligodendroglioma)	Ataxic weak. L. arm, hemianopia
106	L. temp. parietal (glio-blastoma)	Slight ataxic weak. R. arm. Jacksonian fits, transient dysphasia
156	L. int. carotid thrombosis just distal to bifurcation	R. hemiplegia, dysphasia
51	L. temp. parietal (deep-seated) (astrocytoma)	R. hemianopia, slight recept. and express. dysphasia
139	L. thalamus, int. caps. and subcortical white matter (astrocytoma)	R. hemiparesis (ataxic), hemianopia
140	R. parietal (sup. sagittal sinus) (meningioma)	L. hemiparesis and visual inattention

the site of which was confirmed at operation or autopsy.

Hemianaesth. and analgesia	Severe postural sense loss	Postural sense impair. fingers and toes	Sensory neglect	Defect. localis. of stim.	Defect. 2-point discr.	Dystereo-gnosis
o	o	+	o	?	+	±
o	o	±	+	+	+	+
o	o	±	o	?	+	±
o	o	+	o	?	+	+
+	+					
+	+					
o	o	+	+	?	+	+
(Too confused for accurate testing: pin prick blunted L. arm and leg)						
o	o	+	+	o	+	+
o	+	+	+	+	+	+
o	o	±	±	+	+	±
+	+					
o	o	o	+	?	o	o
+	+					
o	o	o	+ (occasional allaesthesia)	+	o	o

hand separately, using large objects at first, e.g. a handkerchief, orange, scissors, comb, pipe, toothbrush, spectacles, and then small ones. e.g. sixpence, pen nib, postage stamp, thimble, small key, bead. Finally, identical objects should be placed simultaneously in the palms of both hands and the behaviour compared. Such tests present no difficulty when the patient is mentally lucid, but in many of our cases the procedure had to be modified. Thus, before applying tests the patient was shown the collection of objects from which selections would be made and he was required to identify them by sight. This was to exclude any possibility of visual object agnosia or, what was more common in organic mental cases—perseveration in thought—which might falsify his answers. Dysphasic difficulties in naming were overcome by removing the object from the patient's hand before his eyes were uncovered and then, when he was allowed to see, getting him to retrieve its double from among the other objects. Many patients, despite being told to close their eyes and rely on the sense of touch alone, would open them and take a look so that the results became hopelessly confused. When this happened the objects were concealed from view in a bag and the patient told to put his hand into it and say what he felt. In point of fact, however, the way in which most astereognosic patients handled objects in their efforts to identify them was very typical. Thus, when a small object was placed on the palm of the hand they tended to close the fingers over it and squeeze it between the muscles of the thenar eminence and the metacarpo-phalangeal joints, instead of pronating the wrist and working the object swiftly into place between the thumb and the first two fingers, as people normally do. Even when they succeeded in making this manœuvre they continued to toy with the object, turning it round and round and utilizing all five fingers in doing so. Further, when identical objects were placed simultaneously in the palms of the hands, the arms being held supinated and outstretched, the patient would often commence to feel the object placed in the sound hand but make no attempt to explore the shape of the other. When his attention was then directed to it he would say: " Oh! I forgot. . . . Oh yes . . ." feeling the object with great care) ". . . I think . . . could this be an apple, too?" This behaviour may be of little moment in patients suffering from diffuse cerebral cortical atrophy with gross amnesia, difficulty in registration, perseveration and possibly some dyspraxia, but when such conditions do not obtain and the disturbances are consistently unilateral they have as much significance as the patient's inability to name the object he is feeling. Indeed, we were struck by the fact, that intelligent patients, later found to have parietal lesions, rarely showed absolute inability to recognize objects by touch. Most of them had little or no difficulty with common objects (beyond what has been said), their defects becoming apparent only when they were presented with unusual objects.

In theory, tests for cortical sensory loss are only required when it can be shown that there is no actual loss of common sensibility. Obviously, the cerebral cortical function of integration and interpretation of sensation must depend on the receptive mechanisms for tactile, and proprioceptive stimuli in particular, being sufficiently intact to provide crude impressions. But, as can be seen from Table 3, some deficiency in postural joint sensibility in the fingers on the affected side was often found in patients with parietal lesions and sensory inattention or neglect was also relatively common. Thus, in case Nos. 51 and 140 it was pronounced, although the situations of the lesions, one being deep-seated in the subparietal white matter, and the other affecting the parasaggital region, probably determined the absence of any recognizable evidence of true cortical sensory loss.

REFLEXES

Critchley,[9] in his account of the neurology of old age, referred to the frequency with which the tendon and superficial reflexes are found to be absent in senile persons. Howell,[93] who examined 200 Chelsea pensioners (only 16 of whom were under the age of 70), noted that although the arm jerks could usually be obtained in men under 70, he was unable to obtain ankle jerks in more than half of all his cases. Plantar responses were normal as a rule, but there was often difficulty in eliciting the abdominal reflexes, the upper quadrants, however, responding better than the lower ones. Relatively few of our cases were over the age of 70, the majority being in the 50–60, 60–70 decades and this probably accounts for the fact that these changes were not often seen.

In a number of cases of diffuse cerebral cortical atrophy with chronic amnesia and other signs of incipient dementia both plantar responses were extensor. Unilateral change in the character of this reflex was only seen in association with contralateral cerebral disease. Absent knee and ankle jerks occurred in only a minority of the cases of general paralysis (taboparesis). In several instances exaggeration of the jaw jerk was of value in suggesting the presence either of a pseudobulbar palsy or of ischaemic infarcts caused by carotico-vertebral stenosis. Another feature which was often of assistance in suggesting a diffuse dementing process was the occurrence of a *snout reflex*. This was obtained by tapping with the finger over the corner of the mouth and observing the lips pursing together in response. A *sucking reflex*, elicited by bringing a spatula or other object into contact with the lips was occasionally obtained in advanced cases of dementia, but was not seen as an early sign, except in one patient in whom there was a chronic subdural haematoma, situated over both frontal regions.

Another reflex often displayed by patients with diffuse cerebral cortical atrophy was forced *grasping and groping*. This had to be distinguished from the (apparently spontaneous) tendency to grasp shown by patients who are perseverating. Thus, if one had been testing the hand grips and then proceeded to other tests the patient might perseverate in grasping at the examiner's hand each time it was brought into contact with him. True reflex grasping and groping, however, were obtainable, without any previous stimulation or background for perseveration, by drawing a smooth round object across the open palm, or by touching the patient's finger tips with an object, the effect of which was to cause him to follow the object with his hand in the direction in which it was moved. As in the case of a unilateral extensor plantar response, the finding of a persistent grasp reflex on one side only should arouse suspicion of a focal cerebral lesion, e.g. a frontal tumour.

Disturbances of *sphincter control* with incontinence of urine (and occasionally of faeces) were of frequent occurrence in patients with diffuse cerebral cortical atrophy whose amnesic state and inactivity led to neglect of natural functions, so that the bladder became distended and overflow incontinence resulted. In one case incontinence was the first clinical indication of a frontal lobe tumour. An elderly woman, she had been admitted to a general surgical ward for obscure abdominal symptoms, and was found one day sitting placidly by the fireside with a large pool of urine on the floor beneath her chair. Although some patients were literally unaware of incontinence, others became emotionally disturbed when they found the bed wet and were inclined to turn the blame on the nurses for their slowness in bringing a bottle.

BIBLIOGRAPHY

68 ELWYN, M. (1946). " Diseases of the Retina." Blackiston, Philadelphia.

69 CRITCHLEY, M. (1953). " The Parietal Lobes." Edward Arnold, London.

70 CRITCHLEY, M. (1939). The problem of awareness or non-awareness of hemianopic field defects. *Trans. ophthal. Soc. U.K.*, **59**, 95.

71 BENDER, M. B. and KRIEGER, H. P. (1951). Visual function in perimetrically blind fields. *Arch. Neurol. Psychiat.*, **65**, 72.

72 MEADOWS, S. P. (1954). *Trans. ophthal. Soc. U.K.*, **74**, 13. Quoted by Parsons-Smith (73).

73 PARSONS-SMITH, G. (1959). Sudden blindness in cranial Arteritis. *Brit. J. opthal.*, **43**, 204.

74 DUKE-ELDER, Sir W. Stewart (1949). "Textbook of Ophthalmology," vol. 4. Henry Kimpton, London.

75 PARKER, H. L. (1928). Tumours of the nervus acousticus. Signs of involvement of the fifth cranial nerve. *Arch. Neurol. Psychiat*, **20**, 301.

76 BLAU, A. (1946). "The Master Hand." *Amer. Orthopsych. Assoc. Inc.*, New York.

77 ELKINGTON, J. ST. C. (1958). Cerebral vascular disease in the light of modern techniques. *Lancet*, **16**, 275–283; 327–333.

78 SYMONDS, SIR CHARLES P. (1957). Occlusion of the internal carotid arteries. In "Modern Trends in Neurology; Second Series" p. 91. Butterworth, London.

79 CRITCHLEY, M. (1956). Neurological changes in the aged. *Proc. Ass. Res. Nerv. Ment. Dis.*, **35**, 198.

80 CURRAN, D. (1930). Huntington's chorea without choreiform movements. *J. Neurol. Psychopath.*, **10**, 305.

81 MARTIN, J. P. (1928). Tumours of the frontal lobe of the brain. *Brit. Med. J.*, **1**, 1058.

82 BING, R. (1925). Sémiologie des affections cérébelleuses. *Schweiz. Arch. Neurol. Psychiat.*, **16**, 3.

83 PEARSON, G. I. (1928). Effect of Age on Vibratory Sensibility. *Arch. Neurol. Psychiat.*, **20**, 482.

84 OPPENHEIM, H. (1885). Ueber eine durch eine klinisch bisher nicht verwerthete Untersuchungsmethode ermittelte Form der Sensibilitätstörung bei einseitigen Erkrankungen des Grosshirns. *Neur. Zbl.*, **4**, 529.

85 BENDER, M. B., SHAPIRO, M. F. and TEUBER, H. L. (1949). Allesthesia and disturbance of the body scheme. *Arch. Neurol. Psychiat.*, **62**, 222.

86 BENDER, M. B., SHAPIRO, M. F. and SCHAPPELL, A. W. (1949). Observation on the extinction phenomenon in hemiplegia. *Trans. Amer. Neurol Ass.*, 74th Ann. Meeting, June 13–15.

87 DENNY-BROWN, D. and BANKER, B. Q. (1954). Amorphosynthesis from left parietal lesion. *Arch Neurol. Psychiat.*, **71**, 302.

88 DENNY-BROWN, D., MEYER, J. S. and HORENSTEIN, S. (1952). The significance of perceptual rivalry resulting from parietal lesions. *Brain*, **75**, 433.

89 JAFFE, J. and BENDER, M. B. (1952). The factor of symmetry in the perception of two simultaneous cutaneous stimuli. *Brain*, **75**, 167.

90 COHN, R. (1953). The role of "body image concept" in the pattern of ipsilateral clinical extinction. *Arch. Neurol. Psychiat.*, **70**, 503.

91 ALLISON, R. S. (1950). Symptomatologie des Sauerstoffmangels im Gehirn und verwandter Zustände. *Schweiz. Arch. Neurol. Psychiat.*, **66**, 1.

92 CRITCHLEY, M. (1950). Discussion on parietal lobe syndromes. *Proc. Roy. Soc. Med., Sect. Neur.*, Dec. 7th.

93 HOWELL, T. H. (1949). Senile deterioration of the central nervous system. A clinical study. *Brit. Med. J.*, **1**, 56.

CHAPTER IV

Organic Mental Testing

THE psychometric methods of estimating intellectual deterioration in organic brain disease, which have been elaborated by Shipley,[94] Brody,[95] Wechsler [96] and others, belong more to the province of the psychologist than to the neurologist and psychiatrist. The best known are the Wechsler-Bellevue, Shipley-Hartford, Mill Hill Vocabulary Scale and Raven's Progressive Matrices.

These tests derive their inspiration from an hypothesis proposed by Babcock [97] that in brain injury or disease vocabulary level and comprehension are little affected in comparison to the capacity for reasoning. In testing such patients Babcock assessed the mental age for these two components by separate series of tests and then used the difference in the scores obtained to form an index of the extent of their deterioration i.e.

$$\text{index of deterioration} = \frac{\text{Vocabulary}}{\text{Reasoning ability}}$$

During the second great war there were unprecedented opportunities for using these tests and of judging how they worked in practice. One of the difficulties encountered was that in primarily backward persons, or those having little educational background, mental ages assessed on vocabulary were apt to be low. As a result the expected difference between mental age scores was not seen and one was placed in the quandary of not knowing whether the low results in reasoning tests were due to primary backwardness or to acquired deterioration. Another difficulty in using vocabulary as a standard measurement, and which led to the development of tests of the synonym selection type, is that in judging patients' answers as to the meaning of words the decisions made by examiners are too " subjective " to be scientific.[98] It should be noted, too, that in later life there is some natural falling-off especially in performance tests designed to estimate reasoning ability, so that in cases in which early organic changes are suspected it may not be possible to say whether or not the results afford positive proof of deterioration. Probably of more value than the actual score is the behaviour of patients under such tests. Thus, one of Brody's [99] subjects, who gained a high score in vocabulary and had no difficulty in repeating the test sentence: " The cricket match yesterday was won in the very last minute," remarked a moment later: " I didn't know there was a match yesterday!", and another patient objected that he was " too old for these childish games ".

Zangwill[100] points out that the two principal pitfalls in carrying out psychometric tests (designed for normal persons) on brain-injured subjects are the occurrence of catastrophic reactions and the influence of superimposed neurosis. In all brain-injured subjects there is some learning or memory defect: of more importance than calculating the extent of deterioration from the previous level is the necessity of finding out whether the patient retains his capacity for learning from past experience and for acquiring new material. Not uncommonly it is found that the former may be well preserved and the latter grossly defective, the condition resembling (although to a lesser extent) the situation seen in Korsakoff's psychosis. As regards the site of cerebral damage in relation to defective reasoning ability Battersby *et al.*[101] conclude, after testing war veterans with a modification of the Maier String Problem, that brain injury in the frontal or parieto-occipital areas, although slowing-up performance, caused less disturbance than was expected. Further, it was found that patients with anteriorly placed injuries fared no worse in their performance with these tests than did those with lesions situated in the posterior part of the brain. However, Meyer and Yates[102] who tested a series of cases of temporal lobe epilepsy both before and after operation, noted that although the intelligence in general was often unimpaired, a year after the operation there was still evidence of defective learning ability.

A number of our patients were referred to the University Department of Psychology, where psychometric tests were made through the courtesy of Professor George Seth. But these were time-consuming and the state of a patient's health did not always permit of their application. So for routine work simple clinical tests were adopted which, although modified from time to time, have been adhered to fairly consistently over the years in the hope that they might prove of value in distinguishing focal from diffuse cerebral lesions. Most, if not all of them, will be familiar as they have been employed by other workers investigating either brain-injured or psychotic patients. No attempt was ever made to score results; these were noted simply in terms of success, partial or complete failure and no time limits were set on performance. Especial care, however, was taken to avoid catastrophic reactions and the tests were not given until time had been allowed for some measure of rapport to be established between patient and examiner.

The choice of tests was determined largely by the belief that the symptoms observed in previously healthy persons recovering from severe anoxia bear a close resemblance to those found in early dementia, caused by diffuse cerebral cortical atrophy. Their mode of presentation is, of course, different, depending upon whether the morbid process is one of reintegration or disintegration, but in both sorts of case impairment of memory, defective grasp and alterations in mood and behaviour are common features. Whether one adheres to the traditional view that in dementia symptoms are caused by diffuse cortical destruction and related to thinly but more or less evenly spread defects in all spheres of intellectual activity, or accepts the hypothesis that disturbance of the centrencephalic system is partly at least responsible, the comparison with anoxia still holds good. In this condition the absence of a circumscribed brain lesion can be assured and in victims dying some weeks or months after exposure the histological changes found are diffuse and symmetrical in the extent to which they affect the cortical neurones, white matter, basal ganglia and other structures in the diencephalon and mid-brain.

The adjective " general " will be used throughout to denote these symptoms, which, it is postulated, are related to global affection of the brain. Specific tests for dysphasia, dyscalculia, agnosia and apraxia were also included, not only to enable their being correlated with the site of the lesion, but to find out how often they occurred in association with, and to what extent they were dependant upon general symptoms. In the past, interest in these specific intellectual defects has centred chiefly around their focal significance, but they have been noted, too, on occasion in post-anoxic patients, e.g. Gillies[103]: finger agnosia and dyscalculia; Adler[104]: visual agnosia, acalculia, dysgraphia; Solomon[105]: visual object agnosia. In diffuse disease of the brain focal symptoms have also been recognized " before their submersion in the sea of mindlessness ".[106]

The tests may be arranged as shown and details of the different procedures are described.

Scheme for Investigation of Organic Mental Cases

1. Mood, appearance and behaviour.
2. Insight.
3. Performance with series.
4. Registration and recall.
5. Factual memory for past events.
6. Orientation.
7. Speech and language.
8. Calculation.
9. Learned memories (agnosia and apraxia).

1. *Mood, appearance and behaviour.*

The importance at the first interview of paying as much heed to appearance and behaviour, as to symptoms has already been mentioned. As practically all our patients were admitted to hospital it was possible to check first impressions by subsequent observation, and in making these reliance for the most part was placed on the nursing staff, reports of the psychiatric social worker, almoner and occupational therapist. The observations made included the following:

(*a*) Day-to-day spontaneous activities: the extent to which patients mixed with and talked to others; took part in simple games, watched television or listened to the radio; engaged in reading and writing; spent their time lying on the bed or keeping to themselves.

(*b*) Personal routine activities: dressing and undressing; behaviour at table, appetite, use of knife, fork and spoon; washing themselves, shaving, brushing the hair; finding their way about the wards and to and from the lavatory or day room; sleep (charts recording hours of sleep by day and night were kept when there was somnolence or insomnia).

(*c*) Prevailing mood: Good-humoured, acceptant, tense, anxious, depressed, agitated, aloof, unconcerned, unduly optimistic, expansive, suspicious, hostile.

(*d*) Abnormal emotional lability, i.e. undue tendency to laugh or cry excessively in the absence of any adequate and appropriate stimulus.

(*e*) Catastrophic reactions (see p. 11).

(*f*) Perseveration (see p. 100). This was often apparent in the behaviour of patients repeatedly asking when they were to be allowed home or in trying to get out of bed.

(*g*) Fits. Circumstances leading up to the fit. Mode of origin, right or left-sided or both sides; turning of head and eyes; alterations in colour; convulsive movements; tongue biting and incontinence; signs of delayed recovery of full consciousness and character of the automatism shown.

(*h*) Incontinence of urine and faeces; degree of awareness on the part of the patient and his reaction to the incontinence.

In appraising the results of such observations attention was directed chiefly to confirming how consistent were changes in mood and behaviour and how these compared with the patient's previous state; also whether there was any indication of progression or of fluctuation from day to day.

2. *Insight.*

The extent to which a patient was aware of the nature and severity of his disabilities and the reasons he gave to account for them were ascertained by putting such questions as: " what is the matter with you?" " what do you feel wrong?" and " what do you think is the cause?" In some, insight was entirely lacking, a patient for example, despite being hemiplegic, declaring that there was nothing the matter with him. In most patients, however, there was some retention of insight, although it was obvious from questioning or watching their behaviour that this was defective and that they were only partly aware of the nature and extent of their disabilities. The term " euphoria " was only used when the patient adopted a persistent attitude of optimism towards his symptoms which, in the circumstances, were of sufficient severity as to have caused him concern. Organized delusional thinking was not seen although patients with defective insight often confabulated freely in their efforts to explain away their defects and avoid admitting them openly. That they did possess some insight was shown by the fluctuations in their mood from day to day and their ability at times to face up to the realities of their situation. An interesting feature in others was the lack of any sign of impairment of insight and the intuition sometimes shown by them that something was seriously wrong.

3. *Performance with series forwards and backwards.*

Patients with organic cerebral disease, strictly speaking, are not inattentive. Their capacity for performance is restricted, however, tasks demanding abstract thought (i.e. referred to the mind and requiring a mental act of judgment) presenting greater difficulty than simple concrete tasks. They appear to be inattentive in that they tend to flit from one activity to another, but when they find one that is within their capacity they become " tied " to it so that it is not easy to get them to do something different. This limited abstract conceptual capacity and difficulty in shifting from one concept to another, unless complicated by co-existing perseveration, can be demonstrated by serial tests. The patient is asked to repeat the days of the week, commencing with Sunday, and when he has done so he is then invited to reverse the process and, starting with Saturday, say them backwards. If this gives him no difficulty one may proceed to try him with the months of the year or with the serial sevens test. In the latter he is required to subtract 7 from 100 = 93, 7 from 93 = 86 and so on. A much simpler test is, of course, to count up to 20 and then count down from 20–1. The only reason for mentioning these alternatives is because in nervous, backward or seriously deteriorated subjects it is important not to make the test too difficult, thereby risking the occurrence of a catastrophic reaction, or to fall into the opposite kind of error of wounding the *amour propre* of a highly intelligent person by giving him something too simple to do. Many persons we found were embarrassed by figures and although they could repeat 6 digits, had great difficulty in reversing more than 4, so that as a rule we kept strictly to serial numbers or names. The occurrence of perseveration was an indication to abandon the test and proceed to others.

4. *Registration and recall.*

In testing learning ability or the capacity to register fresh data, we gave the patient a fictitious name and address to repeat. Before doing so it was explained that this was simply a test of memory, and that it did not really matter if he could not do it: the important thing was that he should try and remember what was said.

The following is an example:

Examiner: " I want you to remember the name of a certain person and his address. If I give it to you, will you try very hard to remember it?"

Patient: " Yes doctor . . . but I'm not very good at this sort of thing . . . being in hospital . . . I used to be all right."

Examiner: " Well then, I want you to say after me: 'Mr. John Gladstone'."

Patient: " Mr. John Gladstone."

Examiner: " That's right! Now, Mr. Gladstone lives at No. 17 Church Road. Will you say that, please!"

Patient: " No. 17 Church Road."

Examiner: " Liverpool."

Patient: " Liverpool."

Examiner: " Now I want you to repeat the name and address I have just given you."

Patient: " Mr. John Gladstone . . . Number . . . Number 17 Church Road, Liverpool."

The name was given first, then the address in the same way, and finally the town. When all three items had been repeated correctly the patient was asked to give the name and address in full. Very often he could not do this at the first attempt and no special notice was taken of this failure, beyond reassuring him that many people had the same difficulty. After a pause, he was then invited to try again, each time the items being said by the examiner and repeated by the patient separately, after which he was required to give the information in full. Inability to register after three or four attempts or persistent mistakes in detail was accepted as evidence of difficulty in registration. Very few patients in whom this technique was followed, and who succeeded finally in registering, failed after the lapse of 5 to 10 minutes to recall part or all of the required information. This was a very consistent feature in our organic mental cases and, as has been mentioned elsewhere, a patient might triumphantly repeat the details a day or a week later, long after the examiner had forgotten all about them!

In the case of patients suffering from expressive speech disorders, but without any gross defects in comprehension, the test was conducted as follows: three objects were exhibited and the patients told to watch carefully whilst each in turn was hidden from view, e.g. in a drawer, in the pocket, under the carpet. They were then asked to indicate where the objects had been concealed. Recall was tested by restoring the objects to their hiding places and by asking the patient some 5 to 10 minutes later to find them.

Factual memory for past events.

No standard procedure was used in trying to determine the extent of memory impairment. In theory, it is desirable to test this aspect of intellectual function in two ways; first, the ability to recall principal public events and personages during the patient's lifetime, and second, his ability to recall events and persons that have had a direct bearing on him personally. In these islands, most people can recall the names of some past and reigning monarchs, prime ministers, other public figures and some details of the two great wars. So, by constructing a series of questions such as that shown below one may compare their ability in these two respects, and also find out whether memory loss is principally for recent events, affects also the " middle distance ", or is global in character.

Distant memory	Personal	Impersonal
	Details of school life, teachers' names, where friends lived, household arrangements, childish interests, first work, marriage.	Boer War, Queen Victoria, suffragettes, King Edward VII, King George V, First world war.
Middle distance	Occupations followed and approx. dates, children, unemployment, holidays, second world war; bombing.	King Edward VIII, King George VI, Munich crisis, 2nd world war, prime ministers, Elizabeth II and Prince Philip.
Recent events	Name of clergyman, baker, grocer, next door neighbour and names of married children, duration of stay in hospital, yesterday's events.	Recent events, current newspaper, T.V. and radio programmes.

This was the method we used at first, but it soon became apparent that differences in primary educational levels and the limited range of so many peoples' interests affected their ability to recall the names of persons or events with which they had had no personal contact. Just as in trying to compare vocabulary levels and reasoning ability, these difficulties often prevented any conclusions being drawn as to the meaning of differences in performance in the two types of test. It was obvious, too, that these natural effects became more pronounced in the presence of organic mental deterioration, such patients when asked if they could recall such and such an event, skating lightly over their inability by declaring that they were " never one for dates " or that they were " not interested in politics ". In other words it was impossible to pin them down to answering questions satisfactorily and, indeed, to continue on such lines was only to invite upsetting them, which was the last thing we wished to do.

Consequently, unless satisfied that the former intellectual status and social position were sufficiently advanced as to make impersonal tests feasible we did not employ them and instead, concentrated on the patient's ability to recall personal events in his life. To do this the relatives were first interviewed and details obtained from them of his work, war service, interests, family, friends and other matters. Armed with this information, which was arranged in chronological order, one then proceeded to question the patient about it, conducting the interview as informally as possible and glossing over any difficulties he might have in recalling events at any particular period of time. In this way it was often possible to show that his recall of recent events was more impaired than that of distant events or that his memory impairment was global in character.

6. *Orientation.*

When there is little or no difficulty in registration, orientation in time should be tested by getting the patient to say the day, month and year. Hospital inmates are usually vague about the actual date, and no significance need be attached to this unless there is repeated failure to name either the day, month or year correctly. On only one occasion was a patient found to be disorientated in place but not in time. Usually, the former was indicative of a more pronounced defect in orientation, the most severe degree of which was seen in inability to recognize persons. In demonstrating these features, however, care must be taken to ensure that apparently correct answers are not due to the combination of chance and the patient's tendency to confabulate, or that failure to give correct answers is not due to amnesia for names or to

6   T.S.B.

perseveration. Thus, the reason a patient fails to respond to the question: " What place is this?" may be because he cannot remember its name. Satisfactory answers may be difficult to get and the required information sometimes may be obtained more readily indirectly through conversation, but it is necessary to find out whether in fact a patient knows he is in hospital or thinks he is at home, and whether he recognizes that the persons visiting him are friends, relatives, doctors or nurses as the case may be.

In addition to assessing " concrete " orientation in time, place and for persons, the extent to which the patient is orientated to his own body should be ascertained, as also his capacity for " abstract " spatial orientation. These are discussed later in Chapter IX.

7. *Speech and language.*

The nature of the relationship existing between anatomico-physiological and psychological factors in aphasia is not fully understood. So, without attempting any lengthy digression, some consideration must be given to the subject before the actual clinical procedures adopted in testing our patients are outlined.

Speech "is the audible expression of language consisting of organized patterns of articulation. When arranged with an agreed (a conventional) symbolic meaning these constitute spoken language . . . written language follows spoken language historically and in normal individual development ".[107]

Language " is a means of the individual to come to terms with the outer world and to realize himself ".[108]

The principle underlying the classical localization theory assumed that language was based on auditory, visual and kinaesthetic images, the sensory and motor components of which were stored in discrete " centres " in the dominant cortex. These centres, it was held, were connected to each other by commissural fibres,[109] and to other centres in which images indirectly related to speech were stored. Protagonists of the theory, such as Broca* and Wernicke, based their conclusions on careful clinical-pathological observations, but there is reason to think that in some of their cases the extent of brain damage was greater than was supposed and that in others lesions were not always found at the sites anticipated. Such experiences, however, only led to modifications

---

* The theory drew its inspiration from the observations of Paul Broca in 1861[110] on two patients with loss of speech, but no other defect in intellect, in whom at post-mortem circumscribed lesions were found in the second and third frontal convolutions. Half a century later, in a critical review, Pierre Marie[111] described his examination of the brains of Broca's two cases (Leborgne and Lelong) which has been preserved in the Dupuytren Museum, and pointed out that the areas of softening were much more extensive than Broca had supposed.

in the pattern of the diagrams that were so much in fashion at the time.

Most clinicians will agree that the " diagram makers " went too far in separating sensory and motor speech centres and in divorcing language from intellect. But anatomical factors clearly play some rôle for, as Symonds (112) points out, many speech disorders are so distinct from one another that it is difficult to conceive how this could be unless they are dependent " upon the loss by disease of separate anatomical arrangements ". He quotes pure word blindness as an example and this is a good point because in genuine cases, although unable to read, the patient comprehends spoken speech and has no difficulty in naming objects, speaking or writing. Neither is his general intelligence impaired. There is usually, however, an associated right homonymous hemianopia. Arguing from the recognized fact that patients with occipital cortical lesions do not show word blindness, Symonds concludes that in this type of aphasia the lesion must involve the optic radiation, before it reaches the occipital cortex and after it has left the parietal lobe.

Support of the view that specialized anatomical mechanisms subserves speech is provided also by the results of direct electrical stimulation of the human cortex. Penfield and Jasper,[113] and their associate Lamar Roberts, have mapped out areas that appear to be essential for its expression. These are: the frontal area, corresponding with Broca's centre; the parietal and temporal areas, which may be distinct or representative only of a single area; and the superior frontal, which lies just anterior to the foot area of the Rolandic motor cortex. " Stimulating arrest " of any one of these regions causes aphasia, but the excision of portions of cortex lying between them has no such effect. They conclude that " The memory of words seems to depend upon a mechanism that includes the cortical speech areas of the dominant hemisphere. If either the temporal or frontal speech area is inactivated the patient becomes aphasic. . . ."

The psychological approach or " organismic " theory of Goldstein owes much to Hughlings Jackson, who emphasized that aphasia is not merely a matter of words being lost but of their being made unavailable to the patient so that he is bereft of the power to propositionize. Jackson held that aphasia could best be understood by considering its different aspects as being expressive of the altered functioning of the remaining intact brain.* His views met with little response until Kurt

---

* Hughlings Jackson accepted that a lesion of the anterior part of the brain " scarcely ever produces any other mental defect than that of (by damage of the left half) affection of speech ". He believed that the revival of images depended chiefly on the posterior part of the hemisphere, but qualified " chiefly " by commenting: " I say chiefly because I do not believe in abrupt geographical localisations. Thus, very sudden or very extensive damage to *any* part of the left cerebral hemisphere would produce *some* amount of defect of speech . . ."[114].

Goldstein and Henry Head began to apply the same mode of approach to the problem. Head [115] directed attention to the extent of intellectual loss, which he believed often occurred, and looked upon aphasia as being the result of the patient's failure to formulate and express symbols. He described four clinical types: verbal, in which the chief difficulty lies in expression, there being little impairment of comprehension; syntactical, in which comprehension is gravely impaired and speech often jargon in character; nominal, in which there is inability to name objects and lack of comprehension of the meaning of words; and semantic in which the patient, although comprehending words is unable to grasp their meaning as a whole. Head's approach, which was so much at variance with traditional teaching at the time undoubtedly marked a turning point in clinical methodology. His classification has been superceded by others, notably that of Weisenberg and McBride,[116] who found both perceptual and expressive defects in all of the 60 cases of aphasia they examined. In some patients the defects were " predominantly expressive ", in others " predominantly receptive ", but in a number of cases gross defects were found in both aspects of speech and language. These authors also proposed the term " amnesic " aphasia for cases in which the principal difficulty lay in the recall of words.

Goldstein has repeatedly stated his belief that the essential and most consistent mental defect to be found in brain-injured subjects is loss of the capacity for abstract thinking. Two kinds of attitude are recognized:[108] " In the concrete attitude . . . our thinking and acting are determined by the immediate claims made by the particular aspect of the object or situation. For instance, we act concretely when we enter a room in darkness and push the button for light. If, however, we desist . . . , reflecting that by pushing the button we might awaken someone asleep in the room then we are acting abstractively ". In his view, concrete aspects of language are represented by the " instrumentalities of speech "; of sounds, words, series of words, sentences, one form of naming* and of understanding of language in familiar situations . . . , and finally of " emotional utterances ". Abstract aspects, on the other hand correspond with difficulties in propositional and rational language. These views on aphasia are supported by the results of statistical methods of investigation with multiple tests. Thus, Schuell and Jenkins[117] have recently reported their comprehensive review of 123 patients with aphasia, whose ages ranged from 19–76 years. Using Guttman's scale analysis technique, they argued that if

---

* He holds that naming demands an abstract attitude, simple association of a word with an object being " pseudonaming ", or naming at a " concrete " level.[108]

sufficient language tests were given to a heterogeneous collection of aphasic patients and the scores were found to be proportionate to the relative difficulty each test presented, one could use this evidence in support of the hypothesis that a " single dimension of language deficit " is present in all cases of aphasia. The data collected by them indicates that this appears to be so. Further, they state that they were unable to find any pure examples of word deafness or blindness, nominal, expressive or receptive aphasia, in all cases there being evidence of co-existing general language deficit. Although they do not say so, the inference seems clear that they are referring to the same thing as Goldstein had in mind when he spoke of loss of the capacity for abstract thinking and expression. With this there should be general agreement but clinical neurologists may not be so ready to accept the view that " concrete " or particulate defects in speech alone do not occur. Aphasia is more than an indication of overall disturbance of intellect and we agree with Heimburger and Reitan[118] that although such patients show loss of intellect, commensurate with the severity of their brain damage, there is also as a rule evidence of specific and variable loss in the " instrumentalities of speech ".

These considerations were taken into account in drawing up the scheme for investigation outlined at the beginning of this chapter. If it has any merit this is probably solely on account of the fact that the same methods were applied to all cases, irrespective of whether or not there was obvious aphasia, the lesion was focal or diffuse or affected the dominant or subordinate hemisphere. The actual speech and language tests used were arranged as follows:

1. Spontaneous speech.
2. Naming of sighted objects.
3. Naming from memory.
4. Writing.
5. Comprehension of spoken speech.
6. Comprehension of written speech.
7. Capacity for gesture and pantomime.

In assessing the capacity for *spontaneous speech*, two aspects were considered: (1) the use made of " small talk " of a concrete kind, e.g. " it's a fine day ", " good morning doctor, are you coming to see me?" repetitive phrases, e.g. " yes, yes ", expletives or other utterances made under emotional stress, and (2) the ability to express propositions or abstract thoughts. The first kind of defect was easier to recognize than the second because many patients took refuge in silence, which they maintained habitually, not talking unless spoken to. Very characteristic was their attitude when approached: they would look up attentively, as if on the point of speaking, but waited for the first remark to come from the other person. Other patients were the reverse. They did not wait until spoken to, but displayed an almost continuous " push " of talk in their endeavour to express themselves. In these one looked especially for difficulties in word finding, mispronouncing, hesitancy in utterance, tendency to break off sentences without finishing them, circumstantiality and repetitiveness in talk. Also, whether as they went on talking their speech became incoherent or meaningless, although sounding from a distance like normal speech (jargon). Patients' awareness of their defects were determined by inference from their demeanour and behaviour. When there was obvious great expressive difficulty, the performance with series was tested, the examiner assisting by saying: " repeat after me 1—2—3 " and counting slowly, and once the patient had begun to follow suit leaving him to do so unaided. In the same way by helping him at the beginning, an otherwise speechless patient might be made to repeat the days of the week, months of the year, or other sequences. This was useful in detecting dyspraxic elements in speech. When it was found that he could not speak, or at the most repeat only " yes, yes ", tests were made for signs of tongue and lip apraxia by requesting him to put out his tongue, lick the lips or purse the lips together as in whistling. Inability to do so was usually indicative of oral or facial apraxia although we had to be careful to make sure by repetition on subsequent occasions that perseveration or lack of comprehension were not responsible for the failure.

Naming of sighted objects. This was tested in three ways: (1) by displaying against a plain dark background a number of objects in turn: a candle, cork, watch, marble, key, matchbox, toothbrush, comb, postage stamp, thimble. The patient was invited to name each object, taking his time and handling the objects as well as looking at them. This was done to exclude the possibility of any difficulty in naming being due to visual object agnosia. (2) by displaying the collection as a whole and asking him to pick out the marble, the comb or the postage stamp etc.

Naming from memory. The patient was asked to give the names of as many cities or towns as he could remember or to name a list of vegetables, fruits, boys' names, girls' names, motor cars etc. This tests the capacity for naming at an abstract level of thought, difficulty in naming sighted objects correlating more with disturbances at a concrete level. The two tests were always used in conjunction so that the relative extent of disability displayed in each might be compared. All replies were recorded verbatim:

Q. " Now, I want you to give me the names of some large towns or cities, please! Mention any cities you like, anywhere!"

A. ". . . well . . . there's Belfast . . . Liverpool . . . Dublin . . . eh . . . Liverpool."

The dots represent seconds approximately. In this example not only is there difficulty in abstract thought, but perseveration occurs. The patient, a middle-aged man, however, did equally badly when trying to recall the names of fruits, boys' names and motor cars. A tendency to mention only the names of cities near the home or in some part of the United Kingdom exclusively was usually indicative of a low educational level. This was also seen (as in the case of young children) in the tendency to confuse the names of countries with those of cities, e.g.: " Belfast . . . London . . . Canada," and by itself was not regarded as having any significance as a dysphasic manifestation.

Other defects in naming which should be looked for are *periphrasis* or circumlocution and *paraphasia*. In the former the patient circumvents his difficulty by describing the use of the object, e.g. Key = "for opening doors ", Tree = " You find it in a field . . . in the country ". The use of such expedients suggests that the patient has insight into his difficulty and also that he possesses some abstract capacity that enables him to formulate an alternative way of expressing the same thing. Paraphasia is less common and often more indicative of defective insight. In the literal variety there is inaccurate use of sounds or change in the sound patterns of words. Thus a Key is said to be a " Kay ". In the verbal form, a different word is given to that required, e.g. Tent = " A camp ", or a neologism is used, which possesses either some similarity in its sound or some quality of association with the object in question, e.g. Bucket = " A buck splasher ".

Writing ability. A dysphasic patient may be hemiplegic and the dominant hand affected so that he cannot write with it. Even with minor defects writing may be handicapped because of the difficulty in performing fine finger movements. This type of writing disability does not constitute true agraphia or dysgraphia, which depends essentially upon loss of the kinaesthetic memories connected with the act. A patient with true agraphia may be unable to write with the unaffected hand, or if he attempts to do so his difficulties are clearly greater than could be accounted for simply on the basis of lack of practice with the hand. This loss of memory for the specific motor patterns concerned with writing is very evident in agraphic patients. When given pencil and paper and asked to write their name, they may take the pencil in the left hand, transfer it to the right, fixing it in the correct position between thumb and forefinger and then pause irresolute with the pencil hovering over the paper. When encouraged to proceed they make ineffectual, hesitant marks on the paper and then, much in the same way as persons unable to draw give up their futile attempts, they put down the pencil with a hopeless gesture and look appealingly at the examiner. This is a common type of response in agraphia and indicative of the patient's own awareness of his disability. Less common is it to find patients who scribble or write nonsensical symbols and appear satisfied with the results. Minor degrees of dysgraphia are common and were investigated by observing the patient's capacity for spontaneous writing, copying and writing from dictation.

(1) To test *spontaneous writing* we got patients to write letters either to relatives, the doctor or nurse. Through arrangement with the relatives some of these were then examined and excerpts put in the case notes. Although in writing patients might confine themselves to concrete expressions, telling how they found things in hospital or simply describing daily events, the very act of doing so indicated that they had some capacity for abstract thought and the test was superior in this respect to copying and writing from dictation, which tested only the instrumentalities of written speech. As fluency in speech and fluency in writing do not go hand in hand, attention was paid also as to how their performance varied in the two fields.

(2) *Copying.* The patient was invited to copy a series of letters of the alphabet. This could be done with paper and pencil, but if there was difficulty sticks were used as in constructional tests (see p. 88). Printed and written words were then given and finally a sentence.

(3) *Writing from dictation.* The same procedures were followed.

In all three tests, but especially in the last two, one examined the writing especially for: evidence of perseveration; constructional difficulties in the formation of letters or reversals in letter forms, i.e. Ǝ for E; spelling mistakes (these were only regarded as being significant when the patient's previous educational standard had been good); faults in punctuation; and difficulties in alignment, the script falling away to the patient's right or not covering the paper evenly.

Comprehension of spoken speech. This was first tested by simple verbal commands, e.g. " touch your nose ", " close your eyes ". When it was clear from his responses that the patient had understood these concrete requests, he was then shown a number of objects and directed to pick out each when its name was called, e.g. " show me the thimble . . . now the cork ". Failure in either of these performances (provided it was not due to perseveration) usually denoted gross receptive verbal defects. If the patient succeeded, however, tests of a more abstract nature were then given. Beginning with the recognition of similarities and differences, the questions we found most useful were:

(1) " What is the difference between a pond and a stream?"

(2) " In what way are an orange and a football similar?"

(3) " When I throw a stone into water it sinks to the bottom. What happens when I throw a piece of wood into the water?"

As the questions were intended to test comprehension of spoken speech, no weight was attached to lack of fluency in replies, but these often provided useful confirmatory evidence of defects in propositional speech, which had not been apparent in casual talk. So far as comprehension is concerned, the important thing to note is whether or not the patient had understood the question. That this might be so, even in the absence of speech, was shown by one man, who was able by miming to indicate that he understood an abstract proposition (see p. 136).

Carrying tests beyond this level in virtually speechless patients is difficult because, although sufficient to convey fairly simple concrete notions, gesture and pantomime cannot take the place of speech in indicating understanding of more difficult abstract propositions. With patients who had little expressive speech disturbance, however, we moved on to more difficult questions such as the difference between a dwarf and a child, misery and poverty, and proverbs, e.g. " persons who live in glass houses should not throw stones ". In testing with proverbs the aim was to determine whether interpretation was at a literal or abstract level. Often patients were only capable of giving literal meanings. Finally, a short descriptive paragraph was read aloud and the patient invited to answer some question that would prove he had understood its meaning. If necessary the paragraph was read a second time and points in it emphasized. The following is an example. It is quoted from the Terman-Merrill Series.[119]

My house was burgled last Saturday. I was at home all of the morning but out during the afternoon until 5 o'clock. My father left the house at 3 o'clock and my brother was there until 4. At what time did the burglary occur?

Comprehension of written speech. A quick method of testing this was to print some simple direction on a card, ask the patient to read it silently and then do what it said:

WHEN YOU HAVE READ THIS PLEASE TEAR UP THE CARD AND PUT IT IN THE WASTEPAPER BASKET.

If he did what was required there was often no need to proceed further, but when reading disability was a conspicuous feature, the tests used were as follows:

Defects in visual acuity were first excluded and the possibility of there being an associated hemianopia was taken into account. Some patients with hemianopia have no difficulty in reading, but in others, especially those with unilateral visual inattention this may be considerable. Thus, with a left-sided defect the patient sees only the right half of a sentence, which in itself may be meaningless.

.THE RAIN IN SPAIN STAYS MAINLY IN THE PLAIN.

When the defect is right-sided only the beginning or left half of the sentence will be seen. Movements of the eyballs should be observed in such cases because the normal scanning movements that occur in reading may be replaced by slow, short-range, hesitant movements, the eyeballs focusing each word in turn. Patients whose difficulty in reading is due to hemianopia can read vertically-disposed type with ease and this observation in itself is enough to indicate that there is no actual dyslexia.

THE	THE
RAIN	RAIN
IN	IN
SPAIN	SPAIN
STAYS	STAYS
MAINLY	MAINLY
IN	IN
THE	THE
PLAIN	PLAIN

(1) *Letters of the alphabet.* The ability to associate visual or written symbols with the actual objects they represent was determined by means of an " Alphabet Picture Book ",* each page of which contained a picture of an object with the first letter of its name, e.g. A with a picture of an apple. Alternately, one could display an assortment of objects together with cards bearing the first letters of their names and try to find out if the patient could match them. Because gross reading disability may be present as a solitary or relatively-isolated expression

* Picture Book Series. E. J. Arnold & Son Ltd., Leeds.

of dysphasia there was usually little difficulty in getting the patient to comprehend what was expected of him, but if he appeared to be puzzled the examiner helped him by miming the required act two or three times. Next, having prepared two identical sets of cardboard letters, one of which was arranged on the table with letters in their proper sequence, the patient was handed a letter taken at random from the second set and asked to match it with its fellow on the table. Failure in these tests was accepted as evidence of literal alexia.

(2) *Words.* Comprehension of written words was tested by exhibiting a series of picture cards* together with other cards upon which only the names of the objects were shown. The patient was required to match the cards. Failure to do so pointed to verbal alexia. When he succeeded, however, and there was little or no associated disturbance of spoken speech, he was shown the Burt Reading Scale,[120] which was found useful in determining comprehension of words of increasing complexity, e.g. SUN, CARRY, SHELVES, TONGUE, DOMINEER, ATMOS-PHERE, INFLUENTIAL.

(3) *Sentences* made up from cards with words written on them were used to test the patients' comprehension of their appropriate place in a sentence and to test his capacity for the use of little words such as the, for, a, on, etc.

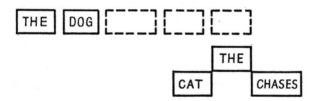

More difficult tests were then given of the " dissected sentence " type in which words are deliberately misplaced so as not to make sense, until they are re-arranged. The following example is again taken from the Terman-Merrill Series.[99]

THIS MORNING FOR A OUR TEACHER US TOOK WALK.

(4) *Reading a paragraph.* The ability to read aloud and to comprehend by silent reading was tested by using short paragraphs from the

* Educational Supply Assoc. Ltd., 233 Shaftesbury Av., London, W.C.2, have prepared group test cards, e.g. series of kitchen and bedroom objects, etc.

Terman-Merrill series of the same kind as that shown on p. 81. This final test often uncovered defects that had not been apparent with simpler methods. Some patients showed a tendency to lose their place in reading or to skip lines so that the meaning of a paragraph as a whole was not understood. Sometimes this behaviour could be related to over-anxiety to complete the task or to " amnesic indifference ", but the manner in which many patients kept their finger on the print, as if feeling their way, suggested that some additional factor of spatial disorientation might be involved.

Gesture and pantomime. Gestures are used naturally to assist in the expression of emotions. Thus, one may shrug one's shoulders and wear a blank look to express disbelief or incredulity, or contract one's brows and shake the fist to express intense anger. In pantomime, however, the intention is not so much to express emotion (indeed emotion may play no part in it) as to effect communication with a person, so that some idea may be conveyed to him. Critchley,[121] who has especially studied the disturbances of gesture that occur in dysphasia, found that with focal cerebral lesions verbal speech suffers much more than gesture language. In severe cases of speech loss, however, although both may be affected, the impairment of pantomime is often greater than loss of the capacity for gesture. It may be, therefore, that the latter corresponds more with speech at the concrete level and the former more with speech at the propositional level. In all our cases attention was paid during the examination: (1) to the extent to which patients employed gesture and pantomime, and (2) to the quality of their performances in these respective fields, i.e. did their gestures appear to be well-executed and convincing or clumsy, inappropriate and meaningless?

8. *Calculation.*

According to Grewel,[122] disorders in calculating ability only began to attract attention at the beginning of the present century, in 1919 Henschen naming and describing the condition known as acalculia. Acalculia or dyscalculia may be found in association with diffuse cerebral disease or with focal lesions of the frontal, parietal and occipital cortex, in the latter instances the dominant hemisphere usually being affected. The symptom is perhaps best known as part of the Gerstmann syndrome, of which it constitutes one of the chief elements (p. 183). Dysphasia may or may not co-exist but when present may contribute to the low level of arithmetical performance.[123] The same applies to hemianopia which, when present in acalculia, may be associated with some visual spatial agnosia and impairment of visual memory in general. In examining patients attention was given to the following points:

(1) Recognition of the meaning and use of common arithmetical symbols: $+$, $-$, $\times$, $\div$; meaning of the cipher o, digits and numbers. This can be tested by giving the patient such simple problems as: $6 + 30$, $7 - 3$, 4×2, $10 \div 5$. When the significance of digits is not understood the patient is unable to say, when shown 6 and 3, for example, which is the greater. Similarly a number such as 286 may be mistaken for 2, 8 and 6 and place value may have no significance, e.g. 26 being wrongly described as 62.[122]

(2) Ability to arrange figures on paper for purposes of calculation. To test this the patient was instructed to write down, one beneath the other a series of numbers, which he was then invited to add:

$$9$$
$$14$$
$$\underline{101}$$

Inability to align numbers correctly so that units, tens, hundreds are misplaced, like inability to recognize digits or place-value in numbers, is often a prominent feature.

(3) Performance with written sums in simple addition, subtraction, multiplication and division. To succeed in these tests memory for the previously learned processes of " carrying over ", " borrowing ", and multiplication is necessary and dyscalculia may be due to their having been forgotten. Joffroy, according to Stoddard,[125] noted failure to " carry over " as a typical feature of the amnesic difficulties of patients suffering from general paralysis.

(4) Mental arithmetic. As this often proves more difficult to the average individual than written sums, care should be taken that the tests set do not exceed the limits of the previous educational level. Persons whose power of mental arithmetic are especially good may possess the faculty of visualizing numbers, and Spalding and Zangwill[123] have described the case of a man in whom a previously well-developed number-form was severely impaired as the result of a gunshot wound of the left occipito-parietal region. This patient showed no lack of understanding of arithmetical principles and signs, but said he " used to have a plan of numbers, but had lost it ". In his case there was an associated hemianopia, residual dysphasia with generalized weakness of visual memory and impairment of topographic sense.

9. *Other learned memories (agnosia, apraxia).*

This subject is considered in Chapter X. Visual object recognition was tested by displaying a number of common objects and getting the patient to demonstrate their use or otherwise indicate that he knew what they were. Colour recognition was similarly tested by displaying coloured blocks and asking the patient to name or match them with other colours. Auditory recognition was tested by covering his eyes

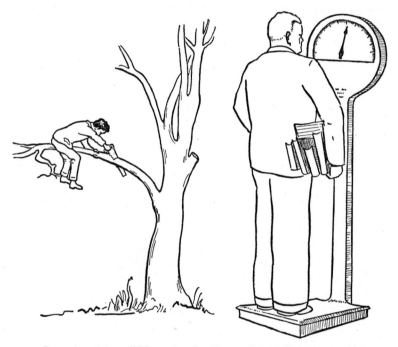

Reproduced from " Measuring Intelligence " by L. M. Terman and M. A. Merrill by kind permission of the Houghton Mifflin Company, Boston, and G. Harrap, London.

and then rattling money, tearing paper, striking a match, turning on water from a tap, pulling a curtain etc., the patient being required to identify the nature of each sound as he heard it. Tactile recognition was examined as already described in Chapter III. Picture recognition was ascertained by showing the patient a series of " Picture absurdities " taken from the Terman-Merrill Series.[119] These are graded for mental age, the simplest pictures (corresponding to a mental age of 7) representing a man sitting on the wrong side of a branch of a tree, which he is sawing; a man walking in the rain and holding his umbrella in the wrong position; a stoutly-built man standing on a weighbridge and carrying a load of books under his arm. More difficult pictures are: the one showing a house, some trees and clothes on a line, with smoke pouring from a chimney in one direction and trees and clothes blowing in the other (M.A. 12); the picture of a man facing the setting sun with his shadow pointing in the wrong direction (M.A. 14). In displaying these examples one noted especially whether the patient interpreted the picture at a literal or concrete level, i.e. simply describing the different items in it or was able to do so at an abstract level, i.e. seeing the absurdity of it.

Tests for *ideomotor apraxia* included (1) folding the patient's coat or dressing-gown and then asking him to put it on, (2) giving him a brush and comb and asking him to brush his hair, (3) watching his performance at meal times and when washing himself, (4) (if a smoker) offering him a cigarette and watching him put it in his mouth and light it, (5) shaving.

The ability to perform acts in pantomime was also tested by asking the patient to (1) pretend to play the piano, (2) wave good-bye, (3) shake his fist, (4) show how he would " thumb a lift " in a motor car, (5) say his prayers. *Constructional Ability (Constructional Apraxia)*. The ability to reproduce or construct one or more dimensional designs was tested by the use of sticks (Goldstein) or matches, Kohs' blocks and drawing tests. Of these the first measures only the ability to construct designs, performances with Kohs' blocks entail recognition of colours (and the test should not be given until one is satisfied that the patient has this capacity), drawing tests, e.g. of a house, entail some " drawing ability or aptitude " and capacity for abstract spatial orientation. Another test used was to draw an arrow on a blank sheet of paper and to invite the patient to copy it. If he could do so, he was then told to draw one pointing in the reverse direction, then to draw arrows pointing to the right and the left respectively. This test was useful sometimes in bringing out perseveration, the patient continuing to repeat the first drawing. Often, too, in organic mental states, although the arrowhead could be drawn pointing in one direction it could not be represented in the reverse position, a typically consistent result being obtained when this was attempted (see Fig. 2). Whatever may be the ultimate conclusion reached, Gooddy[124] believes that failures in this test is often an early and isolated sign of cerebral disease and that it may be present long before there are any classical signs of hemiplegia, hemianopia or attention defects. Drawing of arrows horizontally may, of course, be hampered by the co-existence of a visual field defect.

(1) *Stick tests.* Taking two matches one arranged these in different positions in relation to each other and asked the patient to copy the design, using two other matches and having the original design under observation whilst he did so. Few patients failed in this very simple

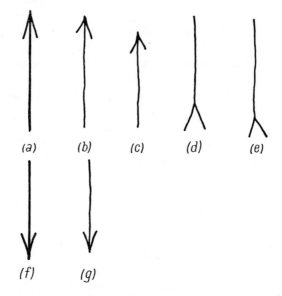

(a)   (b)   (c)   (d)   (e)

(f)   (g)

Fig. 2.—Drawing Arrows

Arrow drawn by examiner (a).
Examiner: " What is this?"
Patient: " An arrow."
Examiner: " Now, will you please copy it!"
Patient's copy (b).
Examiner: " Now, I want you to draw the arrow pointing in the opposite direction—not this way but that way."
Patient responds by drawing as at (c).
Patient's response after further explanation (d) and (e).
Examiner draws arrow then in required direction (f).
Patient's copy (g).

test and one then proceeded to make designs with three, four or more matches, the patient's responses being noted at each attempt. When his ability to construct simple designs had been tested in this way, his ability to construct from memory was tested. To do this he was shown designs made with two, three or more matches, which were then concealed from view before he was asked to reproduce them.

(2) *Kohs' blocks*. This proved a most useful test for uncovering evidence of constructional apraxia and abstract spatial disorientation. The blocks are all the same size, each, however, being painted in different colours on its six sides. Thus, one side is red, others are white, blue

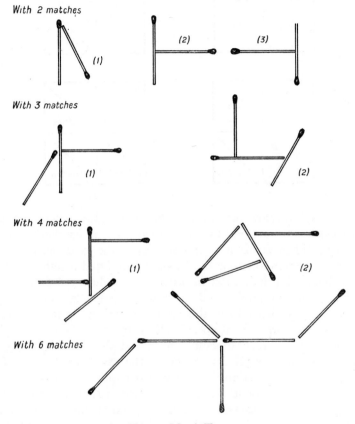

Fig. 3.—Match Tests

and yellow respectively. The remaining two sides are painted one-half yellow and blue, and the other red and white. A number of designs mounted on cards are provided and the object is to reproduce these from the blocks, fitting them together into the required pattern. Detailed instructions for conducting and scoring the test will be found in psychological textbooks. But as we were not concerned in measuring intelligence and obtaining scores, and wished only to find out whether or not the patient had constructional difficulties, only the first four test designs were used. These are as follows:

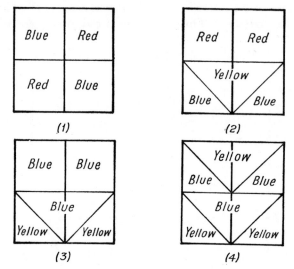

Before displaying the card with the first design the patient was given four blocks and encouraged to handle them so as to familiarize himself with them. Then displaying the first design, the examiner proceeded to demonstrate how the four blocks should be fitted together with the red and blue sides uppermost in order to reproduce the design. The blocks were then reshuffled and the patient invited to repeat the performance on his own. Even this simple task may be impossible for patients with constructional apraxia although as a rule most of them succeeded without much difficulty and looked pleased with their work. They were then given No. 2, 3 and 4, the examiner desisting from helping, but allowing as much time as was required, and noting carefully how they set about the tasks. Many organic mental patients complained that they had never been any good at this sort of thing or that their glasses did not suit them. Some patients could not bring the blocks together to form a square, aligning them as shown below or piling one on top of the other.

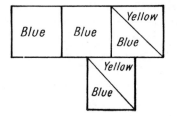

Others brought the blocks into position correctly but after some preliminary turning over and examining the different sides, ceased further work on the design and enquired unconvincingly: " Is that right?" When they are told to make a further attempt they sighed and turned to them again, toying with the blocks and trying the different sides, one after the other, in the hope of finding the correct ones. Many got the simple colours (red and blue) correct but could not manipulate the particoloured blocks into the required positions. In several patients, who succeeded in arranging three of the blocks correctly, we noticed a tendency, after vainly trying to arrange the fourth block, to break up the whole design and start again from the beginning, a feature which has some points of similarity to the " Penelope Syndrome ", which Critchley mentions was described by Pinéas[126]in another connection.

(3) *House drawing tests.* These were also found to be helpful, especially in doubtful cases where the distinction arose between a purely affective disorder or psychoneurosis and an organic mental state. Healthy normal dults, when asked to draw a house, protest that they have no skill in such matters and only comply with reluctance. Children over the age of 9–10 years display the same trait, but children under this age and many brain-damaged subjects lend themselves easily to the test, and their drawings have some points of similarity (see Chapter IX).

BIBLIOGRAPHY

94 SHIPLEY, W. C. (1941). Measurement of intellectual impairment in psychotics. *Amer. J. Psychol.*, **97**, 1313.

95 BRODY, M. B. (1942). The measurement of dementia. *J. ment. Sci.*, **88**, 317, 512.

96 WECHSLER, D. (1939). " Measurement of Adult Intelligence." Williams and Wilkins, Baltimore.

97 BABCOCK, H. (1930). An experiment in the measurement of mental deterioration. *Arch. Psychol.*, **117**, 105.

98 RAVEN, J. C. (1958). " Guide to Using the Mill Hill Vocabulary Scale with the Progressive Matrices Scales. H. K. Lewis, London.

99 BRODY, M. B. (1943). Discussion on the quality of mental test performance in intellectual deterioration. *Proc. Roy. Soc. Med.*, **36**, 243.

100 ZANGWILL, O. L. (1945). A review of psychological work at the Brain Injuries Unit, Edinburgh. *Brit. Med. J.*, **2**, 248.

101 BATTERSBY, W. S., TEUBER, M. L. and BENDER, M. B. (1953). Problem-solving behaviour in men with frontal or occipital brain injuries. *J. Psychol.*, **35**, 329.

102 MEYER, V. and YATES, A. J. (1955). Intellectual changes following temporal lobectomy for psychomotor epilepsy (preliminary communication). *J. Neurol. Psychiat.*, **18**, 44.

103 GILLIES, H. (1945). Mental sequalae in acute carbon monoxide poisoning and brain injury. *J. Roy. nav. med. Serv.*, **31**, 60.

104 ADLER, A. (1950). Course and outcome of visual agnosia. *J. nerv. ment. Dis.*, **111**, 41.

105 SOLOMON, A. P. (1932). Acalculia, other agnosias and multiple neuritis following carbon monoxide posioning. *Med. Clin. N. Amer.*, **15**, 2, 531.

106 WILSON, S. A. K. (1940). "Neurology," p. 913. Edward Arnold, London.

107 "Terminology for Speech Pathology" (1959). Authorized by the College of Speech Therapists, London.

108 GOLDSTEIN, K. (1948). "Language and Language Disturbances." Grune and Stratton, New York.

109 BASTIAN, H. C. (1887). On different kinds of aphasia with special reference to their classification and ultimate pathology. *Brit. Med. J.*, **2**, 931.

110 BROCA, P. (1861). Remarques sur la siège de la faculté du language articulé. *Bull. Soc. Anat., Paris*, **6**, 336.

111 MARIE, P. (1906). Revision de la question de l'aphasie: l'aphasie de 1861 à 1866; essai de critique historique sur la genèse de la doctrine de Broca. *Sem. médicale*, 48.

112 SYMONDS, C. P. (1953). Aphasia. *J. Neurol. Psychiat.*, **16**, 1.

113 PENFIELD, W. and JASPER, H. (1954). "Epilepsy and the Functional Anatomy of the Human Brain." Churchill, London.

114 TAYLOR, J., Editor (1932). "Selected Writings of John Hughlings Jackson," Vol. II, p. 142. Hodder, London.

115 HEAD, H. (1926). "Aphasia and Kindred Disorders of Speech." Macmillan, New York.

116 WEISENBERG, T. H. and McBRIDE, K. E. (1935). "Aphasia, a Clinical and Psychological Study." Commonwealth Fund Publication. Hildrath, New York.

117 SCHUELL, H. and JENKINS, J. J. (1959). The nature of language deficit in aphasia. *Psychol. Rev.*, **66**, No. 1, 45.

118 HEIMBURGER, R. F. and REITAN, R. M. (1955). "Testing for Aphasia and Related Disorders." University Medical Center, Indiana.

119 TERMAN, L. M. and MERRILL, M. A. (1944). "Measuring Intelligence." Harrap, London.

120 BURT, SIR C. (1938). "The Burt (Rearranged) Word Reading Test." University Press, London.

121 CRITCHLEY, M. (1939). "The Language of Gesture." Edward Arnold, London.

122 GREWEL, F. (1952). ACALCULIA. *Brain*, **75**, 397.

123 SPALDING, T. M. K and ZANGWILL, O. L. (1950). Disturbance of number-form in a case of brain injury. *J. Neurol. Psychiat.*, **13**, 24.

124 GOODDY, W. (1956). Personal communication.

125 STODDART, W. H. B. (1919). "Mind and Its Disorders," 2nd Edn. H. K. Lewis, London.

126 PINÉAS, H. (1931). Ein fall von räumlicher Orientierungsstörung mit Dyschirie. *Zbl. ges. Neurol. Psychiat.*, **133**, 180.

CHAPTER V

Acute Disturbances of Consciousness

THE mental symptoms shown by elderly patients with organic brain disease do not lend themselves so readily to classification as do their general physical and neurological signs, but in general, three principal clinical pictures can be recognized:

(1) Acute or subacute states of mental confusion occurring in apparently previously healthy persons, in whom the symptoms are related to gross disturbances of consciousness.

(2) Chronic amnesic syndromes, in which the chief feature is impairment of memory and intellect. In these patients there is usually some clouding of consciousness but this is never so apparent as it is in the first group.

(3) Patients with neurological signs indicative of focal cerebral disease, e.g. hemiparesis, hemianopia, dysphasia, in whose cases symptoms of (1) or (2) are superimposed.

Transient and at times protracted episodes of clouding of consciousness are of especially common occurrence at this age and may be the first indication of the presence of an organic mental state. As they are potentially reversible, their recognition is important both in regard to assessment of the intellectual and behavioural abnormality and to treatment.

NATURE OF CONSCIOUSNESS

Purdon Martin,[127] discussing the theoretical concept of a " seat " of consciousness, reminds us " that in the time of Galen it dwelt in the lateral ventricles; in the seventeenth century it was reputed to be in the pineal body or corpus striatum, and that since the time of Hughlings Jackson and Ferrier it had generally been accepted that consciousness depended on activity of the cerebral cortex, although to some the evidence had not been wholly convincing ". Ferrier[128] was certainly one of those who doubted the contention for he pointed out that, despite the known effects of cerebral cortical ablation on mentation " when we come to discuss the functions of the hemispheres, whole tracts may be completely and irrevocably cut out of the territory of intellectual consciousness without interfering with the integrity of consciousness *qua* others. . . . Hence we are not entitled to say that mind, as a unity (he identified mind and consciousness as being one and indivisible) has a local habitation in any one part of the encephalon, but rather that mental manifestations in their entirety depend on the conjoint action of several parts. . . ." Experience with penetrating head injuries in two world wars amply supported these conclusions, as have the results of excision of one or other frontal lobe, Jefferson,[129] and excision of one whole hemisphere, Krynauw.[130]

Korsakoff, at a much earlier date, had drawn attention to the peculiarly characteristic derangement of memory and orientation that attends permeation of the nervous system with toxins, and Wernicke had described pathological changes in the grey matter around the third ventricle in patients with the same symptoms. But, as Riddoch[131] suggested, it was the epidemic of encephalitis lethargica and the clinico-pathological studies of von Economo (1931) " that first opened the eyes of clinicians " to the importance of the diencephalon in regard to the allied functions of sleeping and waking. One of the first to note this was Simmonds,[132] who reported the case of a woman with hypo-pituitarism suffering from unexplained lapses of consciousness, which ultimately led to her death. In his monograph, on pituitary tumours Cushing[133] described states of pathological sleep and Caughey and Garrot[134] have stressed the danger of precipitating coma in cases of hypopituitarism by giving anaesthetics, insulin or permitting the patient to become water intoxicated. Jefferson,[135] Cairns[136] and other neurosurgeons have remarked on the frequency of altered states of consciousness in lesions of the brain stem and hypothalamus and Cairns *et al.*[137] have reported a peculiar mental state (" akinetic mutism ") in a patient with an epidermoid cyst of the third ventricle. This man lay inert with his eyes open, gazing steadily at the examiner; at other times he slept. Although his gaze could be diverted to passing objects or at novel sounds, in the half-waking state he remained mute and passive, no movements being apparent except on painful stimulation, when reflex withdrawal movements occurred . . . " but usually without tears, noise or other manifestations of pain or displeasure ". In their experimental work on concussion in animals Denny-Brown and Ritchie Russell[138] concluded that the effect on the brain stem was not dependent on forebrain influence since the transient paralysis of the respiratory and vasomotor mechanism noted after blows on the head could be obtained in decerebrate preparations.

Many other clinical observations of the same kind could be cited such as Whitty and Lewin's[139] report of the curious difficulty experienced by patients after anterior cingulectomy in distinguishing between their thoughts and actual events occurring around them, and the lack of awareness of their surroundings shown by cats after bilateral ablation of the cingulate gyrus, Kennard.[140] But experimental proof of the existence in animals, such as the cat and the monkey, of diencephalic and brain stem centres had to await the introduction of electroencephalography and techniques of deep implantation of electrodes, the site of which could be determined accurately by stereotaxic methods. Space precludes a detailed account of the many experiments which have been done but a few may be mentioned. Bremer[141] induced cerebral cortical rhythms characteristic of sleep by division of the brain stem at the intercollicular level (*cerveau isolé*) and Lewy and Gammon[142] found that destruction of the optic thalamus or interruption of the thalamo-cortical fibres in the internal capsule abolished cortical electrical activity. They concluded that this must be dependent on impulses transmitted through the sensory pathways in the brain stem because no such effects were observed after destruction of the cerebellum, excision of both frontal or occipital lobes or of the opposite hemisphere. Forbes and Morison[143] showed that, under anaesthesia, stimulation of a peripheral nerve gave rise not only to a cortical response in the area related to the site of stimulation, but that, after an interval, widespread electrical discharge followed over the whole of the cerebral cortex. Morison and Dempsey[144] obtained experimental proof of the existence between the thalamus and the cortex of " at least two systems . . . (*a*) the well-known specific projection system with a more or less point to point arrangement; (*b*) a second and 'non-specific' system with diffuse connections ". Later, Moruzzi and Magoun[145] showed that this general alerting response was " unquestionably mediated by neural connections between the reticular formation and the cerebral hemispheres ", the special areas concerned in the ascending reticular formation of the cat being: the central core of the brain stem, and through the pons and tegmentum into the caudal diencephalon, the pathway thence being by the diffuse thalamic projection system. Direct stimulation of the sensory pathways in the lemnisci had no widespread effect on cortical rhythm.

In man the application of peripheral sensory stimuli causes reversion in the E.E.G. from sleeping to waking rhythms. When sensory stimuli are repeated at less than 3 sec. intervals the response in the E.E.G. is very small but with stimuli given at 12 sec. intervals much greater responses are obtained. If the same stimulus continues to be repeated the response gradually diminishes, but if a change is made in its quality, larger responses are evoked. Pampiglione.[146] This author concludes that: " below the level of conscious memory there exists an activating mechanism capable both of immediate and delayed signalling to a large part of the brain " and that " the response to a given stimulus is at least in part determined by events which have occurred several seconds or even minutes previously."

Two questions have been asked: how applicable are experimental findings in animals to the problem of human consciousness, and in what way does consciousness in man differ from consciousness in animals? The solution to the first question cannot yet be given but it seems probable that, in the words of Ferrier " mental manifestations in their entirety, depend on the conjoint action of several parts ". Language alone is inseparable from the demonstration in others of fully developed consciousness, Turner,[147] and this fact in itself detracts from the possibility that the reticular formation plays a dominant part in consciousness in man. Penfield and Jasper,[113] whilst recognizing that the activity of the " centrencephalic system " is functionally inseparable from that of the cerebral cortex, believe that there can be little doubt that " it is the reticular system, with its diffuse and separate projections to the cortex, which is the central controlling mechanism for states of consciousness. Anaesthetics, although acting diffusely upon the brain, show a predilection for the reticular activating system, blocking conduction in the ascending medially-situated pathway in the brain stem and leaving conduction in the laterally-placed ascending fibres unimpaired," Feldberg.[148] Walshe,[149] however, insists " it is inconceivable that a lowest level segmental mechanism can subserve the highest level functions . . . when we consider the vast range and infinite variety of the physical content of full human consciousness and the necessarily complex neurological substratum it must call upon. That the cerebral cortex needs to be 'warmed up' as it were, by the reticular or 'centrencephalic' furnaces in the brain stem below, like a Roman Villa by the hypocaust beneath its floor, is likely enough, but the hypocaust is not the villa ".

CLINICAL ASPECTS OF CONSCIOUSNESS IN MAN

This most apt summing-up by Walshe of present knowledge in relation to consciousness leads to consideration of the clinical meaning to be attached to the term and the need for review of the many variations which may be recognizable in man, ranging from profound stupor or coma to full consciousness. Further, it will be obvious that, whereas there may be little clinical difficulty in assessing the degree of awareness in coma, use of the term " full consciousness " implies much more than the occurrence of an arousal or awakening response through which an individual becomes aware of himself and of his environment.

Many writers, following the example of William James, have prudently declined to attempt any definition. Yet, examination of random hospital notes show that there is confusion in the use of such terms as " conscious " and " unconscious ". Thus, one patient may be described as " unconscious, but able to answer his name to insistent demands ", another may be said to be " conscious but disorientated ". Here, the term consciousness will be accepted in the Jacksonian sense as being similar to and parallel with all aspects of mentation, although it will be maintained that certain functions of the latter are more directly concerned than others with its maintenance. Lhermitte[150] attracted to Sherrington's views, discusses the clinical aspects of consciousness in relation to disease under three heads: consciousness or awareness of the environment; awareness of the bodily self; and " la conscience réfléchie "—reflective or contemplative consciousness. This is a useful classification because the principal disease states interfering with consciousness may be correlated with it. Thus, the first kind is seen most often in acute toxic confusional psychoses, the " vigilance " of the patient being reduced but not lost and giving him—" l'aspect d'un dormeur à demi éveillé, égaré dans un univers qu'il ne comprend plus ". Disturbances of the body image are associated with hemisphere lesions and of the last kind with the epilepsies where the patient, although capable of behaving like a fully conscious person, has no subsequent recollection of his actions.

It is necessary, however, for an objective clinical approach to observe the hour to hour and day to day alterations in responsiveness and behaviour that can be seen in patients passing either from states of full consciousness into coma or regaining full consciousness after having been in coma. Symonds[151] did this in a series of head injuries. Equating recovery of full consciousness with restoration of memory, he measured the duration of unconsciousness by the length of amnesia following injury to the head. He concluded that there was no essential difference between the after-effects of simple concussion (where recovery of full consciousness was swift) and those protracted mental states dignified by the title of " acute traumatic psychosis ", in which recovery was delayed for several days or weeks. The clinical features of the latter he likened to a slow motion picture, while in less severely injured patients: " the phases of stupor, confusion and amnestic automatism pass in such rapid succession that the whole sequence is over in a matter of minutes ".

Although Symonds was careful to include only head injuries and patients without focal neurological signs in his series, so that he could " observe the direct effects of the injury upon cerebral function as a whole ", it is difficult in post-traumatic cases to exclude such complicating factors as traumatic subarachnoid haemorrhage, and bilateral subdural haematoma. It was for this reason that one has preferred post-anoxic patients for study of the mode of recovery in unconsciousness, i.e. healthy subjects, the victims of coal gas poisoning, cases of temporary cardiac arrest, dehydration, alkalaemia.[65, 91] In these there is considerable variation, the most severe effects occurring after cardiac arrest. Although death usually results when there is absolute arrest of cerebral circulation for more than a few minutes, one has seen full recovery to the former intellectual level take place in a young man whose heart had stopped for 5–7 minutes.[153] Milder and more transient anoxic effects causing clouding of consciousness result from electrolyte disturbance or dehydration and coal gas poisoning occupies an intermediate place. In experiments with young rats it has been shown that the more recently developed parts of the brain at birth respire at a slower rate than the older parts. But as growth advances their relative positions are reversed.[154] Further, the experimental work of Yant, Chornyak *et al.* on dogs[155] and the conclusions of Hoff, Grenell and Fulton[156] indicate that from whatever cause anoxia may be due, the effects on the brain are very similar. The effect of anoxia on the neurones depends on the extent to which these naturally utilize oxygen. Thus, the cortical neurones are most susceptible and the superficially placed ones more so than those at deeper layers. The thalamus suffers more than the corpus striatum and the red nucleus and oculomotor nuclei are relatively resistant. In the fatal case of cardiac arrest studied by Howkins, McLaughlin and Daniel,[157] in which death occurred on the twenty-sixth day, irregular focal areas of necrosis were found in the putamen and caudate nucleus, and in the thalamus there were fairly large areas in which no nerve cells could be seen. But in the medulla, pons and mid-brain apart from some " powdering " and alterations in shape in the neurones with excentric positions of their nucleoli, there was little change and the substantia nigra was normal. By contrast there was extensive and widespread loss of neurones all over the cerebral cortex, with commencing white matter degeneration.

Initial coma.

When first seen many of our anoxic patients were deeply unconscious, respiration being stertorous or faint, sighing in character, the pulse rapid and the blood pressure low. There was absolute loss of postural tone, the patient lying inert in the position in which he was placed and tendon reflexes being unobtainable. The pupils were equal, rarely contracted, although sometimes dilated, and the eyeballs were seen to make slow conjugate roving movements from side to side. Usually there was no response to light and the corneal reflexes were absent. No response was obtainable on painful stimulation, but on giving the patient a mixture of oxygen containing 10 per cent. carbon dioxide to inhale increased depth of respiration and temporary rise of systemic blood pressure were noted. When respiration was shallow, oxygen was administered and in such cases, if immediate improvement did not take place, death usually resulted. However, in the absence at the time of precise information relating to the duration and extent of the anoxia, it was very difficult to foresee the outcome. Thus, strange as it may appear, one patient, a woman of 60 years, who was deeply unconscious when admitted to hospital (respirations being stertorous and limbs rigid in the decerebrate posture and plantars extensor in type) recovered full consciousness within the space of eight hours.

Drowsy stupor.

The earliest signs of recovery from coma are the reappearance of postural tone in muscle, the patient assuming the lateral decubitus with the limbs semi-flexed in the foetal posture. Roving conjugate movements of the eyeballs still occur but soon cease, the eyelids being closed naturally as in sleep, with the eyeballs rotated upwards. At a later stage, on pulling back the eyelids, the patient may momentarily fix his gaze on the examiner before turning his head away and screwing up his eyes. Pupillary light and corneal reflexes return. Respiration is shallow and often of the Cheyne-Stokes or Biot type. Tendon reflexes can be obtained and the plantar responses are bilaterally extensor, this sign usually persisting for 24–72 hours in patients who have been rendered anoxic. Painful stimulation evokes the beginnings of an arousal response, which is the first indication of the patient's returning awareness of his environment. Simple withdrawal movements or grunting sounds are made. Insistent verbal commands may evoke the utterance of an expletive or semi-inarticulate protest, after which the patient lapses back into stupor.

Gradually, over the next few minutes, hours or days, it becomes less difficult to provoke arousal responses and a change is noted in their character. When a painful stimulus is applied to the face, not only is the head turned away to avoid it, but the hand is brought up to brush it aside, protect the area of skin assailed or to rub the part. Painful stimuli applied to a limb now, not only set up local withdrawal movements, but cause the other limb to come into action, the hand being brought over to ward off the stimulus.

Instead of lying motionless, spontaneous movements are made, the patient turning over in bed or on to his back and making slow flail-like movements at the shoulder joints or occasional flexion and extension movements at the knees. Later, if left alone, he may be observed scratching himself, picking at his nose or working with his finger at his lips, as if trying to remove something adhering there. Whilst being fed he may spit out the contents of his mouth, push away the spoon with his hand or keep his jaws firmly clenched. There is incontinence of urine and faeces.

Delirium.

This stage follows imperceptibly upon that of drowsy stupor, but varies much more in its manifestations. In some cases it may be so slight or transient as to pass unnoticed, in others so pronounced as to make transfer of the patient to a mental hospital expedient. Some writers have suggested that post-anoxic delirium, as compared to other varieties, is especially liable to be accompanied by violent behaviour. But in our experience this has generally not been so; when it has occurred the patient has been under intense emotional stress at the time of being rendered unconscious, and it is possible that the antecedent mood may play a large part in determining whether behaviour is violently aggressive, fearful or suspicious during the delirious phase. Another factor influencing it is the co-existence of visual hallucinations.

The principal features of delirium may be grouped under the following heads:

(1) *Motor restlessness.* Motor activities are often repetitive, misdirected or inappropriate so that behaviour, although purposeful, is often random and bizarre in character. The patient struggles to get out of bed and, if he succeeds, may roam about the wards or corridors. There is a rush of talk, speech being often incoherent and the mood is boisterous and/or aggressive. Thus, one man stalked up and down the ward in a threatening attitude, half-attired and announcing repeatedly that he was a celebrated boxer. After making to attack some of the other patients, he urinated in the corner and then allowed himself to be escorted back to bed. Another case, a woman who had been repeatedly trying to get out of bed, was not restrained on one occasion; instead she was assisted to take a short walk, the course of which was finally directed back to her bed. When she reached it she got in, lay down and promptly fell asleep.

(2) *Distraction.* Chance external stimuli largely determine the trend of activity on arousal from drowsy stupor and the sound of conversation may excite such repetitive retorts as " Is that you, George "

(3) *Perseveration.* This symptom, which first becomes apparent

during delirium, persists as a rule throughout the subsequent phases of clouding of consciousness and, although gradually diminishing, does not disappear until full consciousness is finally regained. In consequence, it is one of the most valuable clinical indicators there are of clouding of consciousness and it is especially useful in distinguishing disorders of behaviour due to this cause from those of hysterical origin. The term "perseveration", according to Kinnier Wilson,[229] was first used by Neisser in 1894 who spoke of a "persevatorische Reaktion". Pick was also aware of the phenomenon but he called it pseudo-apraxia.

In perseveration the patient responds correctly to a stimulus but continues to make the same response after the stimulus is withdrawn and another substituted for it. Thus, when directed to put out his tongue he will do so correctly, but when told to close his eyes, he will keep on putting out his tongue. This behaviour, which is typical of perseveration, may defeat all efforts at further communication but tends to disappear spontaneously in time. So, if one returns to the patient's bedside in half an hour and asks him to perform the second action he will have no difficulty, although if one follows the request by asking him to do something else the characteristic perseverative response will once more become apparent. In the state of delirium perseveration is often global in the extent to which it affects all kinds of responses. Some patients show it more than others but its presence can almost invariably be demonstrated. As clouding of consciousness lightens, however, it tends to become less pronounced and more selective, some activities being affected more than others, and curious effects are often observed. Thus, the patient, having responded correctly to the request to put out his tongue, may succeed in obeying the second order to close his eyes, but whilst doing so may be seen to protrude his tongue simultaneously. Perseveration is also often seen in patients in whom there is little evidence of clouding of consciousness but who have focal cerebral lesions affecting the dominant hemisphere and causing dysphasia. In such cases it is likely to be confined to speech alone. When asked to name different kinds of fruit the patient starts off confidently with " apples . . . oranges . . . apples ", his further efforts to recall other fruits being blocked by the perseveration. That the memory for names is relatively unaffected, is often shown by the way a patient can overcome perseveration, e.g. " apples . . . oranges . . . apples . . . no, I've said that before . . . apples . . . no . . . no . . . bananas " etc. Similarly, he may have no difficulty in saying the days of the week but be unable to repeat the months of the year.

(4) *Defective perception or grasp.* This feature is always pronounced

in the phase of delirium and, although it tends to disappear as the level
of consciousness rises, some difficulty in perception can usually be
demonstrated until consciousness has fully been regained. It is often
obvious during physical examination. Thus, it may be found that a
patient can flex his knee strongly against resistance, but when asked to
lift the straight leg off the bed cannot apparently grasp what is required
of him because he continues to go on flexing the knee. This sort of
behaviour is probably due to perseveration. Similarly, apparent
defective grasp may be related to visual object or auditory agnosia, but
in most brain-injured subjects, as Goldstein has shown, defective
perceptual ability is due to inability to form figure-background concepts
or appropriate " gestalts " out of the perceptual data available. The
effect of this upon behaviour in patients with clouding of consciousness
is at its greatest in the early stages of recovery. One of our patients,
when offered a cup of tea, dipped his fingers in the tea and then rubbed
them in his hair. Archer's[158] patient, when presented with a bowl
of water, soap and towel and told to wash himself, proceeded to wash
the towel.

(5) *Hallucinations*, usually visual in character, are less common in
delirium due to anoxia and trauma than in drug or metabolically-
induced states, but they may be present in cerebral vascular lesions
affecting the posterior part of the cerebral cortex and examples of such
and of toxic metabolic effects have already been given.

Disorientation.

To orient a thing means literally to place it facing towards the east.
Figuratively, it implies placing things or persons in clearly understood
relations to one another. Derived from *orior*, "I arise", it is associated
with the religious act of turning towards the east or rising of the
sun (159). It is characteristic of severe anoxia that in their recovery to
full consciousness most patients pass through a phase of disorientation
both for persons, place and time. This may be of extremely brief
duration and merge with the phase of delirium or be protracted and
persist for some weeks after delirium has subsided. An example of
the first kind was a lamplighter, a man aged 48 years, who had been
accidentally gassed. He was admitted in stupor but regained full
consciousness in 4 hours:

5.30 p.m. Stuporose. Withdrawal movements to pinprick. Oxygen administered.

6.45 p.m. Responds to insistent questions by repeating the question, e.g.
Q. " What is your name?" *A.* " What is your name."

7.15 p.m. Restless, aggressive movements. Resents all interference.

7.30 p.m. Keeps on reiterating: " What has happened to me?" Ignores all explanations.

8.00 p.m. Observed to be feeling himself all over as if to find out if he has been injured.

8.10 p.m. Opens his eyes. Asks where he is and enquires for his son. It is time, he says, to light his lamps. Struggles to get out of bed and cries out that he will be late, if detained.

9.30 p.m. Quiet and rational. Recognizes that he is in hospital and what has happened. Recalls events leading up to his being rendered unconscious.

Another patient, an elderly woman of 70 years, who had been found deeply unconscious with right-sided hemiparesis after more than 24 hours accidental exposure to gas escaping from a broken pipe, was not so fortunate. Although she recovered fully in time, she remained disorientated for 39 days.

2.11.47 Admitted to hospital in coma.

28.11.47 Recovered sufficiently to respond correctly to simple requests although perseveration is pronounced. When asked where she is looks bewildered and makes no reply.

2.12.47 Placid mood. Less perseveration and talks more freely. Hemiparesis no longer apparent. Recognizes and can name any assortment of common objects. No right-left disorientation and can identify her fingers.

4.12.47 More alert, understands simple questions and replies promptly. No evidence of perseveration, but disorientation pronounced.

Q. " What is this place?"

A. (The patient points to the ward and other patients in it): "This is a Home . . ." (turning to the nurse) " she is a lady doctor."

Q. " What year is it?"

A. " It is 1918."

Q. " And the month?"

A. " December."

Q. " How long have you been here?"

A. " I think about a month."

Q. " Do you know why you are here—have you been sick?"

A. (looks puzzled, then points to her right arm and leg): " It is because of my foot and my side. They are all benumbed."

13.12.47 On being questioned, she says that the year is 1900 and the month January, gives her age and date of birth correctly. Able to take meals without assistance and sit out of bed.

16.12.47 Gives her age as 59 years and the year 1888. In very good humour and appears to be most anxious to co-operate.

17.12.47 Talk is very free, circumstantial and she illustrates her remarks by gesture or pantomime. Mood friendly and happy. Knows now that she is in hospital but persists in saying that the hospital is in Armagh (place of her birth and childhood). Says the year is 1963 but knows the month and day of the week. She can repeat the months of the year but cannot say them in reverse. She can repeat 4 digits, has some difficulty in registering a name and an address and after 3 minutes has forgotten them. She remembers the names of her brothers and sisters and can recall some episodes from her childhood.

2.1.48 Remarkable improvement in the last 2–3 days. Orientation in time and place now consistently correct. Has good insight and is able to recall circumstances leading up to the accident, displays appropriate concern.

Many of the features in these cases resemble Korsakoff's psychosis, and as Korsakoff pointed out: " the patient gives the impression of a person in complete possession of his faculties; he reasons about everything perfectly well . . . makes witty remarks, plays chess or a game of cards. . . . Only after a long conversation with the patient one may note that at times he utterly confuses events and that he remembers absolutely nothing of what goes on around him. . . . On occasion the patient forgets what happened to him just an instant ago. You came in, conversed with him, and stepped out for one minute; then you come in again and the patient has absolutely no recollection that you had already been with him," Victor and Yakovlev.[160] Confabulation, as described by Korsakoff, is seen in post-anoxic cases, but visual hallucinations as already mentioned are rare except in drug-induced delirium. On analysis, therefore, the chief features of the state of disorientation are (1) alteration in mood, (2) loss of factual memory for past events, (3) inability to register fresh data or to recall the same, (4) disorientation, (5) defective grasp.

(1) *Alteration in mood.* During the later stages of the phase of disorientation most post-anoxic patients display a fairly constant mood of placid acceptance, readily agreeing to what is said and having little to offer in the way of constructive remarks. They are eager to please and will undertake simple repetitive tasks such as separating peas from beans or pasting a series of coloured pictures on to cardboard. Tense, angry, catastrophic types of reaction are unusual, and when they are confronted with something that is beyond their capacity, e.g. recalling a name or the day, they excuse themselves or confabulate and promise to do better the next time.

(2) *Loss of factual memory for past events.* Learned memories concerned with the recognition of common objects and colours are usually regained with disappearance of delirium, but invariably in disorientation

there is severe factual memory loss for past events. This was so great in one case that the patient, a sailor, who had been rendered comatose as the result of an explosion aboard ship, could not at first recall having been in the navy, and he passed by other shipmates in the hospital ward without any trace of recognition. As a rule, however, such global loss of memory for the past is unusual and patients can recall episodes from their childhood, schooldays or early working life, although these events are at first not clearly recalled in their temporal relations to each other. As they improve, events are recalled with some degree of clarity close up to the time of the anoxic experience, although for the actual event and circumstances following it there is no recollection.

(3) *Inability to register and recall.* This is absolute as a rule in the phase of disorientation, the patient being unable to register any details of a name and an address even after repeated attempts, but gradually, as day by day such tests are repeated, steadily improving until he succeeds in repeating the information given after two or three attempts. Recall presents much less of a problem to him than registration and, indeed, months afterwards he may startle the examiner by his ability to recall names and addresses that formerly he had such difficulty in registering.

(4) *Disorientation.* During delirium the patient (as in the case of the lamplighter) may appear to be trying to orientate himself to his own body. With the disappearance of this phase, disorientation for other persons may persist as it did in the case of the sailor whose amnesia was so great, but usually orientation for persons is the first to be recovered. Persistent disorientation for persons indicates a very severe degree of general cerebral impairment. Following this there may be a relatively long period during which, although orientated to himself and to others, the patient is without spatial or temporal orientation. Again, following the recovery of spatial orientation, some days may elapse before orientation in time is gained, this being the usual sequence of events in post-anoxic cases. Paterson and Zangwill,[161] commenting on the principal characteristics of spatial disorientation in post-traumatic cases with clouding of consciousness, note that at first in answer to questions the patient makes no reply or simply appears bewildered. Then he passes through a stage when correct and false answers are given side by side in the attempt to rationalize his position. Affective influences play a part in determining answers; thus, he will agree one moment that he is in hospital at A, and a moment after declare the hospital is at B, the latter usually being a place that has some particular affective significance for him (this was well shown in the case of the woman who insisted that the hospital was in Armagh, which happened to be the place in which

she had been born and spent her early years). Later, the patient shows
signs of realizing that there is something inconsistent between what he
is being told and what he believes and proceeds to confabulate that
A and B are situated close to each other, or that he has recently been
transferred from B to A. Weinstein and Kahn's[162] three patterns
of disorientation in organic brain disease are comparable. These
authors point out that in recovering orientation this is acquired for
persons and places, as a rule, before time, whereas in the reverse
process, i.e. developing delirium, orientation in time is lost first.

Recovery of spatial orientation in post-anoxic cases appears to take
place from within outwards towards the external world, and is determined by the limited perceptual data available. When the patient
becomes orientated to himself and his bed, his first conclusion often is
that he is at home. When he has assembled further perceptual data
in relation to his immediate environment, the other persons in the
ward, doctors and nurses, he accepts the fact that he is in hospital.
From thence he is likely to equate the situation of the hospital with
his home town or some other place of which he has especially fond
memories. Being unable to register, he shows little or no concern at
the discrepancy between what he is told and what he believes. His
further progress towards recovery depends on his improving capacity
for registration and his acquiring further perceptual data, which
render former beliefs untenable. In this way many false orientations
in space may be effected before correct orientation is achieved. A good
example of this was seen during the last war in an officer who, when he
had fully regained consciousness, was able to reconstruct part of the
pattern of his previous spatial disorientation.

He had been admitted to a temporary U.S. Naval Hospital in the U.K. after
a severe closed head injury. Although, English by birth and upbringing, he
had for many years lived very happily in New York, where he and his wife
occupied an apartment on an upper floor overlooking Central Park. He said
that his first recollection on recovering consciousness was hearing American
voices and this gave him the idea he was back in New York at his old apartment. Then, some days later he noticed trees through the window of the
hospital ward and thought these looked unfamiliar. Later still, he remembered
thinking they must be very tall trees indeed to reach to the window of his
apartment, or alternatively that the apartment building must have acquired a
roof garden in his absence.

(5) *Defective grasp.* Although still present, this is much less pronounced than it is during delirium. The disorientated patient recognizes
common objects and is able to demonstrate their use. He can usually
make shift to dress himself, take his meals and attend to his natural
needs. When asked to shake his fist or wave good-bye, he imitates the

act very convincingly. Similarly, when shown a picture he can pick out individual objects in it and describe them correctly. Perseveration may occasionally interfere with performance but quite clearly these concrete tasks are well within his capacity. It is only when he is presented with an abstract proposition that the difficulty in grasp becomes apparent. Thus, he will recognize an orange and a rubber ball but be unable to say in what respect they are similar. When shown the Terman-Merrill[119] picture absurdity of a fat man standing on a weighbridge and carrying a load of books under his arm, he will announce simply that the man is weighing himself, the point of the picture being overlooked.

The motor equivalent of this conceptual difficulty for abstractions is seen in the presence of some degree of constructional apraxia, which usually co-exists. Essentially this consists of an inability to assemble parts so as to form whole objects or things. It is considered in more detail in Chapter X. Constructional apraxia is often seen in association with focal cerebral lesions, in fact it was first described in connection with such, but its constancy (when sought for) in post-anoxic states can scarcely be doubted by anyone who has taken the trouble to examine these patients during the later stages of their recovery to full consciousness. It has also been observed in cases where clouding of consciousness has been due to other causes, e.g. hepatic encephalopathy.[31, 127, 163]

Recovery of full consciousness.

One of the most remarkable features in the sequence of events leading to recovery of full consciousness is the relative suddenness with which orientation, grasp, ability to register and memory for past events may return. This cannot, of course, always be demonstrated but in many patients it is most striking. Thus, one week progress is apparently at a standstill. The next, or two or three days later, a profound change is observed. The patient has lost his placid air of indifference and is now clearly concerned and anxious to find that he has been so long in hospital and fears something serious must have happened. He is now able to reconstruct past events up to a short time before being rendered unconscious and he can cast his memory back from the present for two or three days to the time when he fully appreciated his situation. He has no difficulty in registering and when shown simple pictures at once sees the point of them. He is correctly orientated both in time and place.

It is difficult to account for these phenomena on the basis purely of cerebral cortical damage. In anoxia emphasis has always been placed on the fact that of neural structures, the cortical neurones fare worst.

But, the brain stem and diencephalic neurones are also affected by anoxia and it seems probable that in these cases of so-called " post-anoxic psychosis " or " post-traumatic psychosis " the mental state is not altogether due to severe cerebral cortical damage. Initially, when the patient is in the stage of delirium and recovering from drowsy stupor it is possible that the anoxic effect on the cortex is still operative, but with the transition to the phase of disorientation or automatism it is likely that the cortical neurones have recovered. This is suggested by two clinical observations. The first is that although in some cases there may be a time lag of some days, in most cases, as already mentioned, the restoration to what Symonds calls " full consciousness " is effected too quickly to be explicable on a purely cerebral cortical basis. The process indeed is somewhat like that seen in patients with subdural haematoma. As is well known, drowsy stupor may be so pronounced in these cases as to render general anaesthesia unnecessary when making burr holes. Yet, as soon as the haematoma is exposed and evacuation of the clot begun, the patient may be able to answer questions, and before he leaves the operating table show other signs of recovering consciousness. This effect is probably due to relief of pressure on the brain stem and hypothalamus. Relief of pressure on the cerebral cortex plays little part. Indeed, increased intracranial pressure may be present without any noticeable disturbance of consciousness in patients with intracerebral tumours, the onset of clouding of consciousness often coinciding with the occurrence of tentorial coning and herniation. It seems probable, therefore, that in these post-anoxic cases in which there is witholding of " full consciousness " for a long period that derangement of the centrencephalic system is responsibile for the memory loss, disorientation and other features. The second clinical point in favour of this view is that the ultimate prognosis in these cases is good. The chance of persistent sequelae or dementia occurring is no greater than in those in which consciousness is fully recovered at an earlier date.

BIBLIOGRAPHY

127 MARTIN, J. P. (1949). Consciousness and its disturbances. *Lancet*, Jan. 1 and 8.

128 FERRIER, D. (1886). " The Functions of the Brain." 2nd Edn. Smith Elder, London.

129 JEFFERSON, G. (1937). Removal of right or left frontal lobes in man. *Brit. Med. J.*, **2**, 199.

130 KRYNAUW, R. A. (1950). Infantile hemiplegia treated by removal of one cerebral hemisphere. *J. Neurol. Psychiat.*, **13**, 243.

131 RIDDOCH, G. (1938). " The Hypothalamus: Clinical Aspects of Hypothalamic Derangement." Oliver and Boyd, London.

132 SIMMONDS, M. (1914). Über Hypophysisschwund mit tödlichem Ausgang. *Dtsch. med. Wschr.*, **40**, 322.

133 CUSHING, H. (1932). " The Pituitary Body, Hypothalamus and Parasympathetic Nervous System." Baillière, Tindall and Cox, London.

134 CAUGHEY, J. E. and GARROD, O. (1954). Coma and allied disturbances of consciousness in hypopituitarism. *Brit. Med. J.*, **2**, 554.

135 JEFFERSON, G. (1944). Nature of concussion. *Brit. Med. J.*, **1**, 1.

136 CAIRNS, H. (1952). Disturbances of consciousness with lesions of brain stem and diencephalon. *Brain*, **75**, 109.

137 CAIRNS, H., OLDFIELD, R. C., PENNYBACKER, J. and WHITTERIDGE, D. (1941). Akinetic mutism with an epidermoid cyst of the third ventricle. *Brain*, **64**, 273.

138 DENNY-BROWN, D. and RUSSELL, W. R. (1941). Experimental cerebral concussion. *Brain*, **64**, 93.

139 WHITTY, C. W. M. and LEWIN, W. (1957). Vivid day-dreaming: an unusual form of confusion following anterior cingulectomy. *Brain*, **80**, 72.

140 KENNARD, M. A. (1955). Cingulate gyrus in relation to consciousness. *J. nerv. ment. Dis.*, **121**, 34.

141 BREMER, F. (1935). Cerveau isolé et physiologie du sommeil. *Soc. Biolog. Paris*, **118**, 1235.

142 LEWY, F. H. and GAMMON, G. D. (1938). The modification of spontaneous cortical activity by sensory stimuli. *Amer. J. Physiol.*, **123**, 127.

143 FORBES, A. and MORISON, B. R. (1939). Cortical response to sensory stimulation under deep barbiturate narcosis. *J. Neurophysiol.*, **2**, 112.

144 MORISON, R. S. and DEMPSEY, E. W. (1942). A study of thalamo-cortical relations. *Amer. J. Physiol.*, **135**, 281.

145 MORUZZI, G. and MAGOUN, H. W. (1949). Brain stem reticular formation and activation of E.E.G. *E.E.G. and J. Clinic, Neurophysiol.*, **1**, 455.

146 PAMPIGLIONE, M. C. (1952). The phenomenon of adaptation in human E.E.G. (a study of K complexes). *Rev. Neurol.*, **87**, 197.

147 TURNER, E. (1955). The seat of consciousness. *Lancet*, Dec. 24.

148 FELDBERG, W. (1959). A physiological approach to the problem of general anaesthesia and of loss of consciousness. *Brit. Med. J.*, **2**, 771.

149 WALSHE, Sir Francis M. R. (1957). States of consciousness in neurology. *Premier Congrès Int. des Sciences Neurol. Rapp. et Discuss.*, **11**, 141.

150 LHERMITTE, J. (1955). Des dissociations des êtats de conscience provoquées par les lesions localisées de l'encéphale. *Rev. Neurol.*, **93**, 233.

151 SYMONDS, C. P. (1937). Mental disorder following head injury. *Proc. Roy. Soc. Med.*, **30**, 33.

152 SYMONDS, C. P. (1938). Traumatic psychosis. In " The British Encyclopaedia of Medical Practice," Vol. X. Butterworth, London.

153 TURNER, H. (1950). Case report: The mental state during recovery after heart arrest during anaesthesia. *J. Neurol. Psychiat.*, **13**, 153.

154   HIMWICH, H. E. (1951). " Brain Metabolism and Cerebral Disorders."
       Williams and Wilkins, Baltimore; Baillière, Tindall and Cox, London.

155   YANT, W. P., CHORNYAK, J., SCHRENK, H. H., PATTY, F. A. and SAYERS,
       R. R. (1934). Studies in asphyxia. *Pub. Hlth. Bull., Wash.*, No. 211.

156   HOFF, E. C., GRENELL, R. G. and FULTON, J. F. (1945). *Medicine*, 24, 161.

157   HOWKINS, J., McLAUGHLIN, C. P. and DANIEL, P. (1946). *Lancet*, 1,
       488.

158   ARCHER, B. C. (1941). *J. Roy. nav. med. Serv.*, 27, 84.

159   GOODDY, W. and REINHOLD, M. (1952). Some aspects of human orien-
       tation in space. *Brain*, 75, 472.

160   VICTOR, M. and YAKOVLEV, P. I. (1955).   S. S. Korsakoff's psychic
       disorder in conjunction with peripheral neuritis. Trans, from *Medizin-
       skioje Obozrenije*, 31, 1899, in *Neurology*, 5, 394.

161   PATERSON, A. and ZANGWILL, O. L. (1944).   Recovery of spatial orien-
       tation in the post-traumatic confusional state. *Brain*, 67, 54.

162   WEINSTEIN, E. A. and KAHN, R. L. (1951).   Patterns of disorientation
       in organic diseases of the brain. *Arch. Neurol. Psychiat.*, 65, 533.

163   JEFFERSON, M. (1955).   Mental confusion after porto-caval anastomosis.
       Brit. Med. J., 1, 786.

CHAPTER VI

Chronic Amnesic Syndromes

In the preceding chapter different stages have been described through which severely anoxic patients may pass before recovering full consciousness. As a rule these merge too freely into one another to permit of their individual recognition, although occasionally as in protracted delirium or disorientation this may be possible. However, they resemble more the projection of pictures in slow motion, the film being unrolled unevenly so that one picture is being projected on the upper half of the screen at the same time as part of the preceding picture on the lower half.

Reviewing the chief features of these different stages it will be apparent that mood and behaviour run parallel. In stupor the patient is inaccessible, resistive and irritable. In delirium behaviour has a purposeful character although determined largely by random stimuli in the immediate environment. Corresponding moods of elation or aggressiveness are seen. In disorientation behaviour is quiet, acceptant and, although still not goal-directed, repetitive tasks can be undertaken. Mood is placid and unconcerned. In full consciousness mood and behaviour are appropriate to the occasion. Perseveration is seen first during delirium and tends gradually to disappear, although its occurrence may still be recognizable from day to day until the patient has fully recovered. The inability to register and recall fresh data correlates with the period of disorientation and is largely responsible for perpetuation of the latter. Although in the final stages of disorientation there may be signs of recovery in the capacity for registration, it is not until full consciousness has been restored that it returns to its premorbid level. Memory loss, initially global in character, is restored first for distant events, the patient being capable of recalling incidents from childhood and later those that occurred up to a few months or years before the anoxic episode, but recovery of memory for recent or day-to-day events is delayed until the fully conscious state is re-established.

In discussing the deterioration of intellect that occurs in slowly developing organic mental states, therefore, the hypothesis will be adopted that this represents the process of recovery of full consciousness in reverse. Thus, as impairment of memory for recent events, perseveration, difficulty in registration and changes in mood and

111

behaviour are the last symptoms to disappear during reintegration, so one would expect them to be the first indications of decline. Chief among them, and often the first symptom to attract attention is impairment of memory.

Memory, says Woodworth,[164] consists of remembering what has previously been learned, and in it three distinct processes can be discerned; learning or registration, retention and recall. Quickness of

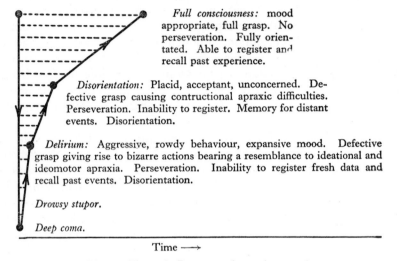

Full consciousness: mood appropriate, full grasp. No perseveration. Fully orientated. Able to register and recall past experience.

Disorientation: Placid, acceptant, unconcerned. Defective grasp causing contructional apraxic difficulties. Perseveration. Inability to register. Memory for distant events. Disorientation.

Delirium: Aggressive, rowdy behaviour, expansive mood. Defective grasp giving rise to bizarre actions bearing a resemblance to ideational and ideomotor apraxia. Perseveration. Inability to register fresh data and recall past events. Disorientation.

Drowsy stupor.

Deep coma.

Time ⟶

Fig. 4.—Phases in Recovery of consciousness in post-traumatic and anoxic patients

perception and individual fatigability influence the capacity for learning, but there are many other factors concerned, among which are motivation and repetition. The former implies the " will " to learn, a greater aptitude as a rule being shown when the new material has some facet of interest for the subject on account of his past experience, or when he can foresee some advantage to be gained by its being learned. Rolleston[3] may have had this in mind when he spoke of the " less agile " minds of the old being comparable to photographic plates " which in course of time have all become occupied by impressions ".

Repetiton also plays a part in registration and learning, spaced repetitions being a more certain method of memorizing than simple repetitions without pause, and these facts are reflected at the physiological level by the tendency displayed by nerve cells " to repeat patterns of activity so that all reactions have a strong tendency to form arrangements which are repeated whenever possible and around which more elaborate processes are built ", Russell Ritchie.[165] This argument, which is in keeping with the Pavlovian doctrine of conditioning, is supported, as Russell points out, by the recent neurophysiological studies of Granit (1953), Eccles (1953) and Bok (1956), who have shown that not only is interneuronal communication facilitated when there has been preceding activity across synapses, but that the opening-up of pathways during learning may be followed by actual structural changes in the respective synapses and filling of the interneuronal spaces in the cortex by numerous traversing nerve fibres, which multiply rapidly, especially in the first two years of life.

These findings provide some hypothetical basis for the long-established belief in " memory traces ", the existence of which psychologists have accepted as axiomatic in order to account for the second aspect of memory; the capacity to retain what has previously been learned. Use of the word " trace " implies some orderly system of storage of memories, such as is adopted for books in a large reference library, but the fashioning in time (as the result of individual personal experience) of interneuronal circuits may in itself provide the basic structure necessary for retention. If this be so, the concept of a centre or site for memory could be dispensed with, although it would still be necessary to postulate intact conducting pathways between the different parts of the brain concerned with their development and organization. At present the specific areas known to play some part in memorizing, i.e. lesions of which may cause profound memory loss, are the diencephalon, the temporal lobes and the hippocampus. Gamper[166] found in chronic alcoholics, who showed the clinical picture of Korsakoff's psychosis before death, that the cerebral cortex showed little of note but degenerative changes were seen in the brain-stem, extending from the medulla oblongata to the anterior commissure, the focal point and most constant site of these changes being in the corpora mammillaria. Williams and Pennybacker[167] have noted memory loss of Korsakoff type in patients with tumours of the third ventricle, and Conrad and Ule[168] in a case of encephalitis, the history of which suggested a toxoplasmic infective origin. There was complete destruction of the mammillary bodies by subarachnoid haemorrhage at the same site. Williams and Pennybacker conclude from study of their own four cases of tumour involving the third ventricle and the records of thirty-two other similar examples that memory loss, confabulation and other features of the Korsakoff syndrome are to be expected (72% of the cases) when the tumour affects the floor and sides of the third ventricle, but that when it is situated more anteriorly so as to implicate the chiasma memory loss is usually not a feature, a point which they regard as significant in emphasizing the purely local character of the effect. As regards the cerebral cortex, it has, of course, long been recognized that impairment of memory accompanies diffuse cortical degeneration and the occurrence in temporal lobe epilepsy of organized hallucinations of past experience, dejâ vue and jâmais vue phenomena and automatism provides strong evidence that this region has special significance. Since destruction of one temporal lobe has no effect and bilateral lesions must be present to disturb memory, Penfield believes that the function is represented in both temporal lobes.[169] Further evidence as to the significance of the anterior and mesial parts of the lobe is provided by this author's evocation of complex and involuntary memories by stimulation of certain points in the temporal grey matter. To these observations must also be added those of Scoville and Milner[170], who have shown convincingly that persistent memory loss is the usual sequel of bilateral damage to the anterior hippocampus and hippo-campal gyrus.

The nature of the processes concerned in the third aspect of memory or recall is also not fully understood. Recall means " remembering something that is not present ", i.e. not presented to the senses at the time, Woodworth.[164] Defective ability to recall past events and other data is often prominent in amnesic patients, and in such the memory loss may be more apparent than real, the chief difficulty lying not in failure of retention but in inability to bring retained facts back to mind, when the occasion requires. Kahn and Thompson[171] referred to this type of memory impairment (failure to use memory " as an intellectual tool ") as being especially characteristic of Pick's disease, in which memory *per se* is impaired only very slowly. Nichols and Weigner[172] also considered that the combination of this kind of memory defect and echolalia is very often seen in Pick's disease. Ajuriaguerra and Rignault de la Vigne,[173] however, noticed the same feature in post-anoxic patients and described their indifference to-wards recalling events as " une sorte d'indifférence mnesique ". Williams and Pennybacker[167] are inclined to correlate " not bother-ing " to use memory with lesions of the frontal area of the cortex. Psychologists, however, have recognized that difficulty in recall implies some sort of interference or competition, which can often be traced to an emotional cause and that it is this interference or competition which is usually at the root of emotional forgetting. But, as neural discharges are constantly occurring in the brain, some physiological inhibitory mechanism must exist to ensure that thought and other activities are not constantly being interrupted by irrelevant memories being obtruded into consciousness, and to enable desired facts to be recalled at will.

Penfield believes that the centrencephalic system in the upper brain stem corresponds with Hughlings Jackson's highest level of functional integration,[113] but whether this is so or not, it may well be that the disturbance in some cases of defective recall may be in these same circuits, which are symmetrically connected with both cerebral hemispheres.

CLINICAL MATERIAL

Among the 198 organic mental patients in this series there were 45 in whom the chief presenting symptom was failing memory. Of these 26 were males and 19 females. The average age when first seen was 58 years, the youngest patient being 37, and the oldest 69. The numbers in each quinquennium rose to a peak at 61–65, thereafter showing a sharp decline.

years	cases
30–35	0
36–40	1
41–45	2
46–50	4
51–55	8
56–60	11
61–65	17
66–70	2
	45

This could have been due to patients over the age of 65 having been referred to Geriatric or Mental Hospital wards, but it is of interest to note that over the same post-war period admissions of patients with presenile and senile symptoms to mental hospitals in Northern Ireland were greater in the 50–60 group than for later decades.[174]

One had expected that impairment of memory would have been a more frequent presenting symptom, but the reason it was not seems clearly related to the fact that, although some impairment of memory was found in most patients, it tended to be lost sight of against other more clear-cut signs and symptoms such as epileptiform fits, hemiplegia or aphasia. The patients selected for review, however, had no obvious physical signs and in their cases impairment of memory was the chief, if not the only, presenting symptom. Further, many of them seemed to be unaware of their defective memory, or were doing their best to hide it. The relatives, although aware, had been inclined at first to attribute it to the natural process of ageing or to overwork or worry. As a rule it was only when some gross or inexplicable blunder was committed, so that the symptom could no longer be ignored, that they decided to take medical advice. Other factors leading to recognition of gross memory impairment were: change of occupation or altered conditions in place of work; promotion; retirement. Chronic amnesic symptoms in elderly people were also sometimes uncovered through their being erroneously treated as " functional " and given barbiturates for purposes of sedation. This practice not infrequently had led to cumulative toxic effects and the unexpected development of an acute confusional state. Similar symptoms had been precipitated in a few instances, where systemic blood pressure was raised, by the incautious use of morphine or by hypotensive drugs.

Typical of the statements of relatives in describing patients' conditions were the following:

" His memory, or rather the lack of it, has been a sort of joke in the family for years—we have all recognized it—it is only since he has begun to forget the day of the week or the month, the names of people he knows well or how to find his way home when he has been down town, that we have begun to worry about it."

" You would tell him to do something and he would forget to do it."

" When he lost something, as he was always doing, he would wander around looking for it, and when I asked if I could help, he could not tell me what he had been looking for, having forgotten what it was."

" She forgets to put on her hat or gloves when she goes out . . . she would make out a shopping list and then forget to take it with her."

" Although he remembers his early life very well, he has to be told what to do, what to eat and when to shave."

" The first thing I noticed was that she could not remember names, and this seemed to worry her greatly."

More specifically, memory defects in women took the form of neglect of housework (usually attributed to loss of interest); lack of attention to personal appearance; loss of imagination in cooking, the same meals being served day after day; and forgetfulness of detail. In the case of men, the first evidence of failing memory was usually noticed in their work. Thus, a previously healthy electrical fitter, aged 45 (whose amnesia had been the sequel of accidental electrocution) was given light repair work at a bench, every consideration being shown to him, but he kept on, as the report said, " making silly mistakes ", forgetting where he had put things and making wrong electrical connections. So distressed was he at these mistakes that he became depressed and had to enter a mental hospital. On resuming work his depression was gone, but he still could not recall where he had put things, and in undertaking even the simplest of tasks he had to " stop and think " what to do next. As a result he formed the habit of carrying technical books of reference to work, but when he put these down he could not find them. So preoccupied might he have been in concentrating on what he was doing that he often returned home in the evening with his luncheon packet untouched, and on more than one occasion, riding home on the bus, he had passed his stop for getting off.

However, the manner in which modern industry is organized often enables patients to continue at work long after amnesic difficulties have become apparent. Thus, a master shipwright of 56, seven years before his death from Alzheimer's disease, had begun to " forget how to do things ", but his mates in the squad in which he worked had " covered up " so well that he had been enabled to continue in employment for three years before finally having to give up. As has already been mentioned, the responses of brain-injured subjects to performance tests depend greatly upon the conditions or setting in which they are conducted and this may account for symptoms of organic mental deterioration only becoming apparent on retirement, although they may have been present before and not have interfered to any considerable extent with the patient's ability to do routine work.

Pathology

Despite the fact that all patients were brought into hospital for observation and had electroencephalography, x-rays, lumbar encephalograms or ventriculograms when the need arose, a firm diagnosis was reached only in 30 cases, or about 66% of the total (Table 4). Those in whom the cause remained in doubt were classified loosely as " presenile dementia ", because the results of electroencephalography and contrast radiography pointed to diffuse cortical atrophy, family history was negative and there was no evidence of arteriosclerosis or other known causes. Angiography was not much used in these cases until 1953 and it may be that the symptoms in some of those so designated were due to carotico-vertebral atherosclerosis. Hurwitz *et al.*[57] have reported a case of carotid artery occlusion in which " the mental state was most suggestive of Korsakoff's psychosis ".

Turning to cases in which aetiology was more clear, *cerebral vascular disease* was accepted as the probable cause of symptoms when there was evidence that minor cerebral vascular accidents had occurred, there was both a pronounced rise of systemic blood pressure and evidence of myocardial changes, or when increased emotional lability with tears, some dysarthria and spastic weakness in the lower extremities suggested an early pseudobulbar palsy. (This condition developed subsequently in one patient.) In one case in which none of the above-mentioned features was present, however, extensive cerebral atherosclerosis was found after death. In five cases the clinical features pointed to *Alzheimer's or Pick's disease*. In two of these the diagnosis of Alzheimer's disease was confirmed at post-mortem examination, the brain showing generalized cortical atrophy and histologically the presence of numerous senile plaques with replacement of nerve cells by tangles of neuro-fibrils. In all five cases global disturbance of memory with loss of initiative and spontaneity were early and pronounced symptoms, topo-graphic memory loss in particular often being so great as to make it

TABLE 4.—*Aetiology of Chronic Amnesic Syndromes*
(45 Cases)

Cause known (30 *cases*):

Tumours (6) . . . . Meningiomata (4)	
	right fronto-temporal (1)
	right frontal (1)
	left frontal (1)
	right parietal (1)
	Pinealoma (1)
	Epidermoid cyst (1), involving third ventricle and chiasma.
Chronic subdural haematoma (1)	
	right parietal
Aerocele, right frontal (1)	
General paralysis of the insane (2)	
Hepatic encephalopathy (1)	
Post. anoxic (6)	
Post. traumatic (2)	
Cerebral Arteriosclerosis (6)	
Alzheimer's disease (5)	

Cause indeterminate (15 *cases*):

" Presenile dementia "   (12)
? Hepatic encephalopathy   (1)
? Myxoedema   (1)
? Jakob-Creutzfeld syndrome (1)

difficult for the patient to find his way out of doors or around his own house. Disturbances in behaviour were also common, being related to memory impairment, perseveration, apraxia or the occurrence of minor fits with transient disturbance of consciousness. Actual convulsive seizures, however, were not seen and, indeed, this observation applies to all chronic amnesic syndromes in this series, excepting those due to cerebral vascular disease or carotico-vertebral atheroma. In the latter, mild convulsive episodes, Jacksonian fits, transient hemiplegia might either be observed or an account of them obtained from the past history. It is not suggested that in diffuse cerebral cortical atrophy convulsive fits cannot occur. Nichols and Weigner[172] and Fuller[175] for example, in their confirmed cases of Pick's and Alzheimer's disease noted them in the later stages, but our experience leads us to believe that they are infrequent, an observation that may be correlated with the relation-

ship known to exist between susceptibility to fits and brain development. As Caveness *et al.*[176] have shown in the macaca monkey, attempts
to produce seizures by intraperitoneal injections of Metrazol in the
neonatal period of their development usually fail, whilst at six months
with the same dose the animal dies in status epilepticus. Even with
intracortical injections of penicillin the young animal is relatively
immune to convulsive seizures, these developing more slowly and less
completely than in the mature animal. It is possible, in a similar way,
that the relative infrequency of convulsive seizures in diffuse cerebral
cortical atrophy may be due to breakdown of the normal adult cortical
mechanism.

A positive family history of other members being similarly affected
with dementia in later life was obtained in only two of these cases, in
most instances the diagnosis of Alzheimer's or Pick's disease being made
on the basis of exclusion of other possible causes and upon the fact
that symptoms had appeared in the presenile period between the ages
of 40–50 years. Stengel's comprehensive review[177] of the symptomatology of these two conditions may enable one to differentiate
between them clinically. This is the experience, too, of Robertson,
Le Roux and Brown,[178] who regard the finding of generalized hyper-
algesia as being very typical of Pick's disease. In their cases, although
the pains complained of were suggestive of thalamic over-reaction,
no lesion was observed at this site after death. Text-books emphasize
certain disturbances of speech that are thought to be characteristic,
i.e. " the tendency to repeat individual syllables or words several
times before getting on with the sentence, somewhat like stammering ",
Stoddart;[125] stereotyped utterances and senseless repetitions of words
and sentences (Henderson and Gillespie),[179] Mayer Gross, Slater and
Roth.[180] Like the dirty and untidy appearance patients may show, these
manifestations are probably more expressions of an advanced state of
disease than of any specific characteristic of the morbid processes. The
general characteristics of speech disorders in chronic amnesic syndromes
due to diffuse cortical atrophy are discussed in the succeeding chapters.
Disturbances of gait when present, however, assist in the diagnosis of
these conditions, the " marche à petits pas " being characteristic, as
also the occasional demonstration of increased muscle tone or inability
to relax muscles so as to enable passive movements to be made freely.
This increase of tone, which affects agonists and antagonists equally,
has an almost hysterical character, being unassociated with either
spasticity of the claspknife type or " cog-wheel " rigidity. In the early
stages of dementia the mistake may easily be made of assuming that the
disturbance of tone and gait is purposively motivated, but when seen

the features are very typical of diffuse cerebral cortical atrophy. The disorder of gait, we believe, is essentially dyspraxic in origin, although at a later stage it may develop an extrapyramidal quality.

Anoxia accounted for six cases. Bedford,[54] Allison[181] and others have commented on its importance as a cause of chronic amnesia in middle-aged subjects. Defective aeration arising during an operation on the neck for the removal of a tumour accounted for one case; in two there had been temporary cardiac arrest during operations for valvotomy; in two others severe haematemesis, and two cases were attributable to accidental carbon monoxide poisoning and electrocution respectively. In accepting the relation between cause and effect in these patients, Donald Hunter's[182] criterion that the period of unconsciousness should be of at least six hours' duration was adopted. In all six instances it was, in fact, much longer, nearly three months having elapsed in one case before consciousness was fully regained. In both *post-traumatic* cases there had been severe closed head injuries with prolonged delay in recovery of consciousness and residual chronic amnesic symptoms.

As regards the four patients with *meningiomas*, reference has already been made to the manner in which these tumours may simulate dementia due to diffuse cerebral cortical atrophy. Headache was severe in one of them but in the others it was either not mentioned or slight. None of the patients with meningioma had had epileptiform fits, which is perhaps noteworthy in view of the cortical situation of the tumours and the fact that in all instances contrast radiography had revealed ventricular shift and there were other signs of cerebral oedema. In all but the case referred to on p. 18 unequivocal signs pointing to a unilateral cerebral lesion could be elicited on careful examination, but these could readily have been overlooked. In only one of the cases was papilloedema observed. The same generalizations apply to the patient whose case is referred to on p. 58 and who at operation was found to have a *chronic subdural haematoma*, situated over the right parietal region; there was no headache or papilloedema and dementing symptoms were even more pronounced. Of space-occupying lesions, however, probably the most striking was the patient with a post-traumatic aerocele:

This was a man of 62, whose forgetfulness, lack of initiative and frequent bouts of disorientation in time and place had been the subject of comment for some months preceding his admission. From his wife it was learned that he had said he could feel " the old bottle " in his head emptying at times and hear " bubbles rising in it ". At these times, she said, fluid ran from his nose. When aged 28 he had fractured his skull and been unconscious for twelve days. For a year after there had been watery discharge at times from the nose, but one day, working in his garden and trying to pull up a rather tough root, he came down heavily on his bottom and the discharge ceased. He had had no further trouble for almost 34 years and, until the recent symptoms developed, had been successfully employed as a manufacturer's agent. On examination his mood was unconcerned and at times facetious, but apart from some coarse tremor of the outstretched arms and hands and a pulsating right exophthalmos there were no physical signs. Radiograms of the skull showed a large aerocele in the right frontal region, which had a patent connection with the frontal air sinus.

Of the two cases in which the tumour was diencephalic in situation, occasional " falling attacks ", recurring headache and some ataxia of gait had been present for years in the patient with a *pinealoma*. But little notice had been taken of these until failing memory, with recurring attacks of drowsiness, had been observed in the preceding six months. In the other case (an *epidermoid suprasellar cyst*, involving the third ventricle) there had been no abnormal drowsiness, but impairment of memory for recent events, confabulation and other features of the Korsakoff Syndrome were most pronounced. Although this patient complained of defective vision no consistent visual field defect could ever be demonstrated. At one time there appeared to be a bitemporal defect, at another an hemianopic defect, but often the fields were full. Her air of unconcern and absent-mindedness, however, made perimetry difficult and it was impossible to draw any firm conclusions from such tests other than that there was some defect in both visual fields. There was no suprasellar calcification, but the cyst was demonstrated by ventriculography and later exposed and drained.

Duration of memory impairment in patients with focal and diffuse lesions.

When attempting to estimate the duration of memory impairment we were, of course, dependent chiefly on relatives and their statements may not always have been accurate, but it is of interest to note that in more than half of the cases in which memory impairment was the principal symptom its known duration was over two years and in about 15% over 6 years:

		cases
1 year or less	....	13
2 years or less	....	7
3 ,, ,,	....	3
4 ,, ,,	....	6
5 ,, ,,	....	6
6 ,, ,,	....	3
7 ,, ,,	....	2
8 ,, ,,	....	0
9 ,, ,,	....	2
10 ,, ,,	....	3
		45

9

Table 5 correlates the duration of symptoms with the underlying pathology. In the six patients with tumours, it will be noted, memory impairment was of relatively short duration; in the diffuse cerebral cortical atrophies due to presenile and arteriosclerotic causes it was more spread out and extended over a greater period of time. This meant that in the former relatives could usually fix within a month or two the date at which memory loss became apparent, whereas in the latter it often stretched back so far into the past as to make it difficult for them to do so. The order of appearance of memory impairment also differed; with focal cerebral lesions other symptoms such as fits, headaches, ataxia usually appeared first, impairment of memory being more of a late-comer, whereas in the diffuse atrophies it was the first symptom to be noted. Further, and this applied especially to cerebral arteriopaths, the steplike character of their decline often allowed them to remain more or less static for a year or more and permitted the development of protective techniques to compensate for their memory loss. These might consist of keeping written notes of what they had to do, restricting their activities to a fixed, regular routine, avoiding controversy, novel or unplanned activities. By contrast, patients suffering from rapidly expanding focal lesions did not use these stratagems to the same extent, probably because dissolution was proceeding at too fast a rate to enable them to do so.

These points are, we believe, of greater importance than any attempt to differentiate between the characteristics of the memory loss shown by patients with diffuse and focal lesions respectively. *Indeed, one should always feel hesitant in accepting a diagnosis of presenile dementia, no matter how much the patient's state at the time might suggest the condition, unless it can be shown that the impairment of memory has been present for some time and certainly before other symptoms were noticed.* Schindler[183] has pointed out that the clinical pattern taken by the symptoms in senile deterioration is influenced greatly by the premorbid personality and temperament so that, as he says: " der Patient reift gewissermassen in seine Diagnose hinein ". Similarly, as regards memory loss, the onset is so vague and the subsequent course of memory loss so insidious that it is difficult to say when it began.

Extent of memory impairment.

In most cases this was global in extent, affecting the ability to recall recent, middle distance and distant events, although the first named were more affected than were memories of childhood and early adult life. Thus, a man, who had recently returned to Ireland from the United States, where he had lived for some years, could remember the

TABLE 5.—*Duration of History and Aetiology* (45 cases ch. Amnesia)

Duration of symptoms in years	No. of cases	Artscl. dement.	Post-traumat.	Post-anoxic	G.P.I.	Alzheimer's disease	Hepatic enceph.	Cerebral tumour	Subdural haem.(1) Aerocele(1)	Presenile dementia
1 or less	13	2	1	–	2	–	1	4	2	1
2	7	1	–	1	–	–	–	1	–	4
3	3	1	–	1	–	–	–	–	–	1
4	6	–	1	2	–	1	–	–	–	2
5	6	2	–	–	–	1	–	–	–	3
6	3	–	–	1	–	–	–	1	–	1
7	2	–	–	–	–	–	–	–	–	2
8	–	–	–	–	–	–	–	–	–	–
9	2	–	–	–	–	1	–	–	–	1
10 or more	3	–	–	1	–	2	–	–	–	–
Total	45	6	2	6	2	5	1	6	2	15

name of the ship (*Leviathan*) and other details of his outward journey in 1924 but had no recollection of his return passage, which had been made only a few weeks before he was interviewed. Another man remembered the names of his teachers and clergyman when he was a boy, and could recall his mother's maiden name, but he stumbled badly when trying to give the names of his wife and children, with whom, of course, he had been in daily contact before his admission to hospital. Good preservation of memory for early events was usually seen in non-progressive post-traumatic and anoxic patients in whom a frequent comment of relatives was that they seemed to dwell in the past and took little or no interest in the present.

In only five patients was impairment of memory strictly confined to recent events. Two of these had frontally situated meningiomas. In the remaining three the explanation lay in the fact that the observer was being privileged to observe a presenile dementia in its earliest stages. One of these was a well-educated woman aged 58 who had had vague digestive disturbances and other symptoms, which may have been due to a " small unrecognized stroke ".[184] Four years later her condition had reached such an advanced state of dementia as to be unmistakable. Yet, initially, it was difficult to distinguish her condition from a purely affective disorder.

She had been referred because of absent-mindedness and forgetfulness for every day matters, giddiness and unsteady gait and had particular difficulty in recalling names. Thus, at parties, when she and her husband were entertaining, she would feel embarrassed because she could not recall the guests' names, a sort of " blank " coming over her mind at these times. This upset her greatly because they were, of course, people whom she knew well. She was inclined to blame it all on worry and was finally persuaded to confide the nature of this, which seemed to provide a reasonable enough explanation for her obvious state of tension and anxiety. On testing, there was no evidence of gross intellectual deterioration but she had difficulty in registering a name and an address and in reversing series. In reading, although she had no trouble in comprehension, she was inclined to mix up lines and lose her place. Memory for distant and middle distance events was very good and when asked to give the names of some cities she reeled off without hesitation: "New York, Chicago, London, Paris, St. Petersburg." A moment later, asked to name two cities in Australia she replied without hesitation: " Brisbane, Sydney." However, she was less fluent in casual conversation (hesitating occasionally over names) than she was in answering questions. Thus, when first encouraged to speak of her worries she replied that she would prefer questions to be

asked rather than that she should attempt to speak about them spontaneously. At the time the significance of this was misinterpreted and
her disinclination thought to be hysterical. However, her house drawing
suggested some spatial disorientation and constructional difficulty and
on neurological examination there was a partial right homonymous
hemianopia. The E.E.G. showed diffuse theta activity, greater on the
left side but non-focal, and on lumbar encephalography there was air
over the convexity of the brain and some cavitation in the left occipital
horn, suggestive of infarction.

Character of Memory Defects

Although occasionally the difficulty in remembering only concerned
names, in most instances multiple defects were present and these were
of four kinds.

(1) *First, inability to arrange or sort former events into their proper
sequence or decide their temporal relation to each other.*

This was well-illustrated in the case of a university graduate and
former teacher, a woman of 62 years with presenile dementia, who was
seen in 1953. Her chief complaint was of tiredness and her sister said
that for some years there had been a gradual falling off in her memory
and range of activities. Formerly a dynamic person and " full of ideas ",
she now had no initiative and was content to " sit around " all day.
When first seen she was in the day room talking to a little girl whom she
was trying to interest in a picture book. So perfect was her poise that it
was difficult to credit that anything was wrong. However, she admitted
that her memory was bad, answering: " I can't remember a single
thing . . . even such a detail as where my bed is in the ward!" As she
said this she laughed in a deprecating way and mentioned that she
supposed it was the consequence of overwork. This patient had no
difficulty with series, but several attempts had to be made before she
could register a name and an address and she had forgotten the information three minutes later. Her spontaneous small talk was most natural
and the naming of objects, both sighted and from memory, presented
no difficulty to her. For example, when asked to name some flowers,
she rattled off: " wallflower, chrysanthemum, dog daisy, marguerite,
hairbell, wild hyacinth, primrose, violet ", and it was the same with
cities. Simple calculations also presented no difficulty and there was no
evidence of agnosia or ideomotor apraxia, but she failed on the match
tests and with Kohs' blocks, remarking: " I don't know what is

wanted; it seems to depend on how you look at it." Picture interpretation was also grossly affected so that when she was shown one of the
Terman-Merrill pictures (suitable for a child of 7) she could not see
the point although she could describe all items in the picture correctly.
When her memory for past events was tested, it was found that names,
places and events were not so much forgotten as their temporal relationships disarranged. This is illustrated in the following excerpt from a
conversation in 1953:

Q. " Miss X . . . do you recall the First Great War?
A. " Oh yes I do . . . I was teaching near Liverpool at the time . . . in Mossley
  Hill . . . the girl's name was G—, a nice child " (she then gave the name
  of the family and other details).
Q. " In what year did that war begin?"
A. " Oh, let me see . . . it was sometime in 1915, or was it 1914?"
Q. " Can you recall who was the Prime Mininster at that time?"
A. " Let me see . . . was it Churchill? . . . Oh no, of course not . . . it was
  Ramsay MacDonald of course!"
Q. " Then there was a Second World War. Do you remember much about it?"
A. " Well, I can't recall the last war . . . I know England is at war now . . .
  at least I think she is . . ."
Q. " Who was Hitler?"
A. " Oh yes . . . of course I recall him . . . how stupid of me . . . what
  happened to him? Is he in prison or is he dead?"

More severe defects in this sphere probably accounted for the peculiar
behaviour of some amnesic patients who did not know when they had
had their last meal, when it was time to stop work or when to commence
work. One man was reported to be rising, dressing himself, and starting
off for his office before six o'clock in the morning. Another man,
who lived in the country first drew attention to his state—he had a
right frontal meningioma—when he set out for town one day to
transact business and only found on his arrival in the city that it was a
Sunday.

(2) *Loss of topographic memory, or inability to remember the spatial
relationships of previously well-known places.*

This curious symptom was a pronounced feature in 13 patients and
it is noteworthy that all of them turned out to have diffuse cerebral
cortical atrophy, this kind of defect (unlike temporal defects) not being
observed in any of the uncomplicated tumour cases. Typical of it was
the tendency to get lost out of doors and to be found wandering in the
streets. Some patients said that they remembered streets looking
vaguely unfamiliar and this *jâmais vue* effect was subsequently traced

to the occurrence of minor fits. However, in others there was no evidence of epileptic seizures and the illusion of unfamiliarity seemed to be related to perseveration, or inability to reorientate themselves to a new scene, owing to persistence of the former scene. That is to say their loss of sense of direction coincided with stopping to window gaze or entering a shop to make a purchase so that when they turned around or came out they did not know which direction to take. One man said that when in doubt he always turned to the left, but this was not determined by his handedness or the existence of either a hemianopic defect or visual inattention to one side. The most severe example of spatial disorientation was in a case of Alzheimer's disease. One night, shortly after being shown to his bedroom, his wife said he was found lying the wrong way round, with his feet on the pillow and his head at the foot of the bed.

Other symptoms associated with this topographic loss of memory included bodily disorientation, particularly the ability to distinguish the right side from the left (see Table 6). This was often present as an isolated symptom, orientation as to place being unaffected, although evidence of abstract disorientation and constructional apraxia could usually be deduced from map and house drawing tests. Visual object agnosia was present in three cases and various forms of ideomotor apraxia in several others. Perseveration was also often demonstrable.

(3) *Inability to remember names.*

This was probably the most common type of defect found and was usually associated with pronounced lack of spontaneous talk, the patient being content to sit " listening in " on a conversation without taking any active part in it—although he might convey the impression of doing so by his habit of looking from one speaker to the other, smiling or making sundry nods of the head. The naming difficulty involved chiefly the recall of proper names. When asked direct questions, patients usually hesitated before replying and then prefixed their answers by an " eh-eh " or they evaded answering by interjecting such remarks as: " Yes, that's right." Another way was to refer the question to the relative accompanying them (see p. 8). When these failed and they had to reply, naming difficulties became apparent. Another point distinguishing the subjects of diffuse cortical disease from patients with focal lesions involving the speech centres was that they were much worse at recalling names from memory than they were at naming sighted objects. These and other features of the disturbances in speech and language seen in chronic amnesic patients are considered further in Chapters VII and VIII.

(4) *Amnesic indifference: failure to employ memory as a tool.*

Although these patients' relatives complained that they were forgetful or absent-minded, there was little evidence on testing of actual failure in retention, the fault appearing to lie more in defective registration

TABLE 6.—*Other signs found in chronic Amnesic Patients with Topographic Memory Loss*

Case No.	Perseveration	Disorientation					Visual object agnosia	Ideomotor apraxia	Construct. apraxia	Diagnosis
		Time	Place	Pers.	Bodily	Abstract				
34	−	+	+	−	−	+	−	−	?	Post. traum.
26	+	+	−	−	+	+	−	−	?	Arterio-sclerotic
183	−	+	−	−	−	+	−	+	+	Alzheimer's disease
60	+	+	+	−	+	+	−	+	?	Presenile dementia
29	−	−	−	−	+	+	−	−	+	ditto
23	+	+	−	−	+	?	+	+	+	ditto
52	+	+	+	+	−	+	−	−	+	postanoxic
121	+	+	+	−	+	+	−	+	+	Alzheimer's disease
104	+	+	−	−	−	+	−	−	+	postanoxic
140	+	+	+	−	−	?	+	+	?	Alzheimer's disease
27	−	+	−	−	−	+	+	+	+	postanoxic
13	−	+	−	−	−	+	−	−	+	Alzheimer's disease.
109	+	+	+	−	−	+	−	+	+	Hepatic enceph.

Note. On investigation, signs of diffuse cerebral cortical atrophy were found in all the cases. All showed defective registration and difficulty in reversing series on formal testing. ? = not tested.

and recall. In this respect and in the characteristic mood of nonchalance they showed, the memory impairment had a Korsakoff quality. Many wore a faintly amused or tolerant condescending expression and, when interviewed, conducted themselves as if they considered the examination to be wholly unnecessary. Confabulation was the usual stratagem adopted to conceal their difficulties. It was often impossible to get them to reverse series and few could be made to register a name and an address, attempts to do so, if persisted in, only resulting in catastrophic reactions. Left to themselves they might sit gazing into space or idly turning the pages of a newspaper. When given a simple repetitive task such as sorting peas from beans, they would begin willingly enough, but if one returned a few minutes later they would be found idle as before, although ready with some excuse to explain why they had not proceeded with the task. One woman was forever " reading " novels, a varied selection of which her husband provided her with each week. They helped her, he said, to while away her time in hospital, and so they did! When she was asked to read a portion aloud she complied at once, reciting it fluently, but a moment later was unable to answer any questions about it, excusing herself by saying that it was not her " type of book ", or that the characters in it did not interest her.

Similarly, when these patients' memory was being tested they would often put up facile excuses to explain their inability to give the desired information, but when prompted might quite unexpectedly supply other related facts gratuitously. The following is an example. The patient, a well-educated woman of 61 years, had a tumour (pinealoma) invading the third ventricle. The conversation related to her childhood, between the years 1892–1907.

Q. " You are old enough to remember Queen Victoria, aren't you?"
A " Yes, I remember her."
Q. " Who succeeded to the Throne after her death?"
A. ". . . was it Albert " (? perseveration . . . prompted: Edward VII) ". . . Oh yes, of course, Edward VII *and Queen Alexandra of Denmark.*"

There is some similarity here to the familiar business of priming a pump in order to obtain an adequate flow of water. Just as with a pump, one may first have to pour a little fluid down the barrel, so in seeking information from many of these patients one has first to supply some fact before other related facts can be recalled. This curious behaviour might be related to the changed affect that usually accompanies it, the mood of unconcern being due to the underlying lesion having a leucotomizing effect on the patient. But patients vary too much in their behaviour and performances from day to day to make this concept readily acceptable, nor will it account for the rapidity with which indifference or inability to use memory as a tool disappears after successful removal of a tumour or subdural haematoma. This type of memory impairment is common and, as in the case of patients with prolonged clouding of consciousness after anoxia, we believe it is comparatively unrelated to co-existing cerebral cortical changes but more dependent on disturbance of brain stem alerting mechanisms.

To summarize, although present in many patients suffering from organic brain disease, advice is not often sought for impairment of memory alone, but when it is other evidence of intellectual disturbance is usually found: difficulty in registration and in reversing series; altered affect; disorientation; perseveration, these symptoms having essentially the same character as those seen in the later stages of recovery of full consciousness after anoxia. Inability to use memory as a tool is particularly common, the impairment of memory being more apparent than real, and its occurrence correlates with other " general " symptoms of clouding of full consciousness, which are usually present. But analysis of the cases shows that cerebral cortical function is also often involved, or may be involved independent of any gross disturbance in the alerting mechanism, and that when this is so memory defects commonly interfere with the recall of spatial or temporal relations or the use of speech and language. Although attempts have been made to distinguish clinically between focal and diffuse cerebral lesions and between the diseases that may be responsible for the latter, focal cerebral lesions often mimic presenile dementia. More reliable guides are the mode of appearance of the amnesia and its duration, when the patient is first seen.

BIBLIOGRAPHY

164   WOODWORTH, R. S. and MARQUIS, D. G. (1952). " Psychology." 20th Edn. Methuen, London.

165   RUSSELL, W. R. (1957). The physiology of memory. *Proc. Roy. Soc. Med.*, **51**, 9.

166   GAMPER, E. (1928). Zur Frage der Polioencephalitis haemorrhagica der chronischen Alkoliker. Anatomische Befunde beim alcoholischen Korsakow und ihre Beziehungen zum klinischen Bild. *Dtsch. Z. Nervenheilk.*, **102**, 122.

167   WILLIAMS, M. and PENNYBACKER, J. (1954). Memory disturbances in third ventricle tumours. *J. Neurol. Psychiat.*, **17**, 115.

168   CONRAD, K. and ULE, G. (1951). Ein Fall von Korsakow-Psychose mit anatomischem Befund und klinischen Betrachtungen. *Dtsch. Z. Nervenheilk.* **165**, 430.

169   PENFIELD, W. (1954). Physiology of memory. 29th Lecture, Roy. Med. Psych. Assocn. rep. in *Brit. Med. J.*, **2**, 1159.

170   SCOVILLE, W. B. and MILNER, B. (1957). Loss of recent memory after bilateral hippocampal lesions. *J. Neurol. Psychiat.*, **20**, 11.

171   KAHN, E. and THOMPSON, L. J. (1934). Concerning Pick's disease. *Amer. J. Psychiat.*, **13**, 937.

172 NICHOLS, I. C. and WEIGNER, W. C. (1938). Pick's disease—A specific type of dementia. *Brain*, **61**, 237.

173 DE AJURIAGUERRA, J. and DE LA VIGNE, A. R. (1946). Troubles mentaux de l'intoxication oxycarbonée. *Sem. Hôp. Paris*, **42**, 1950.

174 McCARTAN, W. (1959). Chief Medical Officer (Mental Health) to Minist. Health N.I., personal communication.

175 FULLER, S. C. (1912). Alzheimer's disease (senium praecox): the report of a case and review of published cases. *J. nerv. ment. Dis.*, **39**, 440.

176 CAVENESS, W. F., NIELSEN, K. C., ADAMS, R. D. and YAKOVLEV, P. (1960). Ontogeny of induced seizures in macaca mulatta. *Trans, Amer, Neurol. Ass., Boston*, June 14.

177 STENGEL, E. (1943). A study of the symptomatology and differential diagnosis of Alzheimer's and Pick's disease. *J. ment. Sci.*, **89**, 1.

178 ROBERTSON, E. E., LE ROUX, A. and BROWN, M. H. (1958). The clinical differentiation of Pick's disease. *J. ment. Sci.*, **104**, 1000.

179 HENDERSON, D. and GILLESPIE, R. D. with assist. of BATCHELOR, I. R. C. (1956). " A Textbook of Psychiatry." Oxford University Press, London.

180 MAYER-GROSS, W., SLATER, E. and ROTH, M. (1955). " Clinical Psychiatry." Cassell, London.

181 ALLISON, R. S. (1952). Psychiatric disorders in later life. *Brit. Med. J.*, **2**, 1286.

182 HUNTER, D. (1955). " The Diseases of Occupations." English Universities Press, London.

183 SCHINDLER, R. (1953). Die psychischen Faktoren der senilen Dekompensation. *Wien Nervenheilk.*, **6**, 185.

184 ALVAREZ, W. C. (1944). Small unrecognized strokes, a common cause of illness in older persons. *J. Mich. med. Soc.*, **43**, 389.

CHAPTER VII

Disorders of Speech and Language

DISTURBANCES of speech and language were often prominent features of organic mental states in older people. They were noted in about one third of all the cases in this series (64 of 198 cases). In 21 of these the signs pointed to a cerebral vascular accident, in 17 an intracranial tumour was found and in the remaining 26 the clinical picture was that of presenile dementia, due to diffuse cerebral cortical atrophy.

As already mentioned in an earlier chapter, previous to recognition of the frequency of internal carotid artery stenosis and occlusion, the sudden occurrence of aphasia with hemiplegia, sensory loss or hemianopia was almost invariably attributed to thrombosis or embolism of an intracerebral artery. One case was proved at autopsy to be due to cerebral embolism, clots having become detached from an atheromatous aorta and causing residual infarcts not only in the left internal capsule but in the subcortical white matter of both hemispheres. In two cases the aphasia and right-sided hemiplegia were due to solitary capsular lesions, but the state of the carotid and vertebral arteries was not ascertained. In a further case in which aphasia was a prominent symptom intracerebral haemorrhage from rupture of a branch of the middle cerebral artery was responsible. No aneurysm was seen on angiography but at operation a large clot in the left temporal region was found and evacuated, the patient subsequently recovering both her speech and motor power. In four other cases the relation of the aphasia to internal carotid occlusion was demonstrated either by angiography or by direct inspection at operation in the neck.

In the other *cerebral vascular accidents*, in which confirmation of the diagnosis was not obtained, reliance was placed on history: that is upon the occurrence over the space of a few minutes or hours of a stroke with transient loss or clouding of consciousness, followed by aphasia, with or without contralateral hemiplegia, sensory loss or hemianopia. In all but 3 of the 21 cases the onset of aphasia had been sudden and few, if any, symptoms pointing to intracranial disease had been observed previous to it. Apart from this " out of the blue " character of the symptoms, other points noted were a previous history of coronary occlusion or of headaches, bouts of vertigo or breathlessness on exertion.

In all 17 cases of *tumour* the site and character of the lesion was confirmed at operation or autopsy. Headache and papilloedema—the classical signs of increased intracranial pressure—were absent in about half of the aphasic patients with tumour and the onset of their dysphasia was more gradual and insidious than it was in cerebral vascular accidents. A common history was of recurring " faints ", " blackouts " or more definite Jacksonian fits with transient dysphasia:

Thus, a retired naval officer, aged 67, who had always been predominantly right-handed, noticed recurring " swooning attacks " in which for some moments he felt faint and had a sensation of stiffness and uselessness in his right arm and was unable to speak. A month previous these attacks had become more frequent and in some of them there had been temporary clouding of consciousness. Clinical examination was negative but during the interview an attack was observed. Suddenly he stopped talking, made blinking movements with his eyelids and nodded his head. Then he reached for a glass of water, took a sip, put the glass down and seized hold of his right hand with his left. Then, rubbing his eyes, he remarked " I can do with it ". When questioned as to what he meant, he went on: " I can do with the umbrella." His behaviour then quickly reverted to normal and the interview proceeded, but he had no recollection of his actions in the interval. At operation some weeks later a left temporal astrocytoma was found.

As in this case, so in a few others, it was remarkable that despite the presence of an infiltrating or expanding tumour in the fronto-temporo-parietal region of the dominant hemisphere persistent disturbances of speech and language did not occur until relatively late in the course of the illness, when other signs indicating the presence of cerebral oedema, displacement and herniation of the intracranial contents had become evident. One patient, an intelligent and well-educated American aged 55, who was undoubtedly right-handed, gave a history similar to that related above. At operation a glioblastoma multiforme was found infiltrating deeply in the left Sylvian fissure into the temporal and parietal lobes. Before operation and therapeutic irradiation of the tumour she had been severely dysphasic for some weeks, but thereafter her condition improved so that in the intervals between fits (which still recurred) it was impossible to detect any speech or language disturbance, her ability to name sighted objects and name from memory, spontaneous speech, reading and comprehension of spoken speech all being perfect. In another patient, a man aged 57, in whom a meningioma (the size of a Tangiers orange) was found compressing the left temporal lobe, there had been recurring vertiginous seizures over the preceding nine years. The only demonstrable sign was a contralateral quadrantic hemianopia. Also right-handed in all activities, disturbances of speech were entirely lacking until three weeks before his death, their late appearance coinciding with signs of rapidly increasing intracranial pressure and clouding of consciousness.

In 3 cases gradual loss of interest, absent-mindedness and increasing taciturnity had at first suggested the onset of a presenile dementia but the history was too short and expressive speech defects too pronounced to be disregarded. In one of these a left temporal meningioma was again found, and in the other two there were multiple secondary deposits in the brain from lung and breast cancers respectively. Of the remaining cases, in a few the onset of aphasia had been so abrupt as to suggest a cerebral vascular accident. In 3 patients whose history was of longer duration time had been lost owing to their condition having been regarded as neurotic.

In all cases of presenile dementia in which speech disorders were observed, the defects were much less conspicuous than were the general falling-away in interest, absent-mindedness and changes in personality and temperament. When pressed, relatives would admit they had noticed that the patient was usually silent unless spoken to or that he often talked nonsense or used wrong words, but in general speech defects appeared to be submerged under the other symptoms of intellectual decline. This generalization, however, was not absolute for there were two exceptions in which isolated dysphasic disturbances were the only symptoms, the patients themselves seeking advice on account of them. One of these has already been referred to (see p. 124). The other was a woman aged 43 (right-handed), whose case was observed over the course of some six years at the end of which she had deteriorated into an advanced state of presenile dementia:

When first seen in 1951 at an ophthalmic hospital she complained solely of " dazzled " vision. There was no defect in visual acuity, fundi were normal and no consistent abnormalities were even found on testing by perimetry or with the Bjerrum screen. As she said herself, her difficulty lay more in reading than in seeing and it made no difference whether she was trying to read big or small print. Short words of three letters were comprehensible but she had to spell longer words, letter by letter, and they looked blurred so that she had often to guess at their meaning. Some days she could read fairly well, other times not. At no time was any disturbance of ocular movements in reading observed. Two years later signs of ataxic paraparesis became evident, the plantars both being extensor and she was becoming absent-minded, her behaviour lacking spontaneity and drive. Catastrophic reactions with tears occurred and she had great difficulty in registering a name and an address but at no time was perseveration observed. Although orientated in time, place and for persons, she had some difficulty in distinguishing right from left and could not read the time or decide on a well-known map which was east and west. Some periphrasis was evident in her naming of sighted objects and it seemed quite impossible for her to recall names from memory. Handwriting was little affected. Simple picture interpretation was faulty, the various items only being mentioned, and constructional difficulties were very evident on testing her with matches and Kohs blocks. There was no difficulty in recognising numbers or in performing simple calculations nor did she show any visual object, auditory or colour agnosia or evidence of ideomotor apraxia, although the last-named became pronounced as her state of deterioration advanced.

General Character of Expressive Speech and Language Defects

The disturbances of speech shown by the 64 dysphasic patients with focal vascular or neoplastic lesions or diffuse cerebral cortical atrophy have been analysed qualitatively, especially towards estimating the extent to which purely expressive and receptive defects occurred and how often mixed forms were seen. Quantitative case to case evaluation of the extent of individual defects was not attempted because of (1) the fluctuations observed in symptoms from day to day, (2) the extent to which the occurrence of catastrophic reactions interfered with performance and (3) the varying states in which patients were encountered, this depending on the nature of their underlying lesions. Thus, some were examined shortly after the occurrence of cerebral vascular accidents, at which times aphasia was usually pronounced. Others were seen at later stages when they were showing signs of recovery, and the same applied to some patients with post-anoxic and traumatic conditions. On the other hand, speech disturbances were often slight in patients with tumours or early presenile dementia and were only pronounced when it happened that they were seen at a relatively late stage.

Capacity for spontaneous talk. In some of the patients with a tumour invading the speech area of the dominant hemisphere no disturbances of speech or language were at first evident, although these appeared later with the development of intracranial complications. But in the great majority the capacity for spontaneous talk was impaired and this impairment took different forms.

(1) *Patients who were entirely speechless, neither attempting spontaneous conversation nor making any attempt to reply to questions.*

The few patients so severely affected had either a focal vascular or neoplastic lesion; absolute speechlessness was not observed in association with a presenile dementia. One of the most typical examples was a woman aged 67, who had a large left temporal meningioma. She sat in bed, folding and unfolding her hands and gazing about her with a bewildered expression. Her failure to respond verbally to any stimuli was more suggestive of a psychological than a physical cause. It was impossible to tell whether she understood what was said to her as she gave no indication and made no use either of gesture or pantomime. This behaviour was in striking contrast to that of 2 other cases, both men with recent cerebral vascular accidents. One of them, although utterly bereft of speech, had clearly no difficulty in understanding because when spoken to he could write an appropriate reply. His handwriting was not normal but sufficiently good to convey his meaning. The other man, rendered hemiplegic as well as aphasic, also had no apparent difficulty in comprehension, a fact which he was able convincingly to demonstrate by gesture and pantomime, both of which he made use of freely, to compensate for his loss of speech. Thus, when asked if he understood the difference between a pond and a stream he nodded his head vigorously and proceeded to draw a circle in the air with the forefinger, after which he placed his hand with the fingers extended in the horizontal plane, palm downwards moving it slowly to and fro. Then, when one said " show me a stream ", he proceeded to make quick repetitive flexion and extension movements of the finger tips, at the same time extending his arm at the elbow. In his case the aphasia appeared to be entirely expressive and to be related to apraxia for tongue and lip movements because he could not protrude the tongue on request, lick or purse his lips.

(2) *Patients who had little or no spontaneous talk, but who attempted to answer questions and take part in conversation initiated by others.*

These showed five types of defect in expressive speech: difficulty in articulation, in word finding, defective sentence construction, inability or difficulty in using abstract or propositional speech, and perseveration.

(a) *Dysarthria.* Liepmann, according to Critchley,[185] was the first to suggest that some cases of motor aphasia were due to articulatory dyspraxia. But as the latter points out, although opinion has changed as to the relationship between dysphasia and dysarthria, " contemporary ideas once again tend to swing away from too rigid cleavage between disorders of speech and disorders of language ". Dysarthria was found in 67% of the cases of Alzheimer's disease and Pick's disease analysed by Sjögren[186] and in 37% of the elderly patients with speech and language impairment reviewed by Joyce Mitchell.[187] The last-named author described mild slurring of compound consonants and scrambling of polysyllable words as sequels of cerebral haemorrhage and gross dysarthria, dysphagia and dysphonia as occurring chiefly after midbrain thrombosis. In other patients with supranuclear bulbar involvement the difficulty in articulation was sometimes accompanied by drooling of saliva, dysphagia and increased emotional lability.

Dysarthria was pronounced in 2 of our cases of general paralysis and, although in the whole series there was only one patient who ultimately developed the full clinical picture of pseudobulbar palsy, the symptom was associated with dysphasia in a number of others with diffuse or focal cerebral lesions. In one of these, syllables were not so much slurred or scrambled as wrong consonants inserted, the effect of which was to distort the natural sound of a word, although it bore some phonetic resemblance to the correct sound. This was well seen in a man of 57 with early arteriosclerotic dementia who had had a recent vascular accident affecting the dominant hemisphere. A matchbox was described as a " patch box ", pictures of a pigeon and a chimney as " didgeon " and " chilney " respectively. Nathan[188] states that in traumatic lesions of the left fronto-parietal region it is common to find that phonation at first is so disturbed that no sound can be obtained from the patient by any means. All the cases with facial apraxia due to wounding, he reported, were at first completely aphonic and one of them later was notably dysarthric, being unable to pronounce consonants, although vowels could be reproduced without difficulty. This man, although he could swallow and whistle, was unable to perform facial movements to command or in imitation. When asked to show his teeth he kept opening and closing his mouth. He could not protrude the tongue on request, lick his lips, blow out his cheeks or raise his eyebrows. Words beginning with consonants, e.g. sister, could not be articulated although when a consonant occurred later in a word he could make an attempt to pronounce it. Thus, the word " sister " was rendered " i—er ". Similarly prisoner became " i—er ". " Yes " was pronounced as " eh ", " no " as " o ". Gradual recovery of the facial and oral apraxia was accompanied by corresponding improvement in his speech.

(b) *Difficulties in finding words (nominal defects).* Inability to name persons and things appeared to play an important part in determining the expressive speech defects of our patients and they compensated for it in a variety of ways.

(i) *By using gesture and pantomime.* Few were as accomplished in this respect as the patient described on p. 136, whose performance was undoubtedly exceptional. Some tried spontaneously to use gesture and pantomime to reinforce their nominal defects but they executed these in such a perfunctory, incomplete or crude fashion as to make it difficult to interpret what they meant by them. Their performance in this respect had indeed an apraxic character. But this was much less commonly seen than total failure to employ such devices on occasions where obviously they would have been of considerable advantage in

10

supplying a missing word or conveying an idea. Occasionally, when the examiner himself used pantomime with the object of illustrating how it could be employed, and provided the patient comprehended his intention, he might subsequently be induced to use the same means to convey his meaning, when stuck for a word. But in many instances, even when there was no evidence of apraxia, difficulties in comprehension, catastrophic reactions or perseveration interfered with the success of such stratagems so that they had to be abandoned.

(*ii*) Many kept on trying to find the word they wanted, uttering a number of related but inappropriate words until they came to the one required or lapsed into silence. Thus one post-anoxic patient with a chronic amnesic syndrome, trying to find the word " tent ", said: " camp . . . no . . . hut . . . eh . . . trench . . . tent ". Another, with carotico-vertebral atheroma and right-sided paresis, whilst we were discussing the weakness of his right hand and how he had tried to use a fork to feed himself, remarked: " I couldn't use the claw at all . . . the clubs . . . aw, the hell . . . I can't find the word for it!"

(*iii*) The most common method adopted to overcome the difficulty in naming was by the use of *periphrasis* or circumlocution. Thus, a thimble would be described as " to put over your finger ": an oil can, " for oiling things ": a calendar, " it dates ": a bottle, " it would have whisky in it ": a box of matches, " it holds lights ": a pair of sun glasses, " a pair for beach . . . beach wear . . . girls wear them on their caps . . . spectacles . . . a special kind ": a hammer, " the off and on ": the trigger of a gun, " the draw back ": a bucket, " what you catch it in ". From these examples it can be seen that when a patient used periphrasis this was an indication in itself that his comprehension was relatively unaffected and the disturbance predominantly expressive in character. Periphrasis is sometimes regarded as being chiefly an expression of a chronic amnesic defect, but it was little used by patients with gross perceptual difficulties and was more common in association with focal than with diffuse cerebral lesions. A not uncommon type of circumlocution adopted by patients with diffuse cerebral cortical atrophy was to describe the object as " the what you call it ", " the so and so ", " that thing there ". Thus, one demented patient, the subject of general paralysis, in describing an action said: " I took the what you call it and tried to lift the so and so."

(*iv*) By the use of *Paraphasia*. Paraphasia, whereby a patient in trying to recall a name substituted some other word or introduced a word not found in the dictionary (a neologism), was much less used than periphrasis and in this series was observed only in patients with diffuse cerebral lesions. Weinstein and Kahn[189] note that the word substituted in paraphasia is nearly always related functionally to the object to which it is intended to refer. For example, a radiator is described as a " stove ", a wheel chair as a " spring wheel ". One of our post-anoxic patients when shown a picture of a bear said: " tiger . . . leopard . . . or beast ". Another woman with presenile dementia not only used words that bore some " clang " resemblance to the right ones, saying " pool " for wool, but made free use of neologisms, a penny being described as a "sixen", a threepenny piece as a "ceyenne", a diary as a " rare paw book ", whilst certain common objects such as a comb, scissors, candle were all correctly named, if allowance were made for her occasional tendency to perseverate. Perseveration and paraphasia were often seen in association as the following example illustrates. The patient had sustained a severe closed head injury so that two months later, when the notes were made, consciousness had not been fully regained. He was shown a series of objects and invited to name them:

A fountain pen: " Is is a minor pen of any description?"
A hair comb: " A No. 2 small pen."
A rubber band: " A rubber boddin."
A handkerchief: " A small hard piece of rubber linen."
A bunch of keys: " Calcium keys."
A pair of shoes: " A pair of Welsh calciums."

This man's performance conveyed the impression that at the beginning of the test, he was able to score " near misses " but that as the examination proceeded his performance fell off and his answers were drawn from random associations. The complacency or satisfied attitude of paraphasic patients is usually in striking contrast to the behaviour of those who struggle to find the right word or seek to convey that they know what it is by pantomime or periphrasis. The latter are aware of their difficulties whereas paraphasic patients often are not. It would be a mistake, however, to assume that paraphasics possess no insight, because in cases we have had repeated opportunities of observing, it has been apparent that at times they answered in a hesitant, unsure manner, as if they knew their choice of words to be wrong but were hopeful at the same time that they might be acceptable. Catastrophic reactions were rare, and we agree with Weinstein and Kahn that paraphasia is usually associated with other defects, in particular a mood of euphoria, anosognosia, disorientation in place and time, and not infrequently some ideomotor apraxia.

(*c*) *Defective sentence construction.* Defective sentence construction was shown in a variety of ways. One of the most common was a tendency to break off in the middle of a sentence and leave it unfinished.

That this was sometimes related to difficulties in word finding was shown by the experience of one man with diffuse cortical atrophy who remarked spontaneously that he would often be so intent in trying to find the word he wanted that he would forget what he had been talking about. Another not infrequent explanation was the occurrence of minor epileptiform fits. Thus, the wife of one patient reported that when he broke off in the middle of a sentence and became confused his eyes would stare and his face assume temporarily a fixed expression. Then he would as suddenly recover and attempt to resume what he was saying—usually unsuccessfully. Grammatical errors were noted in the speech of most of our dysphasic patients but it was difficult to draw any conclusions from them because so many normal subjects under the influence of emotional stress may speak ungrammatically. The primary educational level has also to be taken into account. Hesitancy in speaking and a tendency to prefix remarks by such exclamations as " eh . . . eh ", or " uh ", " well " were also very common in early dementing patients. Less common was the " telegrammatic " type of utterance in which a patient attempted to express his meaning in the fewest possible words.

> *Examiner:* " I see you have a book there . . . what is its title?"
> *Patient:* " Can't remember title or author."
> *Examiner:* " Well, what is the book about?"
> *Patient:* " About a ranch."
> *Examiner:* " What is the name of this hospital?"
> *Patient:* " Can't think."
> *Examiner:* " Is it the Royal Victoria Hospital?"
> *Patient:* " No."
> *Examiner:* " Is it Claremont Street Hospital?"
> *Patient:* " Yes."

(*d*) *Difficulty in discussing abstract topics.* Many patients showed a striking difference between their ability to formulate and discuss concrete ideas and to express themselves propositionally or abstractly and their failure in the latter respect was often recognizable despite the absence of any perseveration, naming defects or difficulties in sentence construction. Thus, they replied easily to questions relating to their home address, neighbours, the weather, their occupation etc. But in response to questions concerning similarities and differences, beginning with the difference between a pond and a stream, and going on to harder propositions as, for example, the difference between poverty and misery or the interpretation of proverbs, expressive difficulties at once became evident. That is to say the patient became either "tongue-tied " or used inappropriate words, perseverating and making grammatical and syntactical errors. A good example of this was seen in a case of post-traumatic encephalopathy in which there had initially been severe expressive and receptive dysphasia. As the day drew near for his discharge home, he composed a letter to his wife in which he wrote: " I am saying enough to thank you for all the things I want to say and to let you know what I will say when I get home as soon as possible." Although this particular example betrays less disturbance of internal thought than of inability to express himself, in many other instances it was evident that there were defects both in comprehension and in expression. Thus, a woman with left-sided parietal signs in addition to a clinical picture of early presenile dementia, when questioned as to the difference between a pond and a stream replied: " A pond is for ducks and a stream a stream." Similarly for rope and chain she gave: " A rope is a cord and chain for a watch." This patient had no difficulty whatever in naming sighted objects or in answering simple concrete questions relating to her family and home.

(*e*) *Perseveration.* Perseveration was practically always an accompaniment of severe dysphasia and was especially noticeable in patients with recent vascular lesions affecting the dominant hemisphere. In these it was clearly one of the principal difficulties interfering with expressive speech. Such patients, when shown an object, might name it correctly, but when presented with a second object would go on repeating the name of the first until forced to give up in exasperation or reduced to tears. The intense emotional reaction induced by such efforts suggested their awareness of these mistakes as did the fact that often, when perseveration was associated with catastrophic reactions, the speech defects were chiefly expressive in type, comprehension being little affected. Even in patients capable of repeating simple series, e.g. days of the week or counting from 1–10, perseveration usually brought such performances to a standstill when one switched from counting to repeating days of the week or vice versa, the patient displaying a persistent tendency to continue in the former activity. When the lesion responsible for causing dysphasia had brought about clouding of consciousness, there was invariably additional evidence of perseveration in the performance of simple actions, such as closing and opening the eyes and mouth. But in ensuing weeks, with recovery of full consciousness, the general tendency to perseverate would disappear although it would persist (in patients with focal lesions involving the speech area) in relation to speech alone.

Perseveration was less noticeable (as were speech defects as a whole) in patients with slowly infiltrating or expanding tumours of the dominant hemisphere. It had to be sought for carefully, but, provided there was no general tendency its presence for speech alone was a valuable sign pointing to the probability of a focal rather than of a diffuse lesion. It was often observed in cases of diffuse cerebral cortical atrophy, but seldom for speech alone, and usually only in conjunction with a much greater tendency to perseverate in actions.

(3) *Patients showing no inhibition of spontaneous talk and responding readily to questions.*

There were relatively few patients in this group and most of them were suffering from recent cerebral vascular accidents, affecting either the dominant or non-dominant hemisphere and post-anoxic or post-traumatic encephalopathy. There was one case of general paralysis of the insane and two of cerebral atherosclerosis. A feature common to them all was clouding of consciousness, which in some cases was greater than it was in others. During waking hours they talked or rambled on, often almost incessantly, the " push of talk " being interspersed with confabulation and nominal or grammatical and syntactical defects of the kind already described, so that incoherence or jargon aphasia often resulted. In the former event utterances lost their meaning and were difficult to follow on account of the tendency to leave sentences unfinished, the lack of pattern in association of ideas and the liberal introduction of irrelevant material. In jargon the patient seemed to know what he wanted to say but periphrasis, mis-pronouncements and the use of neologisms turned his speech into gibberish. Distinctions between incoherence and jargon may be difficult to draw, but if there are any these are probably more qualitative than quantitative. In incoherence the rudiments or " instrumentalities " of speech are not lost, expressive difficulties being more apparent at the conceptual level of thought. In jargon aphasia the rudiments are lost but conceptual thought is disturbed to a much less extent. This is suggested by the purposeful manner in which these patients talk, un-awareness of their faults often giving rise to irritability or exasperation that those listening do not understand what they say. Incoherent patients, on the other hand, are apt to ramble on quite unconcernedly, paying little regard to the responses of their listeners or to their sur-roundings.

Incoherence was noted chiefly in patients with chronic amnesic syndromes, due to diffuse cerebral cortical atrophy in whom an episode of acute confusion (clouding of consciousness) had supervened as the result of a minor vascular accident, inducing cerebral circulatory insufficiency, or of their being given potentially toxic drugs such as opium, barbiturates, blood-pressure reducing drugs or allowed to become dehydrated. It was seen also in patients recovering after severe anoxia or head injury. Jargon aphasia was less common but seen more in the initial stages of recovery from major vascular lesions affecting the dominant hemisphere. It was not remarkable with tumours involving the speech area, but when some disturbance of expressive speech had already been present, further deterioration into jargon aphasia might be precipitated by angiography or air encephalography.

However, the buoyancy of mood and self-confidence of all severely dysphasic patients, who display no inhibition of spontaneous speech, suggests some associated defect in auditory word recognition, interfering with their awareness of defects. But, as in most instances there was clouding of consciousness it would not be right to ascribe this unawareness to that cause alone. Symonds,[112] reviewing the rare syndromes associated with pure word deafness (word-sound and word-meaning-deafness) comments on the odd behaviour of such patients, which is often so pronounced as to make one think they are play-acting. The disorder is almost wholly on the receptive side although inability to name objects may co-exist. Not quite the same as these cases of Symonds, but having certain points of resemblance was the talk of two of our patients, samples of which are given below.

The first was a right-handed man aged 43, who had sustained a severe closed head injury. Initially there was an extensor plantar response on the left side with paresis of the left face and arm. These signs gradually disappeared but for four months he remained disorientated in time and place and had no capacity for registration, his mood being facile and complacent. The E.E.G. showed persistent diffuse slow activity, most pronounced in the left fronto-temporal region. About the fifth or sixth month orientation was regained and he could repeat a name and an address although perseveration was still at times apparent both in his speech and actions. He had difficulty naming sighted objects and in recalling names from memory, but responded correctly to simple commands, could recognize the nature of common objects and sounds and distinguish colours. Familiar actions could be reproduced and he had no difficulty in dressing or feeding himself and was able to reproduce match designs and make a fair showing with the Kohs' blocks. There was no right–left disorientation or finger agnosia and his handwriting was well formed and correct enough although its meaning was obscure (see example on p. 141). He was able to sing " God Save the Queen " and " When Irish Eyes are Smiling " but failed dismally at the simplest sums, not appearing to recognize arithmetical symbols although being able to count actual money without difficulty.

His expressive speech defects represented a sort of intermediate stage between incoherence and jargon, the words and phrases he used being so inappropriate as almost to suggest a paraphasia of expression. For example, after demonstrating correctly the use of a hairbrush, he remarked: " I'm sorry, sir, but my hair is not a great exception, sir." Answers were frequently prefaced with either, " I'm sorry, sir," or " I'm doing the best I can, sir," his manner being curiously obsequious or anxious to please and, according to his wife, quite out of keeping with his usual character! When asked to draw a house he did quite well, remarking as he pencilled in the chimney: " This is the thing to bring in the fireplace bridgings, but I don't know if that is acceptable to you. . . . I'm doing the best I can, sir." In a short question and answer sequence his replies were as follows:

Q. As you were saying, this is a hospital. Now, will you tell me why you are here in hospital?

A. " Well Sir, I suppose it's because I'm an Irishman, Sir."

Q. " Yes, but what is wrong with you? Do you know why you are in hospital?"

A. " Well, it was a man called Campbell who worked in the mill, and I was doing a few jobs for him at the time . . . I was doing some plumbing for the kilns at the far side for the engineers to go inside . . ."

Q. " Thank you. Tell me do you feel happy here?"

A. " Well, I'm very good . . . I'm very good. I like to do the best I can and help the older men because I don't like them to be substitutes."

The other case was a man of 69 who had been in good health until shortly before admission, following the development of mental confusion. On examination he was found to have a left-sided hemianopia with sensory impairment in the left hand and a persistent right grasp reflex. At first he talked incessantly and incoherently, was often rowdy and inclined to break into song. A month later, when he had become more placid, the following conversation took place. He was still disorientated and denied being ill:

Q. " What is this place?"

A. " I do not know the idea . . . what place it is . . . simply for doctors . . . I don't know a great deal about it."

Q. " What do you think it is?"

A. " I consider it was liberally laid out for doctors."

Q. " Do you think, for example, that it is the City Hall?"

A. " If it is the City Hall it would be cheerful in Belfast compared with the town . . ."

Q. " Could it be a hospital?"

A. " It could."

Q. " Can you tell me the date? What month is it?"

A. " I would say it was about twelve months of the year."
Q. " Yes, but what month do you think it is?"
A. " I could not tell you that."
Q. " Is the name of the first month January?"
A. " Yes."
Q. " What is the name of the second month of the year?"
A. " The next thing would be about the second of January."
Q. " If the first month is January, what is the second month called?"
A. " Something similar to what was cleared up at the front."

Here again, the bizarre character of the responses is remarkable. Indeed, the cautious way in which answers were given bears some resemblance to the replies of unsatisfactory witnesses in Court, who convey the impression that either they do not know or are trying to be evasive so as to avoid possible traps set for them by cross-examining counsel.

Naming sighted objects and naming from memory.

Patients were tested for their ability to name objects placed before them, which they could both see and feel as desired, and for their capacity to recall names from memory. Their attempts at doing so have already been described but it may be asked in what ways, if any, did the performances of patients with purely focal lesions differ from those of patients with global cerebral affections? To test this 2 groups of cases were selected. The first comprised 16 cases whose symptoms and signs were caused by a tumour, the site of which was known to be in the fronto-temporo-parietal area of the dominant hemisphere. The second group contained the same number of cases but in all of these disturbances of behaviour and impairment of memory had been the principal presenting features, physical signs either being absent or distributed bilaterally and more or less symmetrically. Some were recovering from anoxia and trauma or had general paralysis of the insane, others had cerebral arteriosclerosis or presenile dementia, associated, as shown by air encephalography and other tests, with diffuse cerebral cortical atrophy.

Table 7 shows the results of comparing the performances in these two groups. As can be seen, patients with tumours had greater difficulty in naming sighted objects than they had in naming things from memory, whereas the reverse was true of patients with global cerebral affections. It would appear, therefore, that the comparisons may sometimes be of value in cases of dysphasia in helping to distinguish between focal and diffuse lesions.

As regards the actual mechanisms interfering with naming, perseveration certainly seemed to play a major rôle in a number of cases. This was evident by the patients' ability to name the first object shown to them correctly but inability to name subsequent objects, owing to persistence of the first response. In a few the naming difficulty was due to facial, oral or tongue apraxia, a fact that could readily be determined by their failure, in the absence of any visual or hearing defects, to reproduce voluntarily words spoken in their presence, although capable of doing so involuntarily at other times, such as on waking or under emotional stress. Naming difficulties in these cases were invariably associated with inability to protrude the tongue on request, lick and purse the lips or perform other voluntary facial movements.

TABLE 7.—*Naming sighted objects and naming from memory*

Nature of lesion	Difficulty in naming sighted objects	Difficulty in naming from memory
Tumours involving fronto-temporo-parietal areas of dominant hemisphere (16 cases)	13 (81%)	9 (56%)
Global cerebral affections, i.e. presenile dementias (16 cases)	9 (56%)	14 (87%)

In the majority, however, the naming inability had an amnesic quality and seemed to bear some resemblance to the difficulties in registration shown by patients recovering full consciousness after cerebral anoxia or trauma. That is to say these patients, when they failed to name an object and had perforce to fall back on periphrasis or paraphasia, could repeat the name correctly if the examiner were first to pronounce it clearly and distinctly in their hearing. A moment later, it must be admitted, when shown the same object, they were unable to comply, but by dint of patient repetition they often succeeded in retaining the names of two or more objects for a whole day or longer, and as their condition improved the period of retention became longer. If amnesia plays a part in determining naming difficulties one would expect such patients to exhibit some defective capacity for registration. Obviously, giving them a name and an address to remember would be unsuitable, but when the test was modified so as to make it non-verbal (see p. 72) patients with purely focal lesions involving the speech centres had no difficulty in finding the objects that had previously been hidden. On the other hand, those with diffuse cortical atrophy were often quite unable to do so, even after the places of concealment of objects had been repeatedly demonstrated to them. This suggests that although superficially resembling defective registration in general, the nominal defects of dysphasics with focal lesions cannot be attributed to general clouding of consciousness but represent some isolated interruption of pathways that are anatomically related to the lesions and the integrity of which is essential for re-learning. Hécaen *et al.*[190] believe that amnesic aphasia is frequently associated with loss of the

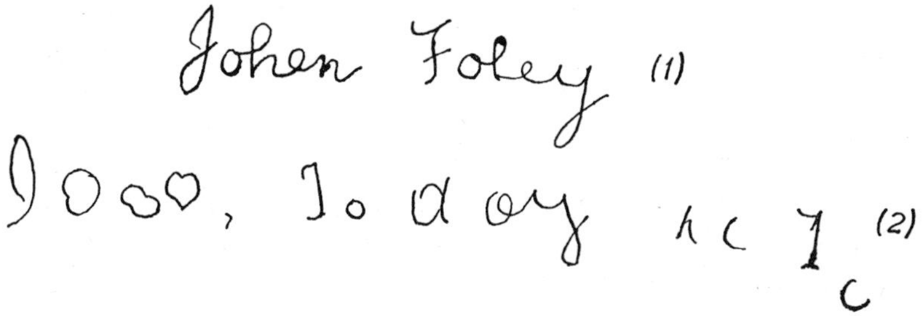

(*a*)

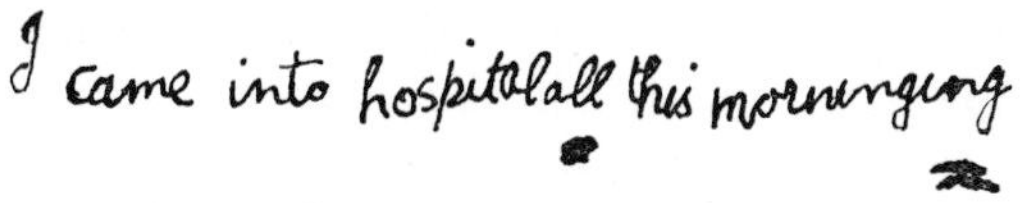

(*b*)

Fig. 5.—Examples of Perseveration in Writing

(*a*) *Case No.* 104. (Atherosclerotic presenile dementia). When asked to write his name, he did so as shown, (1) misspelling John. Then he was asked to write: " Today is Thursday." At (2) the first word begins with " Jo ", as if he were trying to write " John ", and perseverating.

(*b*) *Case No.* 97. Aged 61, this woman had a chronic amnesic syndrome of 2 years' duration. There was papilloedema and bilateral hydrocephalus due to a tumour in the third ventricle, which was obstructed.

capacity for abstract thinking. In certain cases of " conduction " aphasia, however, in which the lesion is interrupting the connections between the parieto-temporo-occipital regions and Wernicke's zone, they suggest that inability to present words and ideas in their proper sequence and syntactical errors in speech may be due to some measure of temporal disorientation (" destruction des possibilités de reproduction des sequences temporalles par incapacité de saisir cette succession, et des possibilités d'expression syntactique par perte de la temporalité de la phrase ").

Writing.

Writing defects were more difficult to appraise than spoken speech defects because of the greater natural variation there is between individuals in the extent to which they employ this method of expression and because the premorbid writing ability depends so much on the primary educational level. Many dysphasic patients, too, were hemiplegic or could not use the preferred hand and were unwilling or unable to understand that they should try to write with the other hand. However, excluding illiterates and difficulties in handwriting due to motor weakness or ataxia, the defects displayed by dysgraphic patients paralleled those seen in the realm of spoken speech. Thus, perseveration was common, although it was never seen solely in relation to writing. Examples are shown in Fig. 5. In the second example there is repetition of the last syllable of the words " hospital" and " morning ". This feature has been described as typical of presenile dementia but as noted in this instance the patient had a tumour.

(*a*) *Spontaneous* (*letter*) *writing and writing to dictation.* Writing a letter demands certain preparation of thought and an abstract attitude much the same as is required in recalling names of persons or things from memory, whereas writing from dictation is a more concrete act, akin to naming sighted objects. Few dysphasic patients could express themselves better in writing than in spoken speech but there were some who could. One such instance has already been referred to (see p. 136). Other examples are given in Figs. 6 and 7. The first patient (Fig. 6), although unimpaired in his comprehension of spoken and written speech, in the later stage of his illness had to choose his words carefully in speaking so that as a result his utterances were halting and conveyed the impression that speaking was an effort. There was difficulty too, in naming sighted objects, periphrasis often being reverted to and he was often emotionally upset. On paper, however, he was much more at ease, his writing flowing smoothly and, although liable to make mistakes, he was capable of correcting these himself. The second patient (Fig. 7) also wrote better than he talked and his distinctive script conveys little impression of the poverty of his spontaneous speech, a record of which has been given on p. 8.

In most cases, however, whether the dysgraphia were due to a focal vascular or neoplastic lesion or diffuse cortical changes the ability to write spontaneously was much more impaired than was writing from dictation. In the latter, words were often left out, misspelt or inappropriate words substituted. One patient, a motor-car salesman with general paralysis, when asked to write: " I regret to tell you that we

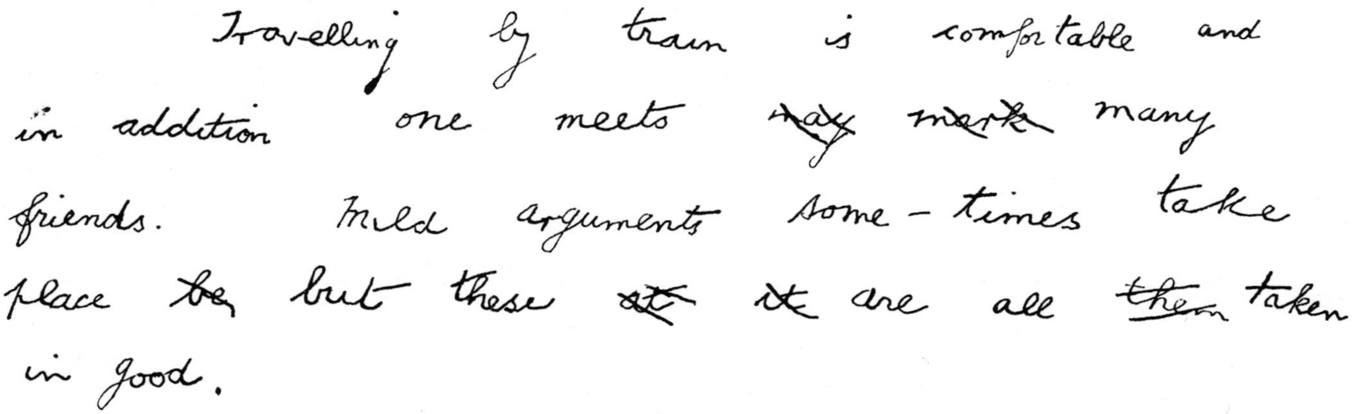

Travelling by train is comfortable and in addition one meets ~~not~~ many friends. Mild arguments some-times take place but these ~~it~~ it are all ~~them~~ taken in good.

Fig. 6.—*Case No. 133* (Meningioma L. Temporal): Expressive Dysphasia
The patient was a well-educated man of 57 years who held a responsible post. The corrections were made by himself

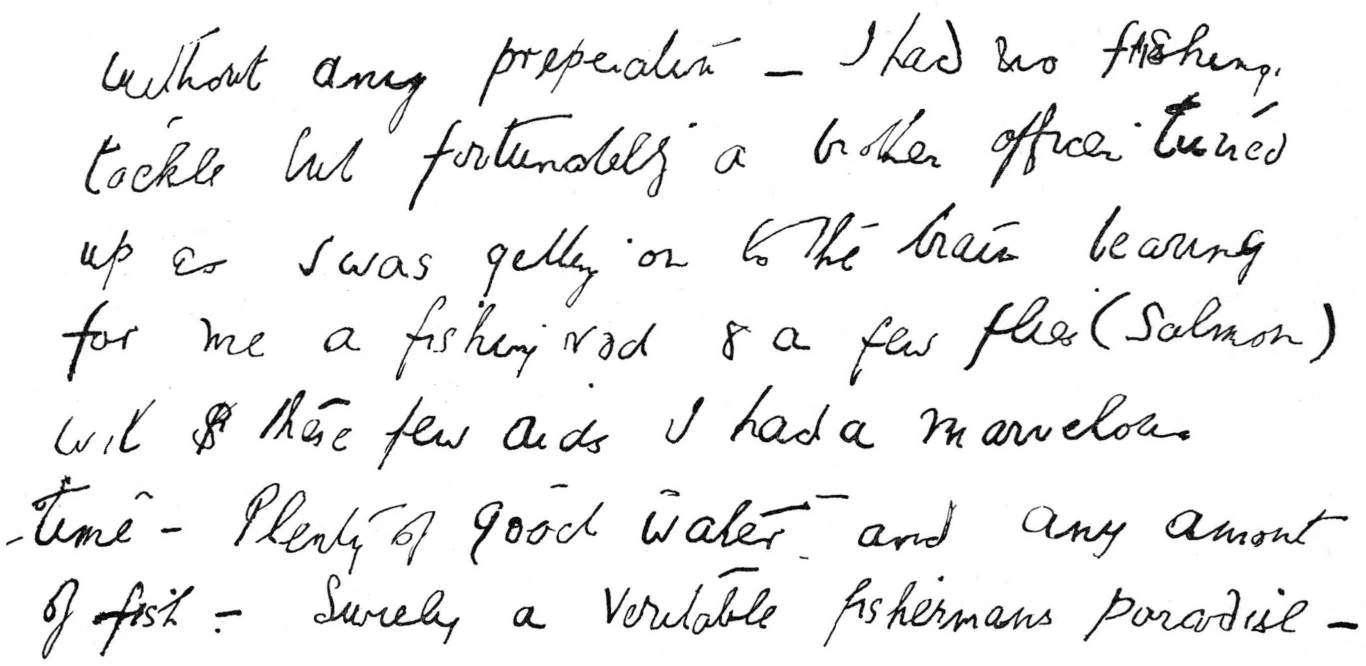

Without any preparation — Had no fishing. tackle but fortunately a butler office.. turned up as I was getting on to the train bearing for me a fishing rod & a few flies (Salmon) with those few Ads I had a marvelous time — Plenty of good water and any amount of fish — Surely a veritable fishermans paradise —

Fig. 7.—*Case No.* 13. Man aged 61, later presenile dementia. In earlier stages writing was better than speech

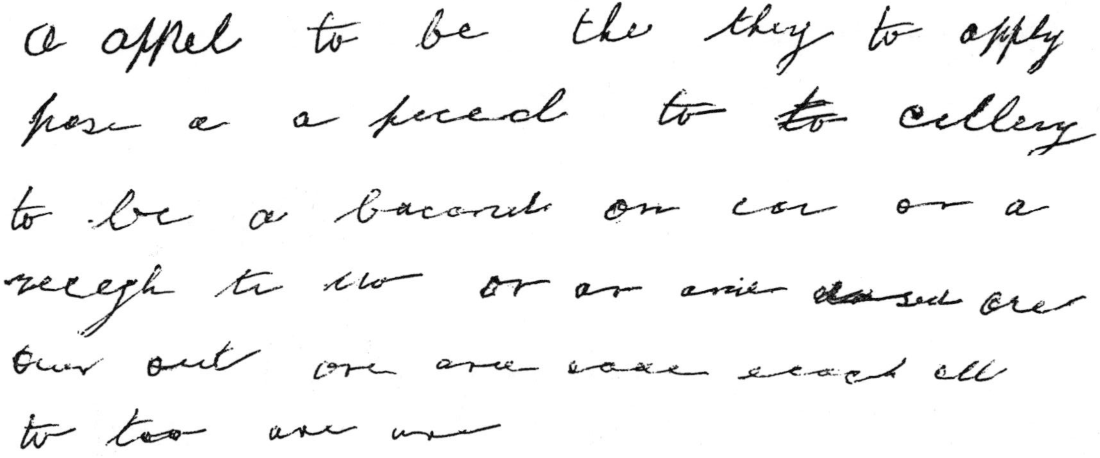

Fig. 8.—" Jargon " Writing

" Jargon " writing in response to the request " write a letter ". The patient, a man of 65, was grossly aphasic but unconcerned and unaware of the extent of his disability.

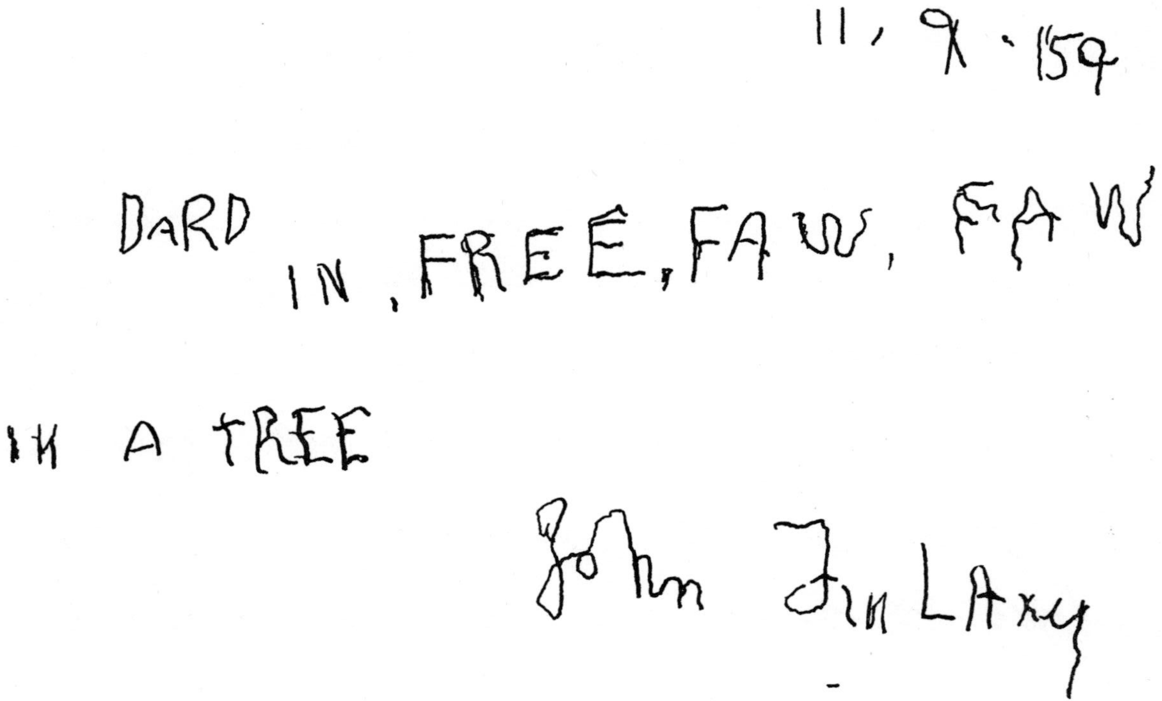

Fig. 9.—Example of Jargon Writing

Case No. 178. The patient was asked to write a letter to a friend

cannot give a firm delivery date for your new car," proceeded: " I regret to tell you that we can not get a firm deliver for your new car." When asked to give his opinion as to the best sea route between Belfast and England, he wrote: " Liverpool the boat are better." Grammatical errors alone, however, are not representative of a specific writing defect, being more amnesic in origin and indicative usually of some general clouding of consciousness, if not due to low primary educational level or perserveration.

As with spoken speech there were several instances of graphical incoherence, the writing of such patients displaying confused association of ideas, verbal omissions, grammatical errors and unfinished sentences, but apart from these faults differing in no essential from normal writing. The following is an example. The patient, an electrician, who had been accidentally electrocuted, was slow in recovering full consciousness and when seen some months later showed signs of early dementia. He was asked to give his opinion as to the relative advantages of electricity over gas for household use, and he wrote: " Electricity can be fitted to both house and factory in such a safe manner, and it is clean and the surroundings easy to switch on without the danger of both matches and smell of escaping gas through the deterioration of lead pipes."* Incoherence in writing was not confined to patients with global cerebral affections. It was also occasionally seen in patients with focal lesions. Thus, one man with an inoperable tumour in the left fronto-temporal region, which had rendered him severely dysphasic, was asked to write a note about the weather. He dated the paper correctly, gave his name and address, the date of his birth and then proceeded: " The weather is born to be warm and I am bound to be in it, fog is particularly suitable and is largely due to the atmosphere effects experienced on the road, however much as it may seem clean." Jargon writing, of which examples are given in Figs. 8, 9, was less common and, as with its equivalent in spoken speech, was usually seen in patients with recent cerebral vascular accidents, or in cases of tumour, when their general state had begun rapidly to deteriorate.

(*b*) *Copying*. The existence of apraxic writing defects, which bore no relation to perseveration, spelling errors and other amnesic features, could usually best be elicited by getting the patient to copy print or script. In the most severely affected cases a curious reluctance in the

---

* This is like the one cited by Bastian.[109] His patient "Charlotte" wrote to her brother: " My dear William, I am glad to see you yesterday, but I hope you are well, it is long since I heard from you last. In February I cannot tell you what we are cannot to do, it is bad. We cannot say what we cannot to do, but we are 81 in January 13 (her correct age and birthday in the previous January). I have nothing to say, but I cannot say what we are going to do, but we are bad. I hope you are well, and the children are well. Yours affectly., Charlotte."

patient's attitude would at once be apparent. When given a pen and told to write he would hold it in an unnatural manner or maintain it poised about half an inch above the surface of the paper. Then he would flex and extend his wrist alternately, the movements being slight and irregular but sufficient to allow the pen to approach the paper and then be withdrawn from it. When further encouraged he might trace lines or symbols that would either be meaningless or bear only a faint resemblance to the letters or words he was required to write. Having done so he would put down the pen, sigh and, if speech were possible, exclaim at the futility of his trying further. Many such patients were equally unable to copy printed letters, or if they made an attempt misrepresented their shape. An example is shown in Fig. 10. This was

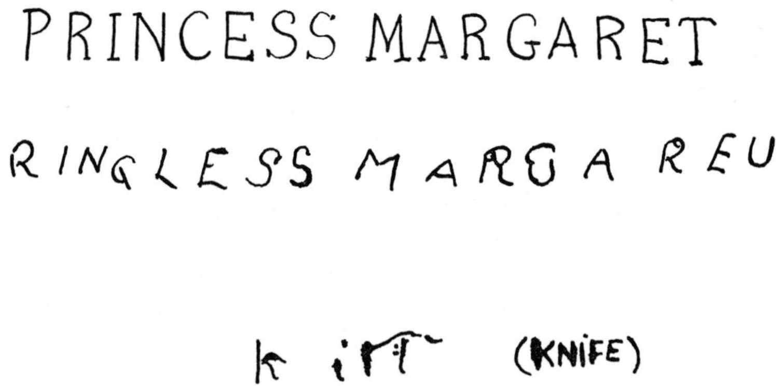

PRINCESS MARGARET

RINGLESS MARGA REU

k i r̃t (KNIFE)

Fig. 10.—Copying from Print

Case No. 57. Woman aged 44. Two years chronic amnesic syndrome with difficulty in reading and writing (presenile dementia)

an educated woman who was suffering from presenile dementia and who had difficulty both in writing and reading. The print was made especially big for her but, as can be seen, she was unable to form some of the letters. Her attempt to copy the word KNIFE is shown at the foot of the illustration. Such defects are often associated with dyscalculia, constructional apraxia, right–left bodily disorientation and finger agnosia and are discussed in Chapter IX.

Dysphasic patients suffering from hemiplegia affecting the preferred hand, who were able to print with the left hand, sometimes showed mirror reversal of letters, E becoming ƎД or the actual letters in a word being transposed, e.g. DOG becoming GOD, this tendency being similar to that often seen in children who are in the process of learning to write.

BIBLIOGRAPHY

185 CRITCHLEY, M. (1959). Broca's contribution reviewed a century later. Disc. at conjoint meeting between Ass. of British Neurologists and Canadian Neurolog. Ass. *Roy. Soc. Med.*, July 15.

186 SJÖGREN, H. (1952). Clinical analysis of morbus Alzheimer and morbus Pick. *Acta psychiat. Neurol., Scand.*, Suppl. 82, 85.

187 MITCHELL, J. (1958). Speech and language impairment in the older patient. *Geriatrics*, **13**, 467.

188 NATHAN, P. W. (1947). Facial apraxia and apraxic dysarthria. *Brain*, **70**, 449.

189 WEINSTEIN, E. A. and KAHN, R. L. (1952). Nonaphasic misnaming (paraphasia) in organic brain disease. *Arch. Neurol. Psychiat.*, **67**, 72.

190 HÉCAEN, H., DELL, M. B. and ROGER, A. (1955). L'aphasie de conduction. *Encéphale*, **2**, 170.

CHAPTER VIII

Disorders of Speech and Language

In the preceding chapter defects in expressive speech have chiefly been considered. Before leaving these to review receptive aspects it should be said that *pure* expressive aphasia or dysphasia was not often seen, occurring as it did in only 16 of our 64 cases. This type of impairment, which implies full comprehension of both spoken and written speech, is usually accredited to fairly circumscribed lesions of the dominant hemisphere, affecting the most anterior part of the cortical quadrilateral concerned with speech. Contralateral paresis may be found in association with it but sensory impairment and hemianopia are not to be expected, being more in keeping with posteriorly-placed lesions involving the temporo-parieto-occipital regions. This being so it is of interest to record the nature and site of the lesions in the cases with purely expressive defects. Seven of these had tumours:

    1. Left frontal—cystic astrocytoma (type III).
    5. Left temporal or temporo-parietal—2 astrocytomas
                                      2 meningiomata
                                        1 glioblastoma multiforme
    1. Third ventricle—ependymoma causing symmetrical dilation of lateral ventricles and obstruction of 3rd ventricle.

Of the remaining 9 cases, four were attributable to cerebral vascular accidents (cerebral thrombosis, internal carotid occlusion) and 5 were due to presenile dementia (1 post-anoxic, 1 post-traumatic and 3 early cases of general paralysis of the insane). In the one anteriorly-placed tumour, the lesion occupied the greater part of the left frontal lobe. On histological examination after autopsy there was no evidence of tumour tissue in the corpus callosum, temporal or parietal lobes, and in the frontal lobe the growth did not extend posteriorly beyond the level of the corpus luysii. Increased intracranial pressure had led to herniation of the brain through the anterior part of the falx cerebri and through the tentorium. Clinically this patient was seen at a relatively early stage in the development of his dysphasia but at a time when there was still no general clouding of consciousness. There was slight contralateral weakness of the face and arm but no sensory deficit or hemianopia. He exhibited marked nominal defects in spoken speech and had greater difficulty in writing than could be accounted for by weakness of the hand, but his understanding of spoken and written speech was un-impaired. However, he had difficulty in performing the simplest calculations although it was noted there was no right–left disorientation, finger agnosia or constructional apraxia.

Clues to the situation of the other more posteriorly-placed tumours were provided by the co-existence of contralateral sensory and motor loss and, in two cases, quadrantic hemianopic defects. One patient, however, from whose posterior temporal lobe a large vascular menin-gioma was shelled out, had neither sensory impairment nor hemianopia, his purely expressive speech defects and slight contralateral weakness in the face and arm resembling in all respects the clinical picture pre-sented by the frontal astrocytoma referred to above. None of the patients with presenile dementia had any unilateral motor, sensory or visual signs, their clinical features being indicative of a chronic amnesic syndrome, to which expressive speech disturbances had been super-added.

RECEPTIVE DEFECTS

The recognition of receptive defects in dysphasic patients is im-portant in determining prognosis and deciding the most appropriate treatment. These, however, are more difficult to analyse than expressive defects, not only because they are often less apparent and less accessible to formal testing, but because it is necessary to decide how much they are attributable to specific lack of comprehension for the spoken and written symbols of speech and how much to defective comprehension or grasp as a whole.

Defective grasp is a prominent feature of the overall disturbance of brain function seen during recovery of full consciousness after anoxia. It is evident in the patient's inability to register or learn fresh data, in his impairment of memory, loss of insight, disorientation, perseveration, ideomotor and constructional apraxia. When we first became interested in the investigation of aphasics it was thought that inability to express themselves would *ipso facto* prevent such general defects being brought to light, but further experience has shown that in the majority of cases this is not so. In fact, one can and should examine all aphasics in the first instance with a view to finding out how much their difficulty in comprehension depends on general lack of grasp. This principle is, indeed, the same as that followed in determining the existence of cortical sensory loss, to do which one must, of course first establish that the inability to recognize objects by touch is not due to gross lack of tactile and postural sensibility.

The tests used for detecting clouding of consciousness in aphasics had to be modified from the usual procedures described in Chapter IV. There was no difficulty in recognizing mood changes towards over-confidence, tension or anxiety and catastrophic reactions. Perseveration was not counted as providing evidence of clouding of consciousness unless it was noted in other activities as well as in speech. For evidence of ideomotor apraxia reliance was placed on day-to-day observations of the nursing staff and matchstick tests and Kohs' blocks were used to test for constructional apraxia. Defective ability in registration was more difficult to recognize when the patient was unable to speak or had gross verbal defects. It was tested for by showing him a number of objects and then hiding them, each in a different place. When a patient watched a comb being hidden under his pillow, a key being placed in the drawer of his bedside locker and a spoon under the counterpane of his bed, he appeared to be registering, but proof of his having done so was only forthcoming when, on being invited to show where they were, he was able to do so correctly. In most instances little verbal explanation was necessary and the patient could be made to grasp what was required simply by gesture and pantomime.

Analysis of the results of such tests indicated that a large number of dysphasic patients showed defective grasp, although in only a small proportion was this confined solely to spoken and written speech. This is not surprising considering the fact that the material contained such a variety of cases at different stages in their clinical course, some only being seen after their condition had begun seriously to deteriorate, while others only after it had commenced to improve. Table 8 gives the percentages of dysphasic patients showing one or other of these defects, the figures in column 1 referring to all cases and those in column 2 to cases of tumour only. General signs of defective grasp are less common in the latter and this, as might be expected, is because of the purely focal character of the lesions and the fact that many cases had not become complicated at the time of examination by rising intracranial pressure. But even in the tumour cases, general defects are sufficiently common to indicate that they must always be taken into account when trying to interpret the significance of receptive speech difficulties.

Difficulties in comprehension of spoken speech.

Provided there was no evidence of impairment of grasp in general, tests were given to assess the patient's ability to comprehend (1) factual or concrete statements and commands, (2) simple abstract propositions involving similarities and differences, (3) well-known proverbs, and (4) the meaning of a short story. Details of the tests used are given in

Chapter IV. Needless to say in interpreting results in terms of success or failure the guides followed were not so much fluency of the patient's replies as his ability to demonstrate by word or gesture that he had understood the import of what had been said. Commands such as " put out your tongue " were not given, as failure to comply might simply have indicated apraxia for tongue movements. Similarly "right and left " directions were not issued, as these might have led to mis-

TABLE 8.—*Occurrence of Signs of Defective Grasp in Dysphasic Patients (60 cases)**

Figures represent the percentage of cases showing the signs in each instance

Signs of defective grasp (Clouding of consciousness)	(1) All dysphasic patients, i.e. cerebral vascular accidents, tumours, global cerebral affections	(2) Patients with tumour of dominant hemisphere
Gross alterations in mood	50	38
Defective registration	65	38
Perseveration	62	53
Ideomotor apraxia	13	7
Constructional apraxia	50	7

conceptions in patients suffering from bodily disorientation. When testing the patient's ability to point to an object which had been named, care was taken to provide a plain background for the objects, only a few of which were put on display at a time. Most of our dysphasic patients had sufficient comprehension of spoken speech to pass this test and to respond appropriately to simple commands. A few clearly had difficulty in linking spoken names with the objects they represented, but of those who failed in carrying out simple commands the majority had signs of defective grasp in general. Perseveration was also very common. A good example of this was seen in a man aged 50 with a recent cerebral thrombosis, resulting in right-sided hemiparesis and aphasia.

* Although there were 64 cases of dysphasia, only 60 were included for this purpose because in 4 information relating to the points at issue was not available.

Perseveration was very noticeable in all activities. He had no spontaneous talk and looked tense and anxious. It was difficult to get him to comprehend but after some preliminary trials it was finally demonstrated that he could recover articles which had previously been hidden from his view. Judging by his behaviour he seemed to be more or less orientated in time and place and he recognized visitors. When told to close his eyes he did so promptly but when directed to touch his nose he kept on repeating the first action. When he was then asked to hold up his " good " arm (the left), he touched his left eye with that hand.* The interpretation put upon these results was that he knew his right from his left and could comprehend simple commands but that his performance was marred by perseveration, a factor that seemed to be largely responsible for his defect in comprehension.

Many patients who comprehended commands or concrete statements were able to grasp the meaning of simple propositions, such as the difference between a pond and a stream and, as has been seen this could sometimes be done even in the presence of severe expressive defects. In others, however, comprehension was too impaired for them to recognize essential points of similarity and difference and any attempt to discover the nature of their defects only served to illustrate the futility of separating receptive from expressive aspects of speech in these cases. For some years we used to go further in testing comprehension of spoken speech by telling the patient a short story with the object of finding out if he could grasp its point, e.g. the fable of the donkey with the load of salt. But repeated experience only showed that the result could be anticipated from previous performances with similarities and differences or proverbs; patients who could grasp the point of these could usually grasp the point of the story, and vice versa.

Difficulties in comprehension of printed or written speech.

Twenty-seven patients had difficulty in reading which could not be attributed to uncorrected errors of refraction, cataract, neuroretinitis or optic nerve disease. In all but 3 there was some associated expressive speech difficulty and in a few others defective comprehension of spoken speech was noted.

(a) *Hemianopia.* The possibility that a visual field defect might be contributing to the difficulty in reading was first investigated. Six of the dyslexic patients had a right homonymous hemianopia and in a seventh, although no actual field defect was found on perimetry, left-

---

* A similar example of perseveration was cited by Claude and Lhermitte.[8] The patient was an old woman with cerebral cortical atrophy: " on lui dit de mettre la main droite sur la tête, elle le fait, mais l'y laisse longtemps, et lorsqu'on veut lui baisser le bras, elle se raidit et résiste. On lui dit de mettre la main gauche sur la tête, elle met la main droite; on lui fait observer que ce n'est pas le mouvement commandé, sa main droite quitte alors la tête et se place sur son épaule gauche ".

sided visual inattention was demonstrable. All 7 were tested for their ability to read simple sentences, arranged first in the horizontal plane, and then in the vertical but in only 2 was reading substantially improved by the latter procedure and one of them was the patient with unilateral visual inattention. A modification of the test mentioned on p. 45 was then given, the 2 patients whose reading had been improved being invited to pick up a line of matches, which had been set before them some inches apart, from left to right. One patient neglected the matches situated to the left of the midline, the other those situated to the right. However, all but one of the other hemianopic patients picked up the matches as readily from one side as from the other. This suggested that, although a homonymous half field defect might be present it did not necessarily contribute to reading disability, unless there were some associated visual inattention.

The exception referred to above proved to be a more complicated problem. This was a woman who was later found to have a left internal capsular infarct invading the thalamus, the result of a cerebral thrombosis sustained some years previously. The cerebral hemispheres were intact on sectioning and the possibility of there being a focal lesion in the cortex or subcortex was excluded. There was right-sided hemiplegia, sensory impairment, and right homonymous hemianopia, without macular sparing. For the first year after the stroke she had been aphasic, but at the time of examination had regained full comprehension of spoken speech, could express herself verbally, although haltingly, and make some attempt to write with the left hand. Her reading ability, however, remained severely impaired and this she attributed to being only able to see to her left side. When she looked " straight " at anyone, she said, she could see " only half of them ". Movements of the eyeballs, when tested in the usual way, were full although there was always great difficulty in coaxing her to look to the right and she could never be persuaded to maintain her gaze in this direction for more than a second or two at a time. This curious feature was associated with aversion of and a tendency to berate her paralysed right arm (see p. 197). But from the standpoint of reading it seemed to have some significance because when she looked at a line of print it was noticed that the natural scanning movements of the eyeballs seen in reading did not occur. Instead, her eyes moved irregularly and slowly from one word to the next, depending on the difficulty she had in interpreting the meaning of individual words. That she had added difficulties in recognizing letters (literal dyslexia) will be seen presently, but whether these were entirely explained by the oculomotor disturbance or were independent of them we were unable to say. Warrington and Zangwill[191] have recently reported a somewhat similar case in which they made a careful study of eye movements during reading. Fixation on print and normal saccadic movements were grossly impaired and the eyeballs made but slow progression along each line of print, small, irregular, backward and forward twitches being observed, which lacked the step-wise character of normal reading movements. As reading ability improved after operation (the patient had a left occipito-parietal meningioma) so did the character of the eye movements.

(*b*) *Difficulty in recognizing letters* (*literal dyslexia*). In seven of our dyslexic patients the fault lay in difficulty in identifying letters of the alphabet, the shape of one letter being confused with that of another or the shape of letters being forgotten. Probably the best example of this form of literal dyslexia was a woman aged 55, a case of Alzheimer's disease. When shown large cardboard letters, which she was permitted to handle as well as to see, she was unable to state what many of them were. When told the name of a letter she had failed to recognize she could retain the information and name the letter correctly when it was shown to her later. But, despite all efforts she could not distinguish an F from an E or an R from a B. When the three letters D, O, G were arranged so as to form DOG, she recognized the word but commented that the letters D and G looked like O. When she was given a longer word, i.e. RAINBOW, she kept on confusing the R with the B, and even when she was assisted in overcoming these mistakes and could at last spell the word correctly, it had no meaning for her. However, immediately when the word was spoken aloud, she declared: " I know . . . it's something in the sky." In her case there was no evidence of visual object agnosia or astereognosis and there were only slight defects in expressive and receptive speech, but she found it impossible to copy the simplest geometric designs. Indeed, in these cases in which there was difficulty in recognizing the shape of letters constructional apraxia was a fairly constant accompaniment.

There were other examples of the same kind in which the principal obstacle to reading appeared to be the tendency to confuse such letters as F, E, R, B, C, G, O, D, P. Patients usually mistook F for E, R for B, C for O, which suggests that they may have been trying to complete what appeared to them an incomplete pattern (F = E). In other words they retained some capacity for " gestalt ", so that when they mistook an F for an E they may simply have been yielding to their natural tendency to form a whole from parts of the whole. At times, healthy subjects make the same kind of mistake (although usually in other activities than reading) and it is possible that dyslexic patients with brain injury make mistakes of this kind more often because of their defective grasp. The habit of guessing a word after recognizing two or more of its constituent letters, which was also common, may be another expression of the same tendency. However, although brain-injured subjects retain to some extent their instinctive tendency in these respects, evidence of disturbance of figure-background relationships can often be demonstrated in those with reading difficulties by criss-crossing the printed or written word with lines. Such patients, although perfectly capable of reading the word " Hospital " are unable to comprehend it when it is represented as ⨉⨉⨉⨉⨉⨉⨉⨉ [192].

The following account suggests a possible means of overcoming this type of defect and illustrates briefly the mode of recovery of reading ability.

The patient was a right-handed woman of 71 who suddenly became con-fused and was found to have difficulty in recalling names. Examination showed a right homonymous hemianopia with visual neglect of the right side of space but no evidence of paralysis or sensory impairment. In naming sighted objects perseveration was marked and she had difficulty in recalling names from memory. There was little or no spontaneous speech but handwriting was unaffected, although she could not read what she had written. Her responses to spoken speech showed that she had no difficulty in understanding pro-positions, proverbs being interpreted on the abstract plane and not literally. However, she was quite unable to read and was disorientated in time and place, could not distinguish the right side of her body from the left or read the time from a clock. Constructional apraxia was pronounced. Blood pressure was elevated and the diagnosis was thought to be cerebral thrombosis with softening in the left parieto-occipital region.

At first she was unable to recognize any letters of the alphabet. But as days passed and these were shown and named to her repeatedly, she gradually began to recognize them, despite her tendency to per-severation. It was about this time that she was observed tracing the shape of letters with her finger (sometimes referred to as Wilbrand's sign), [69] an act which appeared to speed up recognition to a remarkable extent. Thereafter, by providing large print and encouraging her to do this she was soon able to read short sentences, provided these were composed of small words. However, two difficulties made progress slow. Continuous encouragement and stimulation were necessary to get her to trace the letters with her finger. Left to herself she would not bother to do so. The other difficulty was that already referred to: when faced by a long word she would not go on identifying the letters by tracing but guess at its meaning from the first two or three letters. Within a year she was able to read print slowly but still had difficulty in discerning cursive script. Constructional difficulties were still apparent but there was none of the former neglect of the right side of space. Despite these handicaps she resumed light household duties and remained in good health until her death some three and a half years later from a further stroke.

In a few cases there was no difficulty in recognizing the shape of letters and the defect appeared to be more amnesic in character. Although one would expect this to be more a feature of global cerebral affections, it was, in fact, first brought to our notice by the behaviour of a patient with a strictly focal lesion involving the thalamus—the case whose disturbance of oculomotor movements in reading has already been described. When shown single letters separately or arranged to form a word she would look at them without understanding and then proceed to say the alphabet over to herself until she came to the letter required, after which she would triumphantly announce what it was. The next letter, if not immediately recognizable was dealt with in the same way. At first this was all she could accomplish, reading being impossible because of her inability to retain the letters sufficiently long as to enable her to get the word. But as her conscious level, memory and capacity for registration improved, she was soon able to retain the first two or three letters and make a guess at the word. Months were required to wean her off this tendency, at which it must be admitted she became extraordinarily adept, but for some years before her death she had acquired sufficient skill as to enable her to read headlines in the news and the captions under pictures in illustrated papers. Eye movements in reading had also reverted to normal.

(*c*) *Difficulty in recognizing words* (*verbal dyslexia*). There were a few cases in which the difficulty in reading seemed to depend more on inability to recognize words than actual letters, but *per se* this type of defect was less common and more often than not associated with semantic difficulties in reading. A good example, however, was seen in a man aged 59, with recent left internal carotid stenosis, causing right-sided hemiplegia and visual inattention. He was aphasic and also showed constructional apraxia. Comprehension of spoken speech was good for, despite the fact that he was speechless, he could employ a wealth of gesture and pantomime in answering questions so that examination was comparatively easy. He could identify individual letters of the alphabet and pick them out unerringly from among a number of other letters. When the three letters B, P, U, were arranged so as to form the word PUB, he nodded his head and at once set about miming the act of drinking. This made one think he had no verbal dyslexia, but affective influences may have been playing some part—it is difficult to explain the discrepancy otherwise—for when he was shown other short words such as PIN, NIB, BALL, GUN, he failed to recognize them or indicate the objects to which they referred, although these together with other objects were displayed to view. Previously, of course, it had been demonstrated through his use of pantomime that there was no visual object agnosia or apraxia in relation to the same objects. In verbal dyslexia it would appear, therefore, that the defect is chiefly amnesic, although in the case described there was in addition some constructional difficulty. This was shown not only in his performance in copying simple designs with matches and with the Kohs' blocks but also by his inability to arrange cardboard letters in their right order and in the required position to form words. Thus, although he knew the letters G, N, U, and understood the spoken direction to form them into the word GUN, he could not do so but arranged them in incorrect order, placed the G and the U upside down and setting the N mirrorwise so that the result was N G U.

(*d*) *Semantic difficulties in reading*. Even when there was no hesitation in recognizing letters or words and it was possible for a patient to read a simple passage correctly, there was sometimes difficulty in comprehending its meaning. In most such cases the contributing factors were perseveration, failure to register what had just been read and a tendency to lose the place, so that printed lines became mixed up, words or lines were omitted or words taken out of their context. This was well seen in a man with a chronic amnesic syndrome, who had difficulty in recalling names from memory but understood spoken speech and could read and understand the meaning of most of the words on the Burt scale, e.g. unique, microscope etc. There were no neurological signs. When given the excerpt to read about " The School Concert ", Terman Merrill,[119] he proceeded:

" On December 20th, the children of the city schools held a concert in the hall of the big school. All the children had . . . some part of the programme . . . which consisted of . . . singing . . . by the boys' school choir . . . oh, I have lost my place . . . I'm sorry these glasses are not too good."

During the reading one could see that he had great difficulty and from the way he paused to scan the print it was evident that he was continually losing his place. At times he would run his finger along the lines to assist his eyes in fixation, but his visual acuity with glasses was good and there was no evidence of hemianopia or unilateral visual inattention.

CEREBRAL DOMINANCE, HANDEDNESS AND APHASIA

All available clinical evidence suggests that in right-handed persons the pathways concerned with speech are situated in the left cerebral hemisphere, the right playing but a subordinate rôle in this specialized aspect of intellectual function. The original concept of cerebral dominance, however, went further in postulating that so closely was handedness correlated with dominance that precisely the same effects on speech might be expected in left-handed persons from lesions of the right hemisphere. Hughlings Jackson noted loss of speech in association with left-sided hemiplegia,[193] and his observations lent support to this contention. But he was careful to point out that not all left-handers were rendered aphasic by lesions of the right hemisphere, and he was aware, too, that in left-handed persons aphasia might result from lesions of the left hemisphere.[195]

Such examples as the last-named, although rare, have always been difficult to account for on the basis of there being a strict association between handedness and dominance. It is known, however, that although the large majority of persons are right-handed and only a small minority left-handed, a considerable proportion show "crossed" laterality, some skilled activities being conducted by the right hand and others by the left. That mixed cerebral dominance can also occur is recognized and cases illustrating this have been published by Friedman and Nielsen,[194]* Humphrey and Zangwill[195]† and others.

As to the explanation of mixed-handedness, Russell Brain[165] concludes that although handedness is genetically determined (right-handedness being a dominant and left-handedness a recessive characteristic) hereditary influences may be annulled either through the influence of parents or teachers converting naturally left-handed children into right-handers or disease of one hemisphere leading to shift of dominance to the other side.‡ It is probable, indeed, as

---

* Nielsen's case was a left-handed man who, as the result of a stroke developed right hemiplegia and hemianopia. There was no aphasia but he showed right—left bodily disorientation and colour agnosia, limited to the right half visual field. Post-mortem examination disclosed extensive disintegration of the left temporal, posterior inferior parietal and occipital lobes. The authors deduced that the right cerebral hemisphere was dominant for speech and the left for colour recognition and body laterality.

† This was a case of right occipito-parietal penetrating brain injury in a left-handed man in whose case there were symptoms pointing to lesions of both parietal lobes.

‡ Infantile right hemiplegia is not associated with aphasia and this is one reason for believing that in childhood at least shift of cerebral dominance can occur, but in adults, where dominance is more firmly anchored it is more difficult to achieve. Thus, Roberts[197] showed that despite pre-existing damage to the left hemisphere some patients became aphasic after operations on that side, a result, he concludes, which should not have occurred had there already been pre-operative shift of dominance.

Critchley[53] suggests that the 5–10% of so-called left-handed persons is made up of a heterogeneous collection of types which includes:

(1) Naturally left-handed persons in whom not only is the left hand selected for all activities but the left eye and foot are also preferred.

(2) Naturally left-handed persons who have been taught to write and perform certain other activities with the right hand although retaining their preference for the left in some activities.

(3) Naturally right-handed persons who as the result of some disability affecting the right arm have been compelled to use the left arm. In such cases it is often found that although the left hand is used in all activities the right eye and foot may still be preferred.

(4) Left-handed persons who are members of a family in which right-handedness is the rule. When both parents are right-handed this is extremely unlikely to occur. When the mother is left-handed approximately 14% of the childship show similar preference; when the father, the proportion is less, approximately 10%.[198]

(5) Cases of alleged ambidexterity. In such persons it may be as Chesher[199] suggests, that the speech mechanism is not lateralized, but if so, he asks, why does any disability of speech result from a lesion of one hemisphere?

Except for the first group in which one can be reasonably confident that the right hemisphere is dominant, probably in the other groups there is no clear cut dominance and this makes it difficult, if not impossible (in the absence of a lesion) to predict the effects on speech of damage to the supposedly dominant hemisphere. In recent times these theoretical considerations have been put to the test by different workers, notably Humphrey and Zangwill,[200] Roberts,[197] Hécaen and Piercy.[201] Humphrey and Zangwill studied in detail 10 patients showing marked left-handed preference, all of whom had sustained cerebral injuries, in 5 the left hemisphere being damaged and in 5 the right. They found some evidence of language disorder in all 5 cases with left hemisphere lesions and in all but one of the cases with lesions of the right hemisphere and concluded: " If left-handedness were correlated with ' right brainedness ' to the same extent as right-handedness with ' left brainedness ' as has commonly been assumed, then dysphasia would have been expected to occur only in the right hemisphere injuries." From their observations it would appear, therefore, that the dominant and subordinate hemisphere arrangement is not organized in left-handers to the same extent as it is in right-handers and that in the former the pathways concerned with speech are more evenly and bilaterally distributed.

Our cases were too few to enable any valid conclusions to be drawn from personal experience as to the relation of handedness and the site of focal lesions in causing aphasia. In the whole series there were 24 pure right-handers with focal lesions in the right hemisphere and 2 left-handers with similar lesions in the left hemisphere. Both of the latter belonged to the mixed group for, although strongly left-handed since childhood, they had been taught to write with the right hand and preferred it for that purpose. Further, of the 26 cases in only 10 (8 right and 2 left-handers) were the results of tests for speech and handedness adequately recorded. The omissions were almost certainly due to the fact that no dysphasia had been discernible, but as specific points had not been noted these cases were discarded. However, of the remaining 10 cases in which the results had been recorded, in all but one patient, in whom defects were observed both in writing and reading, tests for dysphasia were negative. The difficulty in copying, in writing from dictation and in reading may have been due partly to left-sided visual inattention because this was a conspicuous feature, but other factors contributing were defective capacity for registration and a mood of unconcern. Failing memory over the preceding nine months with numbness and weakness in the left arm and leg had been the principal symptoms and it had been noted that when dressing herself this patient was inclined to put her clothes on the wrong way. After operation for the removal of a right parietal meningioma writing and reading, together with registration, returned to normal.

Each of the 2 left-handed patients had a tumour involving the left temporal lobe. One was a man of superior intelligence. Naturally left-handed (although his other 6 brothers and sisters were all right-handed), he had been taught as a child to write with the right hand and habitually used it for this purpose. But he could write with his left hand and preferred it for most other activities, e.g. cricket, table tennis. But in boxing in his youth, he had adopted a stance with the left foot and shoulder advanced, keeping the left arm outstretched and relying on the right for punching. This, however, was his only variation for when playing cards he dealt with the left hand and he used the left hand for striking matches, brushing his hair and shaving. Often at table he would begin, as he had been taught, by using the soup spoon in his right hand but before long would transfer it to the left, although curiously enough he had never felt any inclination to transfer his knife and fork, being content to use these in the customary manner. At football he could kick only with his left foot, but he preferred his right eye to his left, when required to use one eye only.

Our impression at the time was that the right cerebral hemisphere was almost certainly dominant and this seemed to be borne out by the total absence of any evidence of dysphasia, despite the fact that he had an infiltrating tumour in the left parieto-temporal region. Apart from some difficulty in registration and in reversing series, which struck us as being unusual for a man of his educational status, the only defect found was constructional apraxia, which was most pronounced.

Summary

Disorders of speech and language were found in 64 or about one-third of all the organic mental cases in this series, 21 being accounted for by vascular accidents involving the dominant hemisphere, 17 by tumours, similarly placed in the speech area, and 26 by diffuse cortical atrophy, due to a variety of different causes.

Absolute speechlessness was rare. More common was it to find that patients made no effort to talk unless spoken to, when their defects at once became apparent. These took the form of: slurring dysarthria and distorted pronounciations; difficulties in word finding (chiefly for nouns); defective sentence construction; perseveration, and inability to discuss abstract topics. Ways and means of overcoming nominal defects included the use of gesture and pantomime; the substitution of other related but inappropriate words; periphrasis and paraphasia. Perseveration was more or less a constant feature in these cases and often appeared to be the chief obstacle to expression. A tendency to break off in the middle of sentences and to leave them unfinished was also noted. In a third small group there was no inhibition of spontaneous talk. Most of these had sustained cerebral vascular accidents or were recovering from anoxic or traumatic encephalopathy. Their push of talk was often interspersed with confabulations, nominal or grammatical errors and speech tended to lapse readily into incoherence or jargon.

In contrasting the ability of dysphasics to name sighted objects and to recall names from memory it was noted that patients with focal lesions involving the speech area had almost equal difficulty in performing these tasks whereas patients with presenile dementia or global cerebral affections had appreciably greater difficulty in recalling names from memory. The amnesic indifference so often displayed by the latter may explain this peculiarity, some " priming of the pump " being necessary to get them to draw upon their memory.

Writing disabilities were more difficult to appraise but spontaneous writing was almost always more affected than the ability to write from dictation or to copy, and attempts at composing a letter revealed the same kinds of defect as were found in spoken speech.

12

Pure expressive aphasia was observed in only 16 of the 64 cases. Most of the others showed the same signs of defective grasp as are found in simple clouding of consciousness, i.e. defective registration, perseveration, disorientation in time and place and abnormalities of mood and behaviour. Only in a small number of dysphasics was defective grasp limited to comprehension of the spoken and written symbols of speech. Understanding of spoken speech was often difficult to judge owing to the patient's inability to express himself propositionally. Specific reading disabilities were common and sometimes related to hemianopia, visual inattention or disturbance of eye movements. In other cases letters could not be identified, this being due either to confusion over their shape (a feature often associated with constructional difficulties) or to inability to remember them except by reference to their position in the alphabet. Difficulty in recognizing words was more often amnesic in origin and corresponded to the comparable type of defect seen in naming sighted objects. Many patients with defective grasp showed semantic difficulties in reading and these appeared to be due, at least in part, to a tendency to lose the place, words or lines being read out of their context, or to the patient forgetting the first sentences of a paragraph before he had time to complete reading it.

The chief purpose in reviewing this heterogeneous collection of cases has been to determine how often speech defects occurred alone or in association with clouding of consciousness. The conclusion reached is that, although the importance of a focal lesion interrupting the anatomical pathways concerned with speech cannot be questioned, disturbances of consciousness (in the sense in which we have used the term) play some considerable part both in the development and character of speech and language disorders. This is borne out by those instances, which we have quoted, where an appropriately-situated tumour has failed to cause dysphasia until a late stage, when shift or herniation of the brain has occurred as the result of cerebral oedema and rising intracranial pressure. Such anomalies have sometimes been attributed to the tumour not actually involving the speech " centres ", to its growth being too slow, or to the possession by the patient of mixed cerebral dominance. But in the cases referred to none of these explanations fitted and the dramatic way in which dysphasia supervened pointed to a connection between its appearance and disturbance of subcortical centres which had been brought about by the development of intracranial complications.

In a later chapter the speech and language disturbances seen in patients with global cerebral affections will be reviewed and their features contrasted with those observed in purely focal lesions. In the former speech defects were always less conspicuous than the general falling away in interest, absent-mindedness etc., and an analogy may be drawn between them and an orchestra, the performances of which have been slowly deteriorating over the course of years, due not so much to loss of individual musicians as to the conductor or the members falling short of their goal to produce good music. They, themselves, may not be so aware of their defects as the audience, and even the latter may have difficulty in picking out specific defects, although they will have no doubt that the performances are not what they used to be. On the other hand, the disturbances of speech seen in focal lesions, whether due to destruction of specific paths, the integrity of which is essential for speech or to more widespread effects, may be compared to the situation that would arise should certain members of an orchestra be taken suddenly ill. Although the others are perfectly fit to continue playing, if a sufficient number be affected, the concert must come to a stop until such time as they are replaced, or the score rewritten so as to allow for their lack of participation. It is on these or similar lines that we think the problem of dysphasia should be approached—to assign what aspects of speech and language can be attributed to failure of the conductor and what to individual members. Schuell and Jenkins[117] believe that a single dimension of language deficit is present in all cases of aphasia. This may well be the case and, if so, it is possible that the seat of the " single dimension " is subcortical, and related to those centres which have a regulating influence on consciousness.

BIBLIOGRAPHY

191 WARRINGTON, E. and ZANGWILL, O. L. (1957). A study of dyslexia. *J. Neurol. Psychiat.*, **20**, 208.

192 POPPELREUTER, W. (1923). Zur Psychologie und Pathologie der optischen Wahrnehmung, *Z. ges. Neurol. Psychiat.*, **83**, 26.

193 JACKSON, H. (1915). Reprints of papers published between 1864–1893. *Brain*, **38**, parts i, ii.

194 FRIEDMAN, A. P. and NIELSEN, J. M. (1941). Autopsy in case of crossed partial temporo-occipital dominance. *Bull. Los Angeles Neurol. Soc.*, **194**, 6.

195 HUMPHREY, M. E. and ZANGWILL, O. L. (1952). Effects of a right-sided occipito-parietal brain injury in a left-handed man. *Brain*, **75**, 312.

196 BRAIN, W. R. (1945). Speech and handedness. *Lancet*, **2**, 837.

197 ROBERTS, L. (1955). Handedness and cerebral dominance. *Trans. Amer. Neurol. Ass.*, **80**, 143.

198 CHAMBERLAIN, H. D. (1928). The inheritance of left-handedness. *J. Hered.*, **19**, 557. Quoted by Brain, W. R. (196).

199   CHESHER, E. C. (1935).   Some observations concerning the relation of
      handedness to the language mechanism.   *Bull. Neurol. Inst., N.Y.*, **4**,
      556.

200   HUMPHREY, M. E. and ZANGWILL, O. L. (1952).   Dysphasia in left-
      handed patients with unilateral brain lesions.   *J. Neurol. Psychiat.*, **15**,
      184.

201   HÉCAEN, H. and PIERCY, M. (1956).   Paroxysmal dysphasia and problem
      of cerebral dominance.   *J. Neurol. Psychiat.*, **19**, 194.

CHAPTER IX

Disorientation

DISORIENTATION is a common symptom in organic mental states and its degree varies greatly both in extent and quality from patient to patient. Such gross forms as inability to recognize personal friends and relations, to know where one is and what time it is, will be considered first, next more abstract forms or disorientation at a propositional or conceptual level, and third, the disturbances that come under the head of bodily disorientation.

DISORIENTATION FOR PERSONS AND IN TIME AND PLACE

In the clinical sense orientation refers to a person's awareness of his own spatial and temporal relations in juxtaposition to other persons and the external physical environment. To be correctly orientated implies ability to recall at least some of past experience and the capacity for registration of fresh data. Correct orientation is indeed synonymous with " full consciousness " in the sense that we have used the term and, as has been seen, patients recovering from anoxia or head injury pass through phases of disorientation, some or all of which may be so brief as to pass unnoticed or persist for days or weeks on end. It is possible that the brain-injured subject first becomes aware of his own body, then of his immediate environment (the ward, nurses, visitors, other patients) and then finally of the hospital in which he is, and of its position in relation to his home and other places. This is the general pattern of what occurs but there are many variations. Orientation towards other persons and in space may be acquired and yet traces of bodily unawareness may persist, e.g. right-left disorientation and finger agnosia. Right-left bodily disorientation and finger agnosia are also sometimes seen in patients with purely focal cerebral lesions involving the parietal lobe of the dominant hemisphere, in whom there is little or no evidence either of clouding of consciousness or disorientation towards external things.

In our patients with organic mental states routine testing showed that disorientation was such a common symptom, and so invariably associated with other signs of clouding of consciousness, e.g. perseveration, inability or defective ability to register, change in mood, altered insight, as to have little diagnostic significance in relation to the site of the lesion. However, there were indications of some correlation existing between severity of disorientation and extent of cerebral damage. For example, total disorientation for persons, place and time was comparatively rarely seen and its incidence confined to advanced presenile dementia and certain cases of post-anoxic encephalopathy, in which the inability to recognize relatives and friends, or the tendency to confuse them with other people whom the patient had known in the past was a very striking feature. Disorientation for persons was never seen in patients with focal lesions in whom there was reason to believe that the rest of the brain was comparatively healthy. Thus, one of our first cases was a sailor who had been rendered severly anoxic through inhaling carbon monoxide. Recovery of consciousness was slow and the stage of disorientation prolonged; but even after he had become orientated in place he still could not recognize his other wounded shipmates in the hospital ward, nor could he recall having been in the navy, although he had served in it for four years. His attitude was unconcerned, facile and euphoric.

Prosopagnosia, or inability to recognize faces, occurring as an isolated or relatively isolated disability was not seen but one of the best accounts of this has been given by Hécaen *et al.*[202] The patient was a right-handed man of 52, who had an infiltrating tumour (glioblastoma multiforme) in the right temporo-parieto-occipital region. This man declared: " Je reconnais les gens à générale, mon frère, les voisins, mais si je cherche à fixer les détails d'une personne que je connais bien, à la regarder en détail, j'ai l'impression que ce n'est plus elle, par exemple même mon frère j'ai les difficultés à le reconnaître. . . ." This man was incapable of recognizing pictures of well-known personages, yet his general orientation in space was unaffected and he was only slightly disoriented in time.

General disorientation in place and time was regularly seen in patients recovering consciousness after cerebral vascular accidents, in whom it might persist for some weeks, and it was also seen in post-traumatic and anoxic encephalopathies and cerebral tumours, especially those of infiltrative type and growing rapidly. With slow-growing expanding tumours it was uncommon to find disorientation in place and time until the stage had been reached when increasing intracranial pressure was beginning to cause herniation of the brain, or there was much cerebral oedema. It was observed also in patients suspected of having cerebral vascular disease or space-occupying lesions, who had previously been well-orientated, as a transient consequence of such procedures as angiography or lumbar encephalography.

Disorientation in time alone was not uncommon. As a rule it represented either the beginning of progressive mental deterioration in global cerebral affections, or, in the case of a focal cerebral lesion, increasing intracranial pressure due to shift of the brain, mounting oedema or haemorrhage into a tumour. In testing patients for temporal disorientation we did not attach much importance to inability to name the day of the week because many hospital inmates cannot do so. Failure to get the month of the year correct, however, or fixing the year at a much earlier date that it actually was, was accepted as evidence of disorientation in time.

ABSTRACT DISORIENTATION IN SPACE

Many patients in this series, although correctly orientated towards other persons, the place at the time of examination and day, month and year, displayed an extraordinarily poor sense of direction. They tended to lose themselves when out of doors or even in their own homes, mistaking one room for another. Their topographic memory was poor so that they were unable to say upon which side of a street they lived or describe the route to be followed in going to church, the cinema, or to visit old friends, whose address they knew well. Such persons may have difficulty in localizing objects in space, i.e. in deciding which of two objects is the nearer, and may be quite incapable of selecting a given object from among a number of other objects, although still able to see and recognize its nature. In most cases there is a hemianopic field defect and in some an associated disturbance of oculomotor movements in reading is demonstrable (see p. 161). Originally regarded as being inseparable from disorientation in general, it was not until the first great war that discrete spatial disorientation was described as a result of parieto-occipital brain injuries, Riddoch (1917), Holmes (1918–19) Kleist (1922), Pötzl (1928). Holmes was of the opinion that in such cases there were invariably bilateral hemisphere lesions, but Brain,[203] Paterson and Zangwill[204] have described spatial disorientation, limited to the left half-field of space in right-handed patients, due to right hemisphere lesions alone.

In testing these patients it was useful to ask them to draw a rough plan of the street in which they lived, indicating the relative position of different buildings and other landmarks. They were also shown a map of Ireland and asked to mark on it the position of well-known places. House drawing tests were used for the same purpose and were found to be particularly valuable in providing evidence of abstract spatial disorientation.

In drawing, aptitude, constructional ability and capacity for spatial orientation are all involved and our experience supports Critchley's contention that patients with defective spatial orientation usually have some corresponding degree of constructional apraxia.

Just as in dysphasia, where a patient may comprehend simple spoken commands or written directions and yet be unable to understand more abstract propositions, so in disorientation a patient may know the time and be perfectly clear about his whereabouts but display a surprising degree of confusion when asked to indicate where he lives on a street plan, to mark well-known places on a map or to draw a house. This abstract disorientation we found was invariably associated with some defective memory for recent events. Indeed, a characteristic feature of patients with diffuse cortical atrophy often was loss of topographic memory, a defect that might colour the clinical picture to such an extent as to make it the chief reason for their seeking medical advice.

Fig. 11 illustrates use of the house-drawing test in detecting abstract disorientation. The patient was a woman aged 70, the victim of a severe anoxic exposure, who had been grossly disorientated and amnesic for several weeks. The first drawing was made when she had almost fully recovered consciousness. Although by then all traces of gross disorientation had disappeared, her drawing still showed evidence of abstract disorientation. A week hence, when even this had disappeared her drawing was that of a fully orientated person.

Allowing for possible lack of natural aptitude and lowered motivation, due to the presence of brain injury or disease, if a patient can be persuaded to draw (and quite a number, it must be conceded, flatly refuse to do so), the chief thing to look for is how they deal with perspective. In other words, do their drawings convey the impression of a house as viewed in one particular plane, and are the chief features, i.e. the door, windows, chimneys appropriately sited, as one would expect them to be in that perspective? The results of such tests are of interest because they bear a close resemblance to the drawings of children between the ages of $2\frac{1}{2}$–8 years, in whom orientation is still not fully developed. The performances of adults recovering consciousness after anoxia and some others suffering from diffuse cerebral disease or focal neoplastic or vascular lesions, suggest that breakdown in their normal capacity for abstract orientation has (as a result of brain damage) led to re-integration of drawing ability at a lower level of performance, that is at a primitive or child-like level. Foster Kennedy[205] records such a case. The patient, a nineteen-year-old honours art student had sustained a fractured skull. In her recovery she showed " an aphasia of expression " that did not involve writing but only her capacity to draw, which reverted to a childish level. Examples of childrens' drawings of houses are shown in Fig. 12 and similar drawings of adults with organic mental states in Fig. 13. The children who made these drawings were in hospital suffering from a variety of minor complaints and none of them was the subject of brain disease or injury. Also, so far as one could tell, their mental development was average. The tendency to place the windows on the side walls will be noted. As Dr. W. Flewett, our house-physician at the time, suggested this may be due to the patient or child thinking of the object in two planes of perspective.

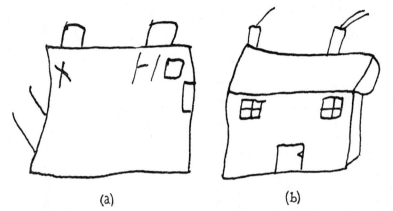

(a)   (b)

Fig. 11.—Abstract Disorientation in Clouding of Consciousness Due to Anoxia

Case No. 12. Woman aged 70; drawing of house. (*a*) was made on 14.2.48 just after she became fully orientated in place and time, able to register and to recall past events. The two lines drawn diagonally upwards from the left side wall are meant to represent the door. The crossed line under the left chimney represents a window as do the lines (oblong and square) on the right upper part of the drawing. (*b*) was made on 21.2.48, a week later, when the patient had improved still further and just before discharge from hospital.[91]

Thus, in the vertical plane the windows and door would appear against the side walls, whereas in the horizontal, or usual perspective adopted in drawing, they would appear away from the walls. Gunzberg[206] discussing this tendency, quotes Kerr's suggestion that such tendencies are indicative of anxiety. This may be so but we feel the above explanation is more basically correct.

Since Carrodo Ricci of Bologna (1887) studied the development of drawing ability in children a considerable literature on the subject has has accumulated, to which the following valuable references may be given: Eng,[207] Claparède,[208] Luquet,[209] Oakley,[210] Ayer,[211] Kerr,[212] Gesell.[213] Luquet noted that children pass through four stages in their

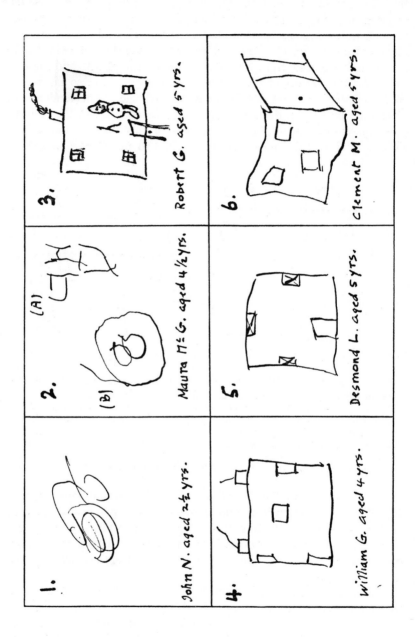

1. John N. aged 2½ yrs.

2. (A) (B) Maura McG. aged 4½ yrs.

3. Robert G. aged 6 yrs.

4. William G. aged 4 yrs.

5. Desmond L. aged 5 yrs.

6. Clement M. aged 5 yrs.

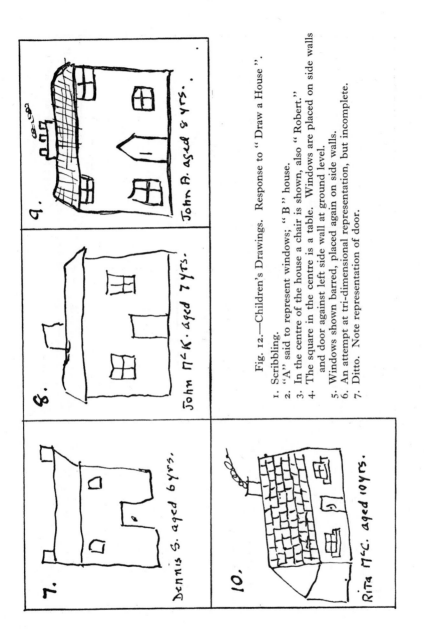

Fig. 12.—Children's Drawings. Response to "Draw a House".

1. Scribbling.
2. "A" said to represent windows; "B" house.
3. In the centre of the house a chair is shown, also "Robert."
4. The square in the centre is a table. Windows are placed on side walls and door against left side wall at ground level.
5. Windows shown barred, placed again on side walls.
6. An attempt at tri-dimensional representation, but incomplete.
7. Ditto. Note representation of door.

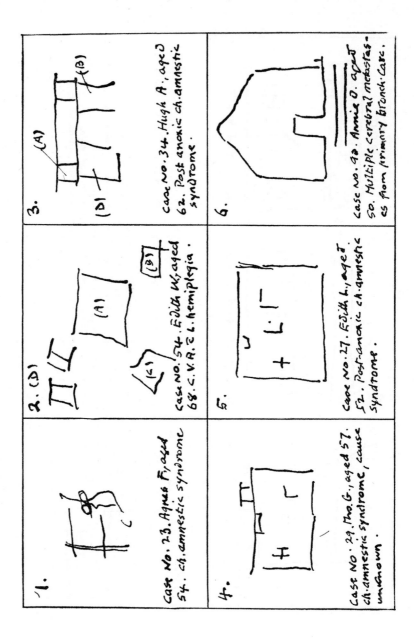

1.

Case No. 23. Agnes F., aged 54. Ch. amnestic syndrome.

2. (D) (A) (B) Case No. 54. Edith W., aged 68. C.V.A. & L. hemiplegia.

3. (A) (B) (D) Case No. 34. Hugh A., aged 62. Post anoxic ch. amnestic syndrome.

4. Case No. 29. Mrs. G., aged 57. Ch. amnestic syndrome, cause unknown.

5. Case No. 27. Edith L., aged 52. Post-anoxic ch. amnestic syndrome.

6. Case No. 90. Annie O., aged 50. Multiple cerebral metastases from primary Bronch. Carc.

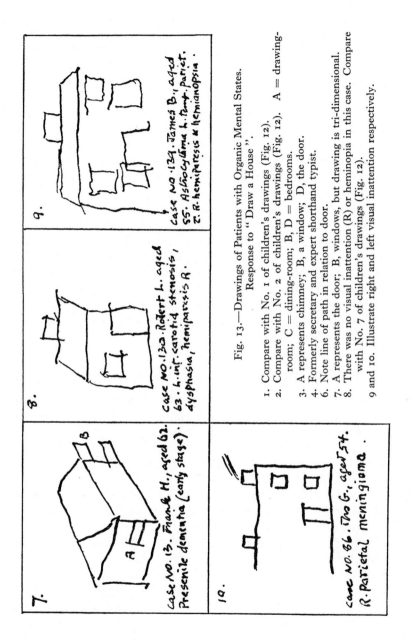

7.

CASE NO. 13. Frank H., aged 62.
Presenile dementia (early stage).

8.

CASE NO. 130. Robert L. aged
63. L. int. carotid stenosis,
dysphasia, hemiparesis R.

9.

CASE NO. 139. James B., aged
55. Astrocytoma L. temp. pariet.
R. hemiparesis & hemianopsia.

10.

CASE NO. 86. Tho G., aged 54.
R. Parietal meningioma.

Fig. 13.—Drawings of Patients with Organic Mental States.
Response to " Draw a House ".

1. Compare with No. 1 of children's drawings (Fig. 12).
2. Compare with No. 2 of children's drawings (Fig. 12).   A = drawing-
   room; C = dining-room; B, D = bedrooms.
3. A represents chimney; B, a window; D, the door.
4. Formerly secretary and expert shorthand typist.
6. Note line of path in relation to door.
7. A represents the door; B, windows, but drawing is tri-dimensional.
8. There was no visual inattention (R) or heminopia in this case. Compare
   with No. 7 of children's drawings (Fig. 12).
9 and 10. Illustrate right and left visual inattention respectively.

181

development. In the first they are capable only of scribbling. In the second they are unable to assemble different parts of an object to form a coherent whole. For example, in drawing a house they represent the rooms separately as they come to mind. In the third stage the child represents in his drawing not only what he is able to see but what he knows the object may contain. Thus, a house may be drawn complete with chimney, windows and door, but a chair, table or person may be represented within it. In the fourth or final stage perspective is developed. These points are brought out in the examples shown in the illustrations and as can be seen the same devices are adopted by patients with organic mental states, especially global cerebral affections, with which loss of capacity for abstract orientation and constructional apraxia are commonly associated.

Map drawing, or getting the patient to mark the position of well-known places on an outline map of Ireland or the British Isles, was another method adopted for showing up abstract disorientation. Mistakes were often made in placing coastal towns inland. Patients suffering from right-left disorientation placed well-known towns on the wrong side of the map. Patients with unilateral visual inattention also tended to neglect the side upon which their visual defect was present and marked places all on the same side, on the right or the left as the case might be (see Fig. 14).

DISTURBANCES OF CORPOREAL AWARENESS

Normal, healthy persons are aware of the chief parts of their bodies and of the spatial relationships of these to each other. Out of these constituents they create what has been called a " body-scheme " (Head) or " body image " (Schilder). Although they may never consciously have attempted to examine this, in health they are capable of doing so and of knowing not only the parts that make up their body, but of distinguishing it from that of other persons, and from the outer world. Head believed that the parietal cortex acted as a " storehouse " of past impressions and that as a result of past experience, various " schemata " were formed and retained there. More recently, Gooddy and Reinhold[159] have emphasized the probable functional significance of body symmetry, the two halves of the body, although anatomically joined, behaving as separate entities. They suggest that "streams of afferent impulses from one-half of the body and formed into complex motor patterns by the cortex are contrasted by the mind (at conscious and unconscious levels) with the motion patterns from the other half of the body ". Orientation in space is achieved " by means of his (the subject's) knowledge of one-half of the body in relation to the other, of the position of one portion of a limb in relation to the other parts". Space, itself, is thought to be a product of the mind and dependent entirely on multiple contrasts and comparisons from these motion patterns, as they are received.

A year or two after birth an infant can identify his mouth, nose, eyes and ears. At 3-4 years he knows his thumb and possibly his little finger. Subsequent acquisition of motor skills is dependent on the sensory apparatus. The body is disposed in the vertebrate pattern along

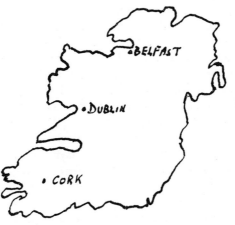

Fig. 14.—Right-sided Visual Inattention

Case No. 41. Right-sided visual inattention with right homonymous hemianopsia

a longitudinal axis from which are derived the symmetrical projections which form the arms, legs and other structures. This symmetrical arrangement, which has a bearing on the capacity for body orientation, is also seen in the nervous system with its two cerebral hemispheres, the one mirroring the other in form and structure, and in the figure of eight arrangement of crossed ascending and descending fibres. The sensory tracts, conveying the data upon which an individual depends in orienting himself traverse and synapse in the ventral nucleus of the thalamus, before passing cephalically to terminate in the region of the supramarginal gyrus of the parietal cortex.

Gerstmann's syndrome.

Jospeh Gerstmann[215] is generally credited with having been the first to describe the symptom complex of: (1) inability to distinguish between right and left, (2) finger agnosia, (3) inability to write spontaneously or from dictation and (4) dyscalculia. Gerstmann's patients could copy, but subsequent reports, Stengel,[215] have shown that constructional apraxia is often seen in association with the syndrome, and, this being so, one would expect copying difficulties often to be encountered.

Gerstmann related these signs to a lesion (vascular or neoplastic) in the dominant hemisphere, affecting the parieto-occipital area. Since then considerable support has been given to this contention and especially of the relation of the syndrome to the dominant hemisphere. Other signs sometimes found in association are contralateral hemianopic defects and loss of opto-kinetic nystagmus. Gerstmann found no evidence in his cases of disturbance of general consciousness, but this has not been our experience for in the majority some general disturbances of cerebral function have been elicited. All the organic mental patients in our series were tested routinely for R–L disorientation and the other signs when conditions permitted and, allowing for certain instances in which notes were inadequate and others in which the signs were too inconstant or fragmentary to be convincing, there were eighteen patients in whom some or all of Gerstmann's signs could be demonstrated. In analysing these we have considered chiefly: the character of the signs, nature of the underlying lesion and how often these signs were seen alone or in association with other emotional and intellectual disturbances.

As Table 9 shows, R–L disorientation and finger agnosia were found in all but 2 of the 18 cases. In only seven cases, however, were all 4 signs present. One case (No. 87) showed only dysgraphia and dyscalculia, 2 (Nos. 69, 92) only R–L disorientation and finger agnosia. Of the remainder, some showed only R–L disorientation, finger agnosia and dyscalculia.

According to Gesell[213] ability to distinguish between right and left is acquired between the ages of 5–8 years. Mentally retarded children may not develop it until later, or they may reach adult status without ever acquiring the sense. It is necessary to bear this in mind when testing for the sign, but none of our accepted cases fell into this category. Affective influences must also be taken into account for in many persons the knowledge of right and left is implicit and they may never have been called upon to demonstrate it deliberately. The well-known example of the recruit turning right instead of left at the word of command illustrates this point, and we found that it was easy to confuse brain-injured persons, when questions were put too rapidly or peremptorily. This applied especially to patients in whom emotional tension, anxiety to please and desire to conceal their defects were pronounced. With moods of unconcern or indifference, one had to contend with the same kind of response that was often seen in testing memory for past events. To the question: " Show me your left arm!" the patient might hold up his right arm and, when corrected and his left arm shown to him, remark: " If you say it is my left arm, I suppose it must be." To distinguish here between the effects of emotional indifference, lowered motivation due to generalized brain affection and true disorientation was always difficult and the point as a rule could only be settled by repeated examination. The co-existence of weakness or sensory impairment on one side added further complications to the difficulty of deciding that genuine R–L disorientation was present.

The same applies to testing for *finger agnosia*. Some people, although they can identify their thumb and little finger, have no preconceived way of referring to their index, middle and ring fingers. Nomenclature varies, some speaking of them in this way, others referring to them as the first, second and third, or second, third and fourth fingers. Allowance must be made for these natural variations before applying tests. As regards these, Critchley[69] recommends (1) telling the patient to point to or hold up different fingers in turn, (2) to name the various fingers when they are touched and, (3) to point to different fingers on the examiner's hand. Other more elaborate tests may be used. Case No. 92 (cerebral thrombosis), which may be selected as typical, was an intelligent man of 60, who had been a works foreman. Mood and behaviour were perfectly natural in his case, but he had some difficulty in registering, memory had been falling off in the previous five years, and there was some expressive speech difficulty. The latter, however, was not sufficiently pronounced to affect his ability to name fingers and he had no difficulty in understanding spoken speech, although reading bothered him. Apart from some disorientation in time he was otherwise fully orientated both at concrete and abstract levels, and he showed no evidence of constructional apraxia or of perseveration.

His responses to questions relating to R–L orientation varied. Some days he had no difficulty, other days even after repeated trials, he could not get the correct answers. So anxious was he to succeed that (when we were not in the ward) he would practise by himself or get other patients to test him. As regards his fingers, he never had any difficulty in recognising the thumb and little finger. But, although he knew the names of the other fingers he made repeated mistakes. Thus, when the examiner touched the left ring finger, he said it was the right middle finger. Similarly he declared that the forefinger was the middle finger.

Agraphia or dysgraphia was present in 10 cases. It varied from complete inability to write, the pen being held in an apraxic fashion (see p. 154), to difficulty in forming letters (literal agraphia) and words

TABLE 9.—*Gerstmann's syndrome in organic mental states* (18 cases)

Case No. Handed	R–L disorientn.	Finger agnosia	Dysgraphia	Dyscalculia	Chief clinical features and nature of lesion
92 (R.)	+	+	—	—	Right hemiparesis and homonymous hemianopia. Naming difficulties c. periphrasis. Dyslexia (literal). Systemic hypertension. L. cerebral thrombosis.
175 (R.)	+	+	—	+	Left homonymous hemianopia. Dyslexia (literal). CO poisoning: anoxic encephalopathy.
26 (R.)	+	+	+	+	Naming difficulties. Dyslexia (semantic). Chronic amnesic syndrome. Presenile dementia—diffuse cortical atrophy.
107 (R.)	+	—	—	?	Spastic paraparesis c̄ extensor plantar reflexes, dysarthria (spastic). Increased emotional lability. Signs old L. hemiplegia. Pseudobulbar palsy and presenile dementia.
60 (R.)	+	+	+	?	R. hemianopia and visual inattention. Dyslexia (semantic). Chronic amnesic syndrome. Diffuse cortical atrophy.
23 (R.)	+	+	+	+	Generalized increase of tone in skeletal muscles (rigidity and mask-like facies.) Presenile dementia–diffuse cortical atrophy.
104 (R.)	+	+	+	+	No neurological signs. Presenile dementia–diffuse cortical atrophy.
29 (R.)	+	+	+	+	"Ataxic", but more apraxic gait. Plantars equivocal, both ? extensor. ? right visual inattention but not confirmed. Dyslexia (semantic). Presenile dementia (diffuse atrophy).

Case					Clinical notes
74 (L.)	+	+	−	+	Choreiform movements. Chronic amnesic syndrome. Family history positive. E.E.G. low amplitude record throughout. Huntington's chorea.
87 (R.)	−	−	+	+	Papilloedema. R. lower facial weakness. R. quadrantic hemianopia. Dyslexia (verbal). Naming difficulties c̄ periphrasis. Left frontal astrocytoma.
130 (R.)	+	+	+	+	Ataxic paresis R. hand and arm. No sensory loss except for impaired tactile sense over R. hand. Naming difficulties c̄ periphrasis. L. int. carotid stenosis.
69 (R.)	+	+	−	?	Plantars extensor. Naming difficulties. Cortical blindness. Temp. cardiac arrest—anoxic encephalopathy.
43 (R.)	+	+	?	+	Right hemiparesis. Prolonged clouding of consciousness, disorientation. Anoxic encephalopathy (carbon monoxide).
125 (R.)	+	+	−	+	Atonic paralysis R. arm c̄ sensory impairment. No hemianopia but right visual inattention. Temp. cardiac arrest—anoxic encephalopathy.
121 (R.)	+	+	+	+	Chronic amnesic syndrome. No neurological signs. Early Alzheimer's disease.
57 (R.)	+	+	−	+	Ataxic or dyspraxic gait. Plantars extensor. Doubtful R. visual inattention, not confirmed. Marked dyslexia (literal). Naming difficulties. Presenile dementia (diffuse atrophy).
50 (R.)	+	+	+	+	Papilloedema. Paresis R. arm. R. homonymous hemianopia. L. parieto-occipital astrocytoma.
90 (R.)	+	+	−	+	Papilloedema. R. upper quadrantic hemianopia and R. visual inattention. Paresis of R. face and arm c̄ cortical type sensory impairment. Dysphasia. Multiple metastases from primary bronchial carcinoma.

(verbal agraphia). In the last-named variety there were numerous spelling mistakes, use of wrong tenses and a tendency often seen, to leave out words, substitute wrong letters or transpose letters in words. The dysgraphia observed in Case No. 50, a right-handed man with a left parieto-occipital astrocytoma, conformed to the description given by Gerstmann: he was quite unable to write spontaneously or from dictation, but had no difficulty in copying letters and words. There was no associated contructional apraxia, but so great was his writing difficulty, that he could not even sign his name. In case, No. 130 (left internal carotid stenosis), writing had to be done with the left hand. In trying to write his name the prefix " Mr " was placed out of line, above and to the left of the first name " Robert ", some of the letters of which were correctly formed, others not (Fig. 15). In writing from dictation he transposed letters and tended to print them mirrorwise, e.g.

TAƆ for CAT

In this case, despite an associated constructional apraxia, there was no difficulty in copying from print.

In Case No. 87—left frontal astrocytoma—" tremendous difficulty in writing " had been remarked at an early stage in the illness. Actually, voluntary power and co-ordination in the right hand were not affected until a much later stage. He could form letters and words but, despite

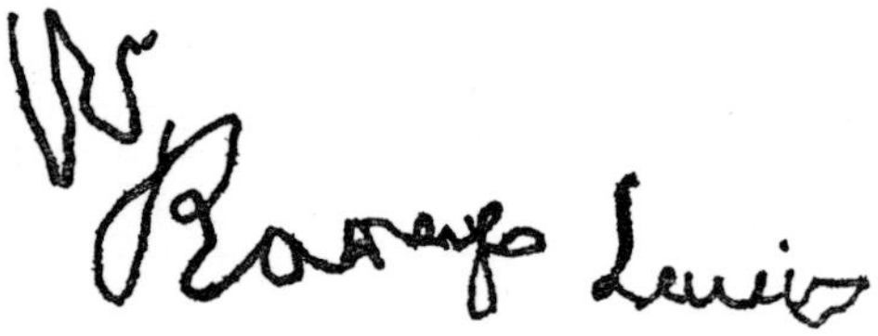

Fig. 15.—Left Internal Carotid Stenosis
Case No. 130. Writing, with left hand, in response to: " Write your name ".

a good educational background, made frequent spelling errors and much of his composition was spoiled by his substitution of other letters for the correct ones. For example, he wrote: " four mounts " when he meant " four months "; " I felt that place " when he meant " I left that place ". In writing from dictation his lines sagged so much to the right as to impede his completing lines further down the page. In this instance, like the foregoing, constructional apraxia was marked but there was no difficulty in copying.

In another patient (Fig. 16) there was well-marked literal agraphia, letters being badly formed or unrecognizable. She had the same difficulty with arithmetical symbols and with digits and was unable to copy. There was also an associated constructional apraxia.

Dyscalculia, amounting to inability to do simple sums was seen in 13 cases. Case No. 87, referred to above, performed " 9 — 3 " correctly, but " 16 — 9 " puzzled him and finally he answered " 6 ". He affirmed with confidence that " 9 × 7 = 72 " and " 8 × 4 = 60 ", changing the latter answer a moment later to " 64 ". In attempting

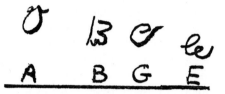

Fig. 16.—Presenile Dementia (Alzheimer's Disease)
Case No. 121. Response to: " Write or make an 'A', 'B', 'G', 'E'."

written sums he wore an air of intense concentration but made mistakes in simple addition and subtraction and was quite unable to divide. He recognized arithmetical symbols, aligned figures correctly for addition, but in trying to multiply, said that he: " couldn't really think how it was done." In case No. 121, also referred to above, the difficulty in calculation stemmed from inability to write arithmetical symbols. Thus, when told to make a " 7 " or a " 2 " she could not do so, but when she was shown figures could recognize them at once and copy them. However, this was not her only difficulty for in mental arithmetic she was unable to add " 2 + 3 " correctly and subtraction was quite beyond her. Case Nos. 74 and 26 had the same difficulty in forming symbols. In case No. 57 the significance of +, —, ×, ÷ was not recognized.

Lesions found in Gerstmann's syndrome.

Table 9 shows that in 2 cases focal cerebral vascular lesions were present, which probably involved the parieto-occipital cortex of the dominant hemisphere. In 2 cases there were solitary tumours, one frontal and the other parieto-occipital, again both being in the dominant hemisphere. Case No. 90 had multiple cerebral metastases from a primary bronchial carcinoma, but clinical evidence pointed to at least one of these being in the parieto-occipital region of the dominant hemisphere. In the remainder the evidence suggested that both sides of the brain were affected. In case Nos. 23, 26, 29, 69, 74, 104, 121, there were no focal neurological signs and the results of air encephalography and other tests had failed to demonstrate any evidence of a focal lesion. In case Nos. 43, 57, 60, 107, 125, 175, in addition to signs pointing to bilateral cerebral cortical atrophy, there were indications of a focal lesion involving either the left or the right hemisphere.

Case No. 50 (the patient with an astrocytoma in the left parieto-occipital region) was the only one that answered to the classical description, both clinically and anatomically. He had all 4 signs and neurological examination was otherwise negative except for papill-oedema and right homonymous hemianopia. Apart from his agraphia, there was no other sign of aphasia and he could register, repeat series forwards or backwards, was fully orientated and showed no per-severation. In the other case with a tumour (No. 87) (see also p. 156) and confined strictly to the left frontal lobe—herniation of the brain was evident at post-mortem, and this had probably already occurred at the time dysgraphia and dyscalculia were apparent. There was some doubt about the right half of his visual field and it appears probable that dislocation downwards of the brain may have accounted for the signs, for there was no tumour tissue in either the temporal, parietal or occipital lobes.

A striking feature of the cases with focal lesions was that these invariably involved the dominant hemisphere. Indeed, a search made through our case material failed to bring to light any example of part or whole of the syndrome being present with a focal lesion in the non-dominant hemisphere. Thus, in one patient, a left-handed man with a left temporo-parietal astrocytoma, there was no trace either of dysphasia or of bodily disorientation, and this observation is in accord with that of Hermann and Pötzl,[217] who reported a Gertstmann's syndrome due to a tumour in the right parieto-occipital region, but the patient was ambidextrous and the right hemisphere probably dominant.

Occasionally, despite the presence of an appropriately-situated lesion in the dominant hemisphere Gerstmann's syndrome could not be demonstrated. Such was the case in a right-handed man aged 64, who was admitted to hospital after a stroke and found to have right hemi-plegia, hemianaesthesia, a homonymous quadrantic field defect and dysphasia.

A week or so later speech had recovered sufficiently to enable him to express himself without much difficulty, and comprehension was unaffected. Mood was appropriate to the situation but he showed no undue anxiety, increased emotional lability or catastrophic reactions. There was no perseveration, he was able to register and was fully orientated in time and place. On testing him repeatedly at this time for signs of bodily disorientation and finger agnosia his answers consistently showed that these symptoms were absent. He knew that his right side was paralysed and that he had no feeling in it, but as the case notes state: " no amount of questioning will get him to alter his opinion in these matters " i.e. in relation to right and left and his fingers. Some months later he died and post-mortem examination confirmed the presence of an organising thrombosis in the left posterior cerebral artery, which had caused posterior parietal and occipital infarction, the ipsilateral thalamus and cerebral peduncle also showing softening.

It could be argued that the focal lesion in this case was too posterior to give rise to characteristic defects in lateralization, or that it was so extensive that it masked any such defects. But the latter is improbable because at the time observations were made speech had largely been recovered and there was no clouding of consciousness. Originally, Gerstmann stated that his syndrome occurred in the absence of any general clouding of consciousness and this may have prompted neurologists to discount its significance when this has been present. However, right–left disorientation and finger agnosia may sometimes be demonstrated in otherwise healthy subjects recovering consciousness after anoxia, Allison.[91] Juba,[218] Benton and Abramson[219] have described them as not infrequent transient phenomena after electric shock treatment.

When our 18 cases of Gerstmann's syndrome were reviewed it became evident (Table 10) that the greater proportion showed signs of clouding of consciousness at the time the syndrome was present. Thus, alterations in mood and behaviour were seen in 10 cases, 8 showed defective insight, 13 had difficulty in registration and only 3 could be said to be fully orientated. The great frequency of constructional apraxia will also be noted. These findings do not detract from the value of the syndrome in recognition of parietal disease of the dominant hemisphere. But we think that without any accompanying signs of clouding of consciousness it is of rare occurrence, and that these same signs play some part in its elaboration, besides helping to bring it into prominence.

Denial syndromes associated with body unawareness.

More gross and bizarre disturbances of body awareness are usually associated with parietal lesions of the minor or subordinate hemisphere. This preference may be due to higher thought processes being disturbed to such an extent in lesions of the dominant hemisphere that agnosia for the opposite side of the body, although present, passes unnoticed. In minor hemisphere affections there is considerably less derangement of thought so that agnosia for the opposite side is more likely to be apparent.

TABLE 10.

Case No. handed	Mood behaviour	Insight	Registratn.	Series	Perseveratn.	Memory
92 (R)	✓	✓	+ −	+ −	✓	+
175 (R)	+	+	+	+	+	+
26 (R)	+	+	+ −	+ −	+	+
107 (R)	?	?	?	?	?	+
60 (R)	+	+	+	+	?	+
23 (R)	+	+	+	+	+	+
104 (R)	+	✓	+ −	+	+	+
29 (R)	+	✓	+ −	+ −	?	+
74 (L)	✓	✓	+	+	?	+
87 (R)	✓	✓	✓	✓	✓	✓
130 (R)	✓	✓	+ −	+ −	+	✓
69 (R)	+	+	+ −	+ −	+	+
43 (R)	+	+	?	?	+	+
125 (R)	✓	+	?	+	+	+
121 (R)	+	+	+	+	+	+
57 (R)	✓	✓	+ −	✓	✓	+
50 (R)	✓	✓	✓	?	✓	+ −
90 (R)	+	✓	+	+ −	+	+

Dysphasia	Orientatn. (Time, place persons.)	Abstract orientatn.	Agnosia*	Ideomotor apraxia	Constructal. apraxia	Case No. handed.
+	T. only	✓	✓	✓	✓	92 (R)
+	Time + place +	+	✓	+	+	175 (R)
+	T. only	+	✓	+	+	26 (R)
✓	Time + place +	?	?	?	?	107 (R)
+	Time + place +	+	?	+	+	60 (R)
+	T. only	+	+	+	+	23 (R)
✓	T. only	+	✓	✓	+	104 (R)
+	T. only	+	✓	✓	+	29 (R)
✓	T. only	+	✓	✓	+	74 (L)
+	✓	✓	✓	✓	+	87 (R)
+	✓	+ −	✓	✓	+	130 (R)
✓	Time + place +	?	✓	✓	?	69 (R)
✓	Time + place +	+	✓	✓	+	43 (R)
✓	T. only	+	✓	✓	+	125 (R)
✓	T. only	+	✓	+	+	121 (R)
+	T. only	+	✓	✓	+	57 (R)
✓	✓	✓	✓	✓	✓	50 (R)
+	Time + place +	+	✓	✓	+	90 (R)

* Other agnosias i.e., visual object, colour, tactile, auditory

The patient may be unaware of one side of his body and when shown his arm deny that it belongs to him. There is often also denial of illness, i.e. of hemiplegia, blindness (Anton's syndrome). Many such cases have been reported in the literature: Ives and Nielsen,[220] Ehrenwald[221] and are to be found in Schilder's[189] monograph on the subject. Lesser degrees of the same thing, patients being aware of their hemiplegia but attaching no importance to it, treating it with indifference, were described by Babinski[223] who applied the term " anosodiaphoria " to the condition. These disturbances may arise either from lesions interrupting sensory tracts or damaging the parietal receiving centres. Important as are the latter, lesions at lower levels may have the same effect, a fact of which we had convincing proof some years ago. The case was that of a man who had been brought to hospital with a minor head injury. Examination revealed nothing remarkable but the surgeon thought it prudent to keep him under observation and placed him on a couch behind a screen. Within a few minutes he called out that there was somebody lying beside him, and on being questioned seemed convinced that his left arm and leg belonged to another person. Shortly afterwards he became stuporose and passed swiftly into coma and died. At post-mortem there was massive haemorrhage into the pons. It appeared probable that the latter was responsible for the disturbance of corporeal awareness and that this had been the initial symptom of the pontine haemorrhage.

Disturbances of corporeal awareness may occur occasionally without there being any focal lesion and a good example of this was seen in the patient with the bizarre illusion that he was wearing two pairs of pyjama trousers and that he possessed two pair of hands and two bowels (p. 24). In the other 5 cases in which gross disturbances of body awareness were seen there were focal signs pointing to a lesion of the right parietal area (Table 11).

Critchley[69] suggests that the occurrence of these symptoms depends chiefly on (1) abruptness of onset of the cerebral lesion, (2) the clarity or otherwise of the sensorium and (3) the question as to whether motor weakness is present or not. Sensory impairment and paralysis are undoubtedly strong contributory factors but we believe that the second condition is even more important, it being rare to find cases in which there is not some coexistent clouding of consciousness. As full consciousness is regained disturbances of the body image tend to disappear, despite the persistence of sensory loss and paralysis. This was well illustrated in a right-handed woman aged 68, who had had a stroke with resulting left hemiplegia. The paralysed limbs were completely toneless on passive movement and there was considerable hemisensory impairment. Although pinprick could be detected it was not felt so acutely as on the right side. Light touch was lost and she was unaware of passive movements at the left wrist and fingers. When

TABLE 11.—*Gross disturbances of body awareness*

Case No. handed	Nature of disturbance	Chief neurological signs: lesion
33 ♂, aged 69 (R.)	Denied that there was anything the matter with the paralysed left side; claimed that he was in hospital for tonsillitis and, when shown his left arm, said it was his right.	L. hemiplegia c. sensory impairment and homonymous hemianopia. Painful stimuli to both sides were only recognized on right. Perseveration +. Incontinent. Plantars flexor. (R. cerebral thrombosis.)
81 ♀, aged 76 (R.)	Insisted for some days that the left arm did not belong to her. Later complained bitterly of severe pains in left arm, and feeling as if wearing a glove.	L. hemiparesis c. extensive hemisensory loss for touch and pain, less for postural sensibility. Sensory ataxia, pronounced on left side. No hemianopia. (R. cerebral thrombosis.)
54 ♀, aged 68 (R.)	see pp. 194–197	see pp. 194–197
112 ♂, aged 73 (R.)	Wondered to whom his left arm belonged because he could not feel anything when he touched it. Later claimed that it was a " temporary " arm, which someone had put in his bed, so that he could do exercises with it. (4–6 weeks.)	L. hemiplegia c̄. extensive hemisensory loss and especially marked loss of joint postural sensibility affecting his appreciation of movement at elbow and shoulder joints. No hemianopia. (R. cerebral thrombosis.)
123 ♀, aged 73 (R.)	see p. 198	see p. 198

her eyes were closed she could not find the left hand in space with the unaffected right hand, and it was noticed that she invariably groped farther over to the left than the actual position of the limb required her to do. There was also a defect in the left half visual field. But signs were not wholly unilateral: there was a grasp reflex on the right side at times, both plantars were extensor, she was incontinent and there was some expressive and receptive dysphasia.

At first she lay inert, picking at the bedclothes and yawning frequently. When spoken to she would reply, but her talk was mostly exclamatory or rambling and her mood fatuous and tearful. Although able to give her name and address, she was incapable of registering and had little or no memory for recent events. Perseveration was marked. Within 72 hours it was noticed that she was more wakeful, although she paid no attention to the hemiplegia. Then about the sixth or seventh day the nurses heard her crying out that there was a baby beside her in bed and that they ought to take it away.

Later, when the paralysed limb was held so that she could see it with the undamaged half of her visual field, repeatedly, day after day, she denied that it was her arm and insisted that it belonged to the examiner. When asked to try and hold up her left arm, she held up her right. She could identify her left and right ears and nose, but when asked to point to her left eye, pointed to the right. Despite these defects she could tell her right side from her left and name the fingers of her right hand.

About a month after her admission Dr. Claudia Blagden, house physician at the time, recorded the following conversation:

Q. " How are you, Mrs. W—?"
A. " Very well . . . feeling very well, thank you."
Q. " Is there anything wrong with you?"
A. " Nothing wrong with arms."
Q. " Move them for me!"
A. (Patient lifted only the right arm.)
Q. " Where is the other one?"
A. (Patient points to her left arm.)
Q. " Is there anything wrong with the left arm?"
A. " No."
Q. " Why are you not moving it?"
A. " Not using the left because I'm well used with using the right . . . my husband says it never rests, morning, noon or night . . ."
     (Examiner holds up the patient's arm (left) so that she can see it.)
Q. " Whose arm is this?"
A. " That's your arm."
Q. " Think carefully, Mrs. W—, which arm is it?"
A. " The left arm."
Q. " Now tell me what's wrong with it?"
A. " Neuritis."
Q. " Whose arm is it?"
A. " Mine."
     (After an interval.)
Q. " Which leg is this (holding up left leg)?"
A. " Your own."
Q. " Are you sure?"
A. " Yes."
Q. " Why do you think it's mine?"
A. " Because I don't feel it."

At this time denial of the left half of the body and of her illness was becoming less pronounced. The inconsistencies in her replies to questions relating to these were strongly reminiscent of those given by disorientated patients recovering consciousness after anoxia and head injury. The upshot was seen when she was readmitted for review 5 months later. There was no vestige of recovery of motor function in the arm or leg and sensory impairment was the same, as was the left-sided visual inattention. Despite these signs, however, she exhibited none of the former disturbance of body awareness. Insight was now good, she was orientated in place and time, could register fresh data and was no longer incontinent. The right extensor plantar response and grasp reflex had disappeared.

In this case the disturbance of body awareness and anosognosia flourished at a period when there was marked general spatial and temporal disorientation, perseveration, defective registration, expressive dysphasia and emotional changes, and the signs faded away as the level of consciousness rose, despite persistence of hemiplegia and gross sensory impairment.

Weinstein and Kahn[244] suggest that strong perfectionist drives in the pre-morbid personality and temperament of these patients may influence their reactions to hemiplegia and sensory loss. Normally such tendencies do not overstep the boundaries of reality, but in the presence of appropriately placed lesions and clouding of consciousness they may be brought to the surface. These authors have actually been able to induce transient disturbances of body imagery in hemiplegic patients by the use of sodium amytal.[225] Two of our cases may be mentioned. Both were highly intelligent women who had formerly been noted for their extreme conscientiousness and exactitude in all their daily transactions.

The first, R. K., aged 46, had sustained a right hemiplegia, sensory impairment and other disabilities as the result of a thrombosis in the dominant hemisphere. Her abnormal eye movements during attempts at reading have already been described (p. 161). After recovering sufficiently to make detailed examination possible, it was noted that she displayed a persistent hypercritical and gloomy attitude towards her paralysed right arm. For the leg, however, which was similarly affected, she showed little or no concern. Repeatedly she declared that the arm was useless and likely to remain so, and would demand " why not get rid of it?" As it was thought this remark had been made facetiously, it was not taken seriously. But, week by week, her mental state deteriorated, the depression increasing and suicidal thoughts becoming apparent. Her intense despair was frequently interrupted by bouts of acute agitation, when she would weep uncontrollably and rail at the futility of going on any longer. The depressive symptoms were, indeed, so pronounced that we considered giving her electric shock treatment, or even performing a leucotomy. Gradually, however, over the following year the depression lifted and was replaced by a steady mood of ironical good humour, which persisted until her death.

The other case, G. P., a single woman of 73, who before her retirement had held a responsible post in the Inland Revenue, was also right-handed. She presented with the same picture of hemiplegia, sensory impairment and hemianopia, but in her case all the signs were left-sided and due to a lesion of the subordinate hemisphere. Three months after a stroke she was still disorientated in time and place, and shewed other signs of clouding of consciousness. Her restlessness and irritability knew no bounds. Persistently incontinent of urine and faeces, she had to be kept in a cot with the bars raised to prevent her trying to get out of bed. Bed-clothes were constantly soiled with excrement and it was impossible to keep them in place for no sooner was her bed made up than she disarranged them again. She wore a tense worried expression and was repeatedly observed smacking her left hand with her right and admonishing it much in the same way as one would a naughty child. When asked about this she replied peevishly that her left hand would not do what she told it; it would move of its own accord and this was her reason for trying to control it.* Each time it moved she would arrest its progress abruptly by seizing it with her sound hand and on one occasion when the left hand was grasping the rail of her cot, she was seen belabouring it frantically in her efforts to tear it free and calling out at it, as if she were addressing another person. However, she did not deny that it was part of her person and no persistent grasp reflex could be obtained. As in the other case these symptoms did not herald a progressive dementia because after several months all traces of them had disappeared and she was able to return home, where she remained reasonably adjusted until her death some years later. There was no recovery, however, from the hemiplegia and sensory loss.

Discussing these curious phenomena, Critchley[227] notes that hemiplegic patients may show a diversity of attitudes towards their disability:

(1) They may apparently be unaware of it or only admit it grudgingly.

(2) They may deny ownership of the paralysed limbs or suggest that they belong to some other person.

---

* A similar observation is reported by Hécaen *et al.*[226] in the case of a man, who had had a right parietal cortical excision on account of recurring fits: "with eyes closed, while trying to think of what his left hand looked like, the patient said that his left hand seemed to be moving towards the right side of his body. . . ."

(3) They may exhibit morbid revulsion towards the limbs; an " almost insane hatred couched in exaggerated language " (misoplegia), or they may attempt to conceal the limb.

(4) They may display morbid concern and feeling for the paralysed limb, " looking upon it as a cherished pet or plaything—an integral part of the body schema. . . ." This phenomenon he has termed " personification ". Nicknames often are attached, to which the patient refers as if he were speaking about another person.

As regards the meaning of these attitudes, Critchley is unwilling to implicate any particular pre-morbid personality or temperament and attaches more importance to the rôle played by intellectual deficit and inadequate insight. Having followed some of these cases over a period of years we are inclined to agree. Persistent attitudes of this kind must be extremely rare.

In conclusion, it may be said that, although disorientation in time and place was a common symptom in organic mental states, it had little diagnostic significance to the site of the lesion, being more a manifestation simply of clouding of consciousness. However, there was some relation between severity of the disorientation and the extent of cerebral damage, disorientation for persons not being seen with purely focal lesions and being more indicative of diffuse cerebral disease. Many patients, although correctly orientated in the concrete sense, displayed abstract spatial and temporal disorientation and of especial value in the recognition of the former were drawing tests. In their drawings these patients exhibited the same tendencies as young children in being unable to acquire correct perspective.

Gerstmann's syndrome was noted in 18 patients. In some of these there were focal lesions in the parieto-occipital region of the dominant hemisphere. No instance was encountered of the lesion being limited to the minor hemisphere, but it was common to find, additional to neurological signs of a focal lesion in the dominant hemisphere, others pointing to bilateral disease, and in a few cases definite signs of a focal lesion were lacking. It was also noted that fragments of the syndrome might sometimes be elicited in anoxic subjects and that occasionally appropriately-placed lesions did not give rise to it. As most of our patients showed some signs of clouding of consciousness at the time the features were demonstrable it is concluded that this must play some part in their elaboration, as well as assisting in their clinical recognition.

More pronounced disturbances affecting the body image as a whole were seen in 7 cases, one of which had a pontine lesion and another simply acute clouding of consciousness of toxaemic origin. In the remainder a focal lesion in the subordinate hemisphere was responsible, but here again the dependence to some extent of the symptoms on clouding of consciousness is remarked. Two cases are described in which strong perfectionist tendencies in the premorbid personality appeared to determine abnormal behaviour in the face of hemiplegia.

BIBLIOGRAPHY

202 HÉCAEN, H., ANGELERGUES, R., BERNHARDT, C. and CHIARELLI, J. (1957). Essai de distinction des modalitiés cliniques de l'agnosie des physionomies. *Rev. Neurol.*, **96**, 125.

203 BRAIN, W. R. (1941). Visual disorientation with special reference to lesions of the right cerebral hemisphere. *Brain*, **64**, 244.

204 PATERSON, A. and ZANGWILL, O. L. (1944). Disorders of visual space perception associated with lesions of the right cerebral hemisphere. *Brain*, **67**, 331.

205 KENNEDY, F. and WOLF, A. (1936). The relationship of intellect to speech defect in aphasic patients. *J. nerv. ment. Dis.*, **84**, 125.

206 GUNZBERG, H. C. (1950). The significance of various aspects in drawings by educationally subnormal children. *J. ment. Sci.*, **96**, 951.

207 ENG, H. (1931). " The Psychology of Children's Drawings." Int. Liter, of Psych. Philosoph, and Scient. methods. Trans. from Norwegian by Hatfield, H. S. Kegan Paul, London.

208 CLAPARÈDE, E. (1907). Plan d'expériences collectives sur le dessin des enfants. *Arch. de Psychol.*, 276.

209 LUQUET, G. H. (1913). " Les Dessins d'un Enfant." Paris.

210 OAKLEY, C. A. (1931). The interpretation of children's drawings. *Brit. J. Psychol.*, **21**, 256.

211 AYER, F. C. (1916). " The Psychology of Drawing." Warwick and York, Baltimore.

212 KERR, M. (1937). Children's drawings of houses. *Brit. J. Med. Psychol.*, **16**, 206.

213 GESELL, A. (1946). " Infant Development. The First Years of Life." Methuen, London. " The Child From Five to Ten." Hamish Hamilton. London.

214 GERSTMANN, J. (1940). Syndrome of finger agnosia, disorientation for right and left, agraphia and acalculia. *Arch. Neurol. Psychiat.*, **44**, 398.

215 GERSTMANN, J. (1924). Fingeragnosie: Eine umschriebene Störung der Orientierung am eigenen Körper. *Wien. klin. Wschr.*, **40**, 1010.

216 STENGEL, E. (1944). Loss of spatial orientation, constructional apraxia and Gerstmann's syndrome. *J. ment. Sci.*, **90**, 753.

217 HERMANN, G. and PÖTZL, O. (1926). " Über die Agraphie und ihre lokaldiagnostischen Beziehungen." Berlin.

218 JUBA, A. (1949). Beitrag zur Struktor der ein-und droffelseitigen Körperscheinsstörungen: Fingeragnosie, atypische anosognosien. *Monatschft. f. Psychiat. Neurol.*, **118**, 11.

219 BENTON, A. C. and ABRAMSON, L. S. (1952). Gerstmann symptoms following electroshock treatment. *Arch. Neurol. Psychiat.*, **68**, 248.

220 IVES, E. R. and NIELSEN, J. M. (1937). Disturbance of body scheme: Delusion of absence of part of body in two cases with autopsy verification of the lesions. *Bull. Los Angeles Neurol. Soc.*, **2**, 120.

221 EHRENWALD, H. (1931). Anosognosie und Depersonalization. Ein Beitrag zur Psychologie der linksseitig Hemiplegischen. *Nervenarzt*, **4**, 681.

222 SCHILDER, P. (1935). " The Image and Appearance of the Human Body." London.

223 BABINSKI, J. (1914). Contribution à l'étude des troubles mentaux dans l'hemiplégie organique cérébrale (anosognosie). *Rev. Neurol.*, **1**, 845. Quoted by Critchley, M. (227).

224 WEINSTEIN, E. A. and KAHN, R. L. (1953). Personality factors in denial of illness. *Arch. Neurol. Psychiat.*, **69**, 355.

225 WEINSTEIN, E. A. and KAHN, R. L. (1950). The syndrome of anosognosia. *Arch. Neurol. Psychiat.*, **64**, 772.

226 HÉCAEN, H., PENFIELD, W., BERTRAND, C. and MALMO, R. (1956). The syndrome of apractognosia due to lesions of the minor cerebral hemisphere. *Arch. Neurol. Psychiat.*, **75**, 400.

227 CRITCHLEY, M. (1957). Observations on anosodiaphoria. *Encéphale*, 5-6, 540.

CHAPTER X

Agnosia and Apraxia

To perceive an object or apprehend it with the mind involves both physiological and psychological processes and these are initiated by the arrival at the cortex of crude sensory stimuli which excite " memories of sensations derived from other sensory channels during previous experience of the object . . ." Russell Brain.[228] Memory plays an important part and agnosic and apraxic defects* may be regarded as specialized forms of memory impairment in the same way as bodily disorientation, for example, may be looked upon as a selective form of disorientation. The region essential for visual perception is the convex part of the occipital and posterior parietal cortex, for auditory perception it is the first and second temporal convolutions and for tactile perception the parietal lobe. Although one hemisphere is often " dominant " for visual and auditory perception, this is not necessarily the same as that which is dominant for speech; thus, in certain cases the right hesmisphere is dominant for visual perception and the left for speech, and vice versa. No such arrangement, however, exists for touch, tactile agnosia or astereognosis being equally liable to result from destructive lesions affecting either parietal lobe or its connections with the thalamus.

The classical teaching has been that objects, persons or things are recognized by a process of " apperception ". That is to say an orange is recognized by successive registration of its colour, shape, size, texture, these giving rise, through already existing transcortical associational pathways, to a constellation of memories which appears in conscious thought as the percept of an orange. This may be important when the purpose is to identify unfamiliar objects, but the Gestalt school maintains that to perceive it is necessary only to register a fraction of the sensory data available. It emphasizes that more important in every day activities is the ability to pick out relevant objects from their background, and disturbances of figure-background relation-

---

* Kinnier Wilson[229] defined agnosia as " failure of intellectual recognition where there is integrity of primary identification " and apraxia as " inability to perform certain subjectively purposive movements or movement complexes, with conservation of motility, of sensation, and of co-ordination ". He states that Freud (1891) suggested the word " agnosia " for defect in object recognition and that Kussmaul, Starr and Pick (1892) were the first to use the word " apraxia ", although " not in the present-day sense ".

ships are regarded as being some of the most important contributory causes of imperception. Young children do not possess this, essentially mature, faculty of distinguishing objects from their background and when shown pictures fail to " see " their meaning although they may be able to describe correctly the different objects depicted in them.

Also overshadowing traditional belief that the cerebral cortex is solely concerned in perception is recent work on the part played by the ascending reticular formation of the midbrain and diencephalon in providing pathways other than the thalamotemporal, parietal and occipital point-to-point connections, the purpose of which is to ensure general cortical alerting, Magoun,[195] and the failure of which, it is now recognized, may be responsible for alterations in consciousness.

Criticizing traditional belief that agnosia is a specific disturbance of gnostic function, Bay[231] states that: " there is no need to search for any mystical gnostic activity to be disturbed. Mind-blindness, or visual agnosia for objects, is due to an impaired primary visual system combined in most cases with general mental deterioration ". He thinks that in trying to analyse cases of dementia into their component parts, the rôle of the general mental state has been underestimated and that conversely, for theory's sake, every author has been anxious to minimize the mental deterioration of his agnosic cases. This could be true, but it is unlikely that it applies to recent observations in the literature, in most of which the general mental state has certainly been taken into account. Indeed, it is axiomatic that one should be cautious in attaching focal significance to apparent agnosic and apraxic defects in cases where there is co-existing evidence of general intellectual impairment. Bay, however, using special perimetric methods and tachistoscopic tests, was able to demonstrate in patients, in whom testing by conventional means had revealed no visual defect, that such did in fact often exist. Ettlinger,[232] whilst confirming this observation, was unable to show any correlation between the extent of such defects and the occurrence of visual agnosia, and thought it unlikely that various disorders of visual perception could be attributed to intellectual defect of a global character.

CLINICAL ASPECTS OF AGNOSIA

Impairment of memory, as has been noted, was a common feature of patients with organic mental disease. Behaviour was not disturbed to any great extent because the kind of information these patients had forgotten—names, past events and topographic details—was seldom required and should the need arise for them to remember something they could always plead that they were not interested or invent some other excuse to explain their inability to do so. Such evasions could not be used to disguise agnosic or apraxic defects, the effects on behaviour of which were much more apparent. These were observed occasionally at an early stage in the development of a chronic organic mental illness, e.g. Alzheimer's disease, but in the great majority of chronic amnesic patients it was remarkable how often such signs were absent, memories connected with every day visual, auditory and tactile sensations being preserved until relatively late in their deterioration. Indeed, the clinical impression was formed that when either agnosia or apraxia were prominent features in a patient, the onset of whose mental symptoms had been sudden and recent, one should suspect a global disturbance of brain function, due to some toxic cause, e.g. drugs, hypoglycaemia, anoxie, hepatic encephalopathy. The comparative freedom of chronic amnesic patients from these defects was very striking and we have attributed it to the fact that perceptual activities (once they have been learned and their pattern well-established through constant use) become automations for the exercise of which no conscious effort of recall is necessary.

Tactile agnosia. A number of patients with focal vascular or neoplastic lesions involving the parietal area were unable to recognize by touch the nature of objects placed in the contralateral hand, but it is only right, in view of what has been said, to mention that it was nearly always possible by careful testing to demonstrate on the affected side some evidence of sensory impairment, however slight, i.e. impairment of two-point discrimination, defective capacity for tactile localization or some difficulty in interpreting direction when fine passive movements of individual finger joints were made. Only one instance was encountered of pure unilateral tactile agnosia, although there were some cases in which it was apparent bilaterally, these being usually patients with advanced signs of intellectual deterioration and bilateral affection of the hemispheres.

Auditory agnosia is usually associated with some receptive defects in speech and with inability to recognize musical tones. As an isolated phenomenon it has been described in connection with lesions of the temporo-sphenoidal lobe of the dominant hemisphere, but if patients with gross dysphasia were excluded there was only one answering to this description. This was a young man, recovering from an acute encephalitis, which was probably of virus origin although the cause was never determined. In his case, when recovery was sufficiently advanced to make testing possible, it was found that he had no difficulty in recognizing objects by touch or by sight. Audiometry and other tests revealed no gross defect of hearing, yet he could not recognize sounds such as those made by tearing up or crumpling a piece of paper, turning on a water tap or manipulating an electric light switch. He could hear the sounds but either said he did not know what they represented or guessed at their meaning, the sounds of tearing paper and running water not being different to him. However, an unexpected loud noise produced a startle effect and he could respond appropriately to simple spoken commands and express himself in reply to simple concrete questions. For months afterwards his understanding of propositional spoken speech was affected so that, despite the fact that he was considered fit to resume work, he found it necessary to write down instructions or have them carefully repeated to him before he could fully comprehend. He was still unable to hum well-known airs from memory or to recognize tunes. Speaking on the telephone caused him particular embarrassment. None of these features could at any time be said to be constantly demonstrable. At times one had the impression he could " hear " better than at others, but being an intelligent person and his work being of a skilled nature, it was difficult for him to cover up his defect, despite his efforts to do so. Reinhold's case[233] is much better documented. She notes that her patient, who had formerly been an ardent pianist, could not recognize " The Blue Danube " waltz when it was played over to her. However, when she was asked was it a waltz she said: " Is it not the Blue Danube?" This type of response is again reminiscent of those we received from chronic amnesic patients. However, it was the persistence of a relatively isolated defect, which was as pronounced in our patient as it was in Reinhold's case, that prompted the belief that there must be a focal lesion causing it. But no proof of this was ever obtained and after a year or two the auditory dysgnosia disappeared and there have been no further symptoms of any kind.

Cortical blindness and visual object agnosia. In seven patients the features were indicative either of cortical blindness or visual agnosia, no refractive error being found and fundoscopic examination revealing no abnormality (see Table 12). Many were post-anoxic in origin and similar to the cases reported by Wechsler,[234] Von Hagen,[235] Adler[236] and others.

In examining these cases, it must be admitted, difficulty was sometimes experienced, first in distinguishing them from hysteria and second, in separating cortical blindness from visual agnosia. Thus, in one case, a woman whose symptoms had followed the surgical operation of valvotomy for mitral stenosis, consciousness was partly regained on the day after operation but on the next she complained of inability to

TABLE 12.—*Cortical blindness*

Case No. Sex Age	Aware-ness of Blind ness	Appreci-ation of light	Associated hemianopic defect	Associated visual inattention	Fundi	Pupils	Ocular move-ments
23 (♀ 54)	yes *	yes	—	—	Normal	Normal	full
47 (♂ 60)	No	Yes			Normal	React sluggishly to light. L>R no response on convergence	defective conjugate move-ments upwards
49 (♀ 68)	Yes (parti-ally)	Yes	—	+ (left)	Normal	Dilated, otherwise normal	Full
67 (♂ 41)	No	No	—	—	Some bitemporal pallor	Dilated otherwise normal	Full
120 (♂ 75)	Yes (parti-ally)	Yes	+ (right)	—	Normal	Normal	Defective conver-gence
123 (♀ 7)	No	No	—	—	At first pa-pilloedema and retinal congestion, later, nil	Dilated, unresponsive to light	no fixation, roving move-ments
124 (♀ 22)	Yes	Yes	+ (left)	—	Normal	Dilated, sluggish re-sponse to light. No response on convergence	Full
144 (♂ 56)	Yes *	Yes	—	—	? Bitemporal pallor	Normal	Defective conver-gence

* An early symptom, in Case No. 144 first noted 7 years before death

see and became greatly distressed. Those in charge of her case were inclined to think her hysterical as, indeed, seemed possible at the time but the pupils were dilated and reacted only sluggishly to light. She could tell when light was flashed in her eyes but was unable to see objects. Consciousness at that time was still clouded because she perseverated both in her actions and speech and was disorientated in time. Vision recovered within a week sufficiently to enable her to recognize objects but she was left with a permanent defect, chiefly in the left half field. A somewhat similar case was reported by François.[237]

and visual agnosia (7 cases). For case No. 123 see p. 208.

Recognition of objects by sight	Figure-background difficulties	Astereognosis	Recognition of auditory sensations	Recognition of colours	Diagnosis
Impaired +	Yes	—	—	—	Presenile dementia ? Jakob–Creutzfeld syndrome.
Impaired +	Yes	—	—	?	Post-anoxic encephalopathy.
Impaired +	Yes	—	—	—	Presenile dementia.
Absolute loss + +	No	—	—	?	Post-anoxic encephalopathy.
Impaired +	No	+	±	+	Cerebral vascular accident, post-cerebral thrombosis (left).
Absolute loss + +	No	—	—	—	Post-anoxic encephalopathy. Failed to recover consciousness. Lived 8 months in state of torsion dystonia. P.M. Widespread cerebral cortical damage.
Absolute loss + +	No	—	—	+	Post-anoxic encephalopathy.
Impaired +	Yes	—	—	?	Alzheimer's disease (confirmed at p.m.)

On the basis of the criteria referred to in Chapter III it is probable that 4 of our cases (Nos. 23, 47, 49, 144) had visual agnosia whilst in the remainder (Nos. 67, 120, 124) the features were more in keeping with cortical blindness. In case No. 47, however, some characteristics of both kinds of defect were present. Five of the 8 patients possessed some degree of awareness of their disability, in two of these (both suffering from presenile dementia) " bad eyesight " having been the first symptom to draw attention to them. Ocular movements appeared to be normal in half of the cases but it was often difficult to be sure about this because of lack of co-operation. The fact that a patient would not, or could not, fix his gaze on objects was sufficiently apparent in itself to suggest blindness, but it was difficult to persuade these patients to make voluntary movements of their eyeballs. In one instance upward and downward movements were defective, upward gaze especially being impaired, and in 2 others there was defective convergence. In all reading was impossible. In 3 there was absolute loss of visual recognition of objects, which was a constant feature from day to day, but in the 5 remaining cases objects were recognized some days but not on others. It was thought that these fluctuations in ability might be due to general fatigue effects, but whilst the performance in visual recognition varied from day to day, there was no corresponding fluctuation in recognition by touch or hearing. Case No. 23 was a good example: when required to identify by ear (e.g. water running, paper being torn up) she never had any difficulty. Indeed, with the exception of No. 123, a little girl who died some months after cardiac arrest without ever regaining consciousness (and cannot be accepted as a case of cortical blindness) perception by touch and hearing was unaffected in all these cases.

Cases No. 23, 47, 49, 144 showed marked disturbance of figure-background relationships in their inability to select relevant from irrelevant objects. Thus, when an object was held in front of a patient and he was asked to identify it, he would respond by peering intently in the general direction of the examiner, stretching out his hand exploringly, and taking another object such as a handkerchief from the latter's coat pocket. This was well illustrated in case No. 23, a woman aged 54 with presenile dementia.

When shown a large coloured piece of toilet soap (she could recognize red, blue and green) she said it was a " cover ". Not knowing what to make of this answer, she was told to point to the object, the soap being conspicuously displayed as before. Ignoring the soap, she pointed to the examiner's white coat, which was obviously what she had been referring to when she said " cover ". The piece of soap was then held to her nostrils and she was told to smell it, when she immediately declared " soap ". On another occasion she identified some objects but not others. For example, she recognized a yale key, a tulip and a daffodil. A half-crown piece, however, she said was a " watch " until it was placed in her hand, when she immediately identified it.

Affective influences may possibly play some part in determining which objects are recognized and which not, and where blindness is transient and recoverable, as in some cases of anoxia, a stage may be reached when an object may be recognized without difficulty against a plain background, but not against an assortment of different objects.

Of other signs shown by these blind patients, ideomotor apraxia was observed in 3 (case Nos. 23, 47, 144), anosognosia in 2 (Nos. 47, 67) and in 1 case (No. 47) right-left bodily disorientation and finger agnosia. Expressive speech had been severely affected originally in case No. 47, but at the time of examination (2 months later) this had almost fully recovered. None of the others showed any appreciable speech defects, but without exception there was difficulty in registration and in reversing digits and days of the week, together with global impairment of factual memory for past events. In only 1 case (No. 120) was there evidence of a focal cerebral lesion.

Strictly speaking, the term visual agnosia implies a defect in one aspect of perception alone and it may not be justifiable to apply it to these cases as all of them showed signs of general intellectual impairment. Nielsen[238] recognizes this difficulty when he stipulates that for visual agnosia to have any value as a localizing sign of disease of the occipito-parietal region of the dominant hemisphere, cerebration should be " relatively " unimpaired;* but we should hesitate to accept the view that the difficulties our patients had in visual recognition were due to their being unable to fix their gaze upon objects, owing to unawareness of their surroundings. Pick, according to Nielsen, described a similar condition in 1902 under the title of " apperceptive blindness of the senile ". The chief points against accepting this explanation in our patients were that visual agnosia was occasionally an early symptom and that their ability to perceive by other senses was unaffected.

Picture agnosia or inability to grasp the meaning of simple pictures, unlike visual agnosia, was a common feature in organic mental states. It was often seen in patients with simple chronic amnesic syndromes and occasionally with focal lesions, but only when there were co-existing signs of general clouding of consciousness. Thus, in 1 case, a right-handed woman aged 59 with a large right parietal meningioma, picture agnosia was pronounced but disappeared shortly after the tumour was removed, as did her other signs of general intellectual impairment. Pictures were chiefly of value in picking out minor disturbances of figure-backgrounds relationships, a feature which many organic mental patients seemed to possess in common. They had no difficulty in describing individual elements in a picture, such as the man sawing the branch off a tree in the well-known Picture Absur-

* One of the best examples in recent literature of a visual agnosia is the case reported by Hécaen.[240] This was a right-handed man of 64 with aphasia, right hemiparesis and hemianopia. There appeared to be visual object agnosia but his mental state was too confused to make detailed examination possible. At operation a tumour was found in the left occipital lobe extending into the parietal and temporal lobes. An occipital lobectomy was performed and as a result mental confusion was relieved, speech improved but he still remained unable to recognise either objects or colours. Of interest, however, was the fact that he could recognize human faces.

dities of Terman-Merrill Series[119] but they were unable to point out the risk involved to him in doing so. Their comments on the man weighing himself whilst holding a pile of books was that he seemed to be " a great reader " or " on his way to work ". In other words, it was apparent that patients who responded in this way had a similar but less severe disturbance of figure-background relationships than others who were unable even to select a given object from among other objects, although quite capable of doing so when the object was presented to them against a plain background.

APRAXIA

As with agnosias, in the past interest in apraxia has centred round its possible value as a localizing sign. The defect has been correlated with lesions involving either the parietal lobe in the dominant hemisphere, in which it is thought are stored memories of movement patterns, or with lesions of the paths connecting the dominant parietal lobe with the motor cortex on the same side and the subordinate hemisphere on the opposite side through the anterior part of the corpus callosum. Liepmann, whose name is associated with the bilateral form of " ideomotor apraxia ", as a result of clinico-pathological studies ascribed apraxia to the effect of subcortical lesions isolating certain areas of the cortex from other parts or to destruction of the corpus callosum, leading to the cutting-off of connections between the right hemisphere and the left.[241] Apraxia was classified into three types: limb-kinetic (now often known simply as motor apraxia), ideokinetic or ideomotor and ideatory apraxia, and this arrangement was widely accepted until Kleist,[242] described a further type—constructional apraxia. Brun[243] noted that typical symptoms of apraxia sometimes were seen in patients with multiple lesions affecting both hemispheres. Thus, in his seventh case there was a large haemorrhagic lesion in the right parieto-occipital region and two similar lesions in the left—one near the occipital pole and the other (the larger of the two) in the neighbourhood of the fusiform gyrus. Indeed, as Critchley[69] remarks: " The terms ' limb-kinetic ', ' ideomotor ', and ' ideatory ' are not altogether satisfactory in that they suggest clear-cut specific entities, with different localizing significance; both assumptions may well prove to be unwarranted. Nevertheless, it would be unwise to dispense altogether with these working hypotheses for they still serve some purpose in clinical diagnosis. Disease of the parietal lobe in the dominant hemisphere certainly tends to be followed by a bilateral disorder of motility which includes elements of an imperceptive or agnosic type, and which can conveniently be described as an ideomotor or ideokinetic apraxia." Constructional apraxia he believes to be " most readily demonstrated in cases of parietal disease of the subordinate hemisphere. But when the dominant side of the brain is at fault, then both conditions—ideomotor apraxia and constructional apraxia—may occur in combination and be difficult to distinguish ".

Limb-kinetic or motor apraxia. In this form voluntary purposive skilled movements cannot be made although the patient can perform the same movements involuntarily. The best examples were seen in certain aphasic patients whose inability to speak was due to apraxia of their tongue, lips or face. This could readily be shown by requesting them to put out the tongue, run its tip over the lips or purse the lips. Motor apraxia was also sometimes evident in the ipsilateral arm in patients with temporo-parietal or parieto-occipital lesions of the dominant hemisphere. It could be demonstrated by getting them to mimic such actions as shaking the fist, waving good-bye or pretending to play the piano. Interpretation of the results of such tests, however, was often difficult in the presence of an associated dysphasia, when perseveration was pronounced or when the patient was known to have always shown strong right-sided preference in his handedness.

Ideatory and ideomotor apraxia. In ideomotor apraxia " the patient does something entirely different from what he intends. He may make a fist instead of putting his finger to his nose, may in dressing put his arms into his trouser legs, may try to write with a pair of scissors ", Neilsen.[238] This author correlates such behaviour disorders with focal lesions of the posterior part of the dominant hemisphere, but regards Liepmann's other type of ideatory apraxia* as being more an expression of extreme absentmindedness, and as such having no focal significance. Theoretically this is sound enough, but in actual practice, although it was not uncommon to observe ideomotor apraxia in patients with posteriorly-placed vascular lesions involving the dominant hemisphere, the symptom when present was invariably complicated by general signs of clouding of consciousness. Similarly with tumours; ideomotor apraxia was never observed in uncomplicated cases although it might be noted after an epileptiform fit or at a later stage when it was evident that increased intracranial pressure was depressing the level of consciousness. On the other hand ideomotor apraxia was comparatively common in global cerebral affections, especially when

---

* An example given by Nielsen is: " trying to light a safety match by stroking it on the sole of the bare foot ". Similar behaviour was seen in a number of our chronic amnesic patients: one man when given clean underwear, putting these on on top of his old dirty ones; another man at table pouring salt in his tea, and a woman undressing to get into a bath, forgetting to take off her shoes.

these were of recent and rapid onset and of toxic origin. It could readily be precipitated, too, in patients with simple chronic amnesic syndromes, in whom there was no reason to suspect a focal lesion, by the incautious use of sedative or narcotic drugs or by the supervention of an upper respiratory or urinary infection. Hepatic encephalopathy was also a fruitful source of ideomotor apraxia, as the following case illustrates, Hurwitz and Allison.[239] The patient, formerly a merchant seaman, was referred to us some months after a portacaval anastomosis had been performed for repeated haematemesis, due to advanced multilobular cirrhosis of the liver.

His wife said that shortly before admission to hospital, on retiring to bed one evening, he had wandered up and down the corridor, looking for the W.C. When he explained his difficulty to her she thought he was joking and paid no attention, but during the night she awoke to find him in a miserable state because his bladder was full and he still could not find the W.C. She got up and showed him. He went in and locked the door but shortly afterwards called out that he could not unlock it to let himself out. As a result she had to fetch a stepladder and get in through the window to assist him. The next morning he took 1½ hours to dress himself and became very angry when she offered assistance. In trying to put on his trousers he first stuck his arms into the legs and finally put them on back to front.

Constructional apraxia. This form of apraxia, which is analogous in many respects to picture agnosia, was encountered more often than either motor or ideomotor forms. It is characterized by inability to construct objects or things from their component parts. In the same way as a patient with visual agnosia can describe correctly individual objects in a picture and yet be unable to grasp its meaning, so in constructional apraxia the patient understands the separate components of the design he is required to construct but cannot join or place them in their correct relationships to one another. As a result his attempt at copying a design is either meaningless or bears only a slight resemblance to that which it is intended to represent.

Gross intellectual deterioration is obviously a bar to such tests, but provided there was no visual-object agnosia and the patient could comprehend what he had to do, these were given as described on p. 88. Simple designs with two or three match sticks were given first, these being arranged against a plain dark background and the patient invited to copy them. If he succeeded the designs were then gradually increased in complexity and up to 6–10 sticks used.

The behaviour of patients with constructional apraxia was very characteristic and, indeed, reliance was placed as much upon this as upon their performance in determining the results. It has been described by Mayer-Gross[244] as follows:

". . . I asked the patient to arrange matches in simple figures such as a square, a triangle, a rhomboid, a house; or as Roman numerals. Then I placed before them rectangular figures, gave them the corresponding number of matches and asked them to copy the pattern. The patients always began readily enough but, even in the mildest cases, failed if the figures were complicated. The difficulties they were struggling with were expressed in a very typical manner. As soon as the patient was unable to go on, he brought his own matches as near as possible to the pattern or tried to build his copy into it . . ."

In addition to this " closing-in " phenomenon, patients showed a tendency to make mirror reversals of simple designs. Others showed a tendency to invert their copies or to omit details from one or other side of it, Critchley.[69] This last-named defect was usually seen in association with a homonymous visual field defect or with corresponding unilateral visual inattention.

Other tests used were the Kohs' blocks and house-drawing tests. Many patients with constructional apraxia were unable to arrange the blocks so as to form a square and would place three end-on in line with the fourth set at right-angles to the line, or place the blocks one on top of the other. Others tried to superimpose the blocks over the card displaying the pattern they were required to copy, and the "Penelope" syndrome was often seen (see p. 91). All of them addressed themselves to the task with great seriousness and most recognized their difficulties, this being evident by their repeated assertions " I'm stupid " . . . " Oh dear, dear " . . . " such a silly thing and I can't do it ". A few, after fumbling vainly with the blocks, would draw them together in a final gesture, as if they had found the correct solution and then ask: " Is that right?" But when told that it was not they would express no surprise or concern but go on trying as before. However, it was neither desirable nor necessary to proceed to such extremes, constructional apraxia when present being usually at once evident from the patient's performance with matches or with the first four designs of the Kohs' blocks. In interpreting results allowance must be made for slowness in performance, forgetfulness and perseveration. These are often seen in amnesic patients and should not be confused with true constructional difficulty. In the latter condition assisting the patient by showing him how designs are made has little or no effect, constructional difficulties persisting and being constantly demonstrable both with stick and block tests.

Although the literature contains many references to the value of constructional apraxia in the diagnosis of focal cerebral lesions, its *significance in global cerebral affections is often discounted and, yet it may be one of the first symptoms to draw attention to the presence of an organic mental state.* In housewives constructional apraxia may be

suspected when there is difficulty in laying the table, preparing a meal
or in doing embroidery. In men it is usually first apparent in their
work. Thus, in the case of a master shipwright, aged 56, subsequently
proved at autopsy to have Alzheimer's disease, one of the first things
noticed was that he had " begun to forget how to do things ". His
mates in the yard, recognizing this, had done their best to cover up his
inefficiency, which they attributed to increasing nervousness. His wife
recalled that at about the same time, she had asked him to replace an
electric light fuse but, although he had the wire and a screw-driver and
knew how to use them, he could not do it. He had not worked for
over a year and in the six months preceding his admission to hospital
had reached the stage when he could not turn on a tap, wash or shave,
use a hairbrush or dress himself. Another patient, a milling machine
operator, whose memory had been falling-off and temperament more
irascible in the preceding two years, said: " If I had a job to do, I
couldn't carry it through . . . certain things I did not understand . . .
I had to go up to another man and get his help."

Q. " What sort of things would muddle you?"

A. " There were certain dimensions I could not work out . . . if I had to drill
a hole 1" away from one side of a plate and had to allow for $\frac{3}{8}$" . . . then
you had to take $\frac{3}{8}$" from the 1" to get the centre from the side . . . (gestures)
. . . this worried me . . . was I doing right or wrong? . . . so I gave up
the job and took an easier one."

This man also volunteered that he had had difficulty in reading
blueprints, especially in two dimensions. It is possible, but unlikely,
that his troubles were determined emotionally. He had never been
very bright, leaving school in Standard V. After clerking for many
years, he had worked in a munitions factory from 1939, and later served
in the London Fire Service. But throughout these difficult times, he
had had no breakdown and at 38, had felt every confidence in trans-
ferring to the milling machine job, at which he had been employed until
the symptoms described above were first noted. His admission to
hospital was determined by sudden visual disturbances (left homonymous hemianopia with visual inattention). Blood pressure was elevated
and a clinical diagnosis of arteriosclerotic presenile dementia with
recent cerebral thrombosis was made. Detailed examination of his
mental state showed only slight difficulty in registration and defects in
memory for past events, and apart from these and constructional
apraxia, there were no other signs of deterioration.

There were other similar examples among the patients with presenile
dementia, in some of whom constructional difficulties had first been

mistaken for psychoneurosis or a purely affective disorder. The Merchant Navy Officer, with hepatic encephalopathy, already referred to, responded promptly in hospital to reduction of his protein intake but when this was increased and day to day watch kept on his mental state it deteriorated slowly and the first evidence of this was his inability to construct simple designs with matches, the appearance of this sign corresponding with changes in the electroencephalogram.

In global cerebral affections, therefore, when onset is gradual and progress of the malady slow, the development of constructional disability may precede that of other forms of apraxia, indeed, the apparent early occurrence of ideomotor apraxia would indicate either more rapidly developing pathology or that the initial phases of an illness had been overlooked. This argument is in keeping with the facts known about the occurrence of apraxia in previously healthy subjects recovering consciousness after severe closed head injury or anoxia. Ideomotor apraxia may be apparent in delirium and early in the stage of disorientation, but usually disappears when the patient becomes fully orientated again, although constructional difficulties may be recognizable until full consciousness is regained.

The significance of constructional apraxia in patients with *focal cerebral lesions* is shown in Table 13. There were 14 patients in this series in whom it had been possible to make full mental and physical tests and in whom constructional apraxia was readily demonstrable. In 11 of these the site and nature of the lesion was confirmed either at operation or autopsy. In 5 it lay in the dominant hemisphere, in 9 in the subordinate hemisphere. This difference in incidence may be due, as Critchley suggests,[69] to apraxia in left-sided lesions being masked by other more blatant defects. With right-sided lesions these are less and constructional defects more apparent. Piercy, Hécaen and Ajuriaquerra[245] analysed a series of 67 cases of constructional apraxia due to unilateral lesions with respect to the side upon which the lesion was found. Excluding patients who showed general disturbance of consciousness at the time of examination and all left-handers, they concluded that the right cerebral hemisphere in right-handed persons has a special non-subordinate rôle in the cognitive factors involved in normal constructional activities. Constructional apraxia may result from a lesion of either hemisphere but in effect they found that it occurred twice as frequently with right-sided lesions as with left, and that it was more severe when the right hemisphere was involved. Indeed, as was our experience, the sign may be the only recognizable mental defect in a patient with a focal lesion of the subordinate hemisphere.

TABLE 13.—Site of lesion and associated mental and neurological signs in 14 cases of constructional apraxia, due to a focal lesion

Case No.	Age	Sex	Handedness—R. or L.	Dominant or subordinate hemisphere affected	Lesion (*Confirmed at operation †Confirmed at p.m)	Abnor. mood and behaviour	Impaired Insight	Perseveration	Series forward and back (unable to repeat)	Registration difficult	Memory for past events defective	In time	In place	For persons	Right—left	Fingers	Speaking	Writing	Understanding Sp. Sp.	Reading	Dyscalculia	Clock telling time	Ideational	Ideomotor	Constructional	Drawing	Tactile	Colour	Visual object	Auditory	Pictures	Hemiplegia (contralateral)	Hemihypaesthesia (contralateral)	Cortical sens. loss (contralateral)	Hemianopia (contralateral)	Visual inattention (contralateral)	Motor neglect (contralateral)	Fits	Papilloedema
100	53	M	R	S	Right parietal-occip. (C.V.A.)	no	no	no	no	no	yes	—	—	—	—	—	—	+	—	—	—	—	—	—	+	—	—	—	—	—	—	+	—	+	+	—	+	—	—
99	54	M	L	S	Left temporal * (astrocytoma)	no	no	no	yes	yes	no	—	—	—	—	—	—	—	—	—	—	—	—	—	+	+	—	—	—	—	—	+	—	+	—	—	+	—	—
86	63	F	R	S	Right parietal * (meningioma)	no	no	no	yes	yes	yes	—	—	—	—	—	—	+	—	—	—	—	—	+	+	+	—	—	—	—	—	+	—	+	+	+	+	—	—
117	50	M	R	D	Left Parietal * (meningioma)	no	no	no	yes	no	yes	—	—	—	—	—	+	+	—	—	—	+	—	—	+	+	—	—	—	—	?	+	—	+	—	—	+	+	—
94	58	M	R	S	Right frontal * (oligodendroglioma)	no	no	no	no	no	yes	—	—	—	—	—	—	—	—	—	+	?	—	—	+	+	—	—	—	—	+	+	—	—	—	—	—	+	—

216

Age	No.	Sex			Diagnosis	1	2	3	4	5	6	7	8	9	10	11	12	13	14	15	16	17	18	19	20	a	b	c	d	e	f
59	159	M	R	D	Left temporo-parietal (C.V.A.)	–	–	+	+	–	+	–	+	–	–	–	–	+	–	+	+	+	–	–	?	no	no	yes	yes	no	no
62	92	M	R	S	Right temporo-parietal (infarct calc.)	–	–	+	+	+	–	–	+	+	–	–	+	+	–	–	–	–	–	–	–	yes	no	no	no	no	no
42	140	M	R	S	Right fronto-parietal * (meningioma)	+	–	+	+	+	+	–	+	–	–	–	+	+	–	–	–	–	–	–	–	no	no	yes	no	no	yes
56	142	M	R	S	Right parietal * (astrocytoma)	–	+	+	–	+	+	–	+	+	–	–	+	+	–	–	–	–	–	–	–	no	no	no	no	no	no
62	130	M	R	D	L. int.-carotid stenosis (angiography) *	–	–	–	+	–	+	–	+	–	–	–	+	+	–	+	–	+	+	–	–	yes	yes	yes	yes	no	no
67	88	M	R	D	Left temporal * (astrocytoma)	–	+	–	–	+	–	–	+	?	–	–	+	+	–	–	+	+	+	–	+	no	no	no	no	no	no
42	41	F	R	S	L. int. capsule and post. lateral thalamus * † infarct	–	+	+	+	+	+	+	+	–	–	–	+	+	–	–	+	+	+	–	–	yes	no	no	no	no	no
64	143	M	R	S	Right frontal metastasis * from bronch.-carcinoma	+	–	–	–	–	–	+	–	+	–	–	–	+	–	+	–	–	–	–	+	no	yes	yes	no	yes	yes
	182	M	R	S	Right temporal * (astrocytoma)	+	+	–	+	+	–	–	–	?	–	–	–	+	–	–	–	–	–	–	–	no	no	yes	no	no	yes

As regards situation of the focal lesion in the 11 cases in which its site was confirmed, this was as follows:

Case No.	Left Hemisphere	Right Hemisphere
99	Temporal	—
86	—	parietal
117	parietal	—
94	—	frontal
140	fronto-parietal	—
142	—	parietal
130	fronto-temporo-parietal	—
88	temporal	—
41	int. caps. and post. lat. thalamus	—
143	—	frontal
182	—	temporo-parietal

The lesion involved the temporal or parietal lobes or both lobes in 8 instances, although in only 3 was it confined to the parietal area. A possible reason for the occurrence of constructional apraxia in the 2 other patients with frontal lobe lesions is that in both there was evidence of cerebral oedema, which could have disturbed function well beyond the confines of the tumour. This explanation, however, will not account for its occurrence in case No. 41, in which no cortical pathology was found, the lesion being in the thalamus.

Analysis of other mental defects shown by these patients with focal lesions indicates that there was only slight evidence of clouding of consciousness. Gross abnormalities of mood and behaviour, impairment of insight, disorientation in place and time were uncommon, and none of the patients had any severe defect either of registration or of memory. Gerstmann's syndrome was present in one case in which, as might be expected, the lesion lay in the dominant hemisphere. Mayer-Gross[244] observed that many of his patients with constructional apraxia could not tell the time but this feature was noted in only one instance. Inability to add numbers owing to failure on the part of the patient to arrange them correctly beneath each other (so-called parietal acalculia) was seen in 4 cases. Thus, one of these, a man with a right frontal oligodendroglioma, when told to write down and add up the numbers "seven", "ten", and "one hundred and sixty", proceeded to set them out as shown, so that although his subsequent addition was correct the answer he obtained was wrong:

$$
\begin{array}{r}
7 \\
10 \\
160 \\
\hline
330
\end{array}
$$

Drawing ability was also often impaired and 4 of the patients were unable to see the point in the picture absurdities (Terman-Merrill) designed to test the intelligence of normal children between the ages of 7–14.

In a number of cases there was an associated hemianopic defect or visual inattention, a circumstance that could, of course, have been coincidental but which may lend support to the theory that in constructional apraxia there is abstract spatial disorientation. The two may possibly be interdependent. Certainly there appears to be some correlation between constructional apraxia, spatial disorientation and posteriorly-placed lesions of either hemisphere. But the apraxia cannot be attributed solely to disturbance of parietal lobe function for, as has been shown, it is often recognizable in global cerebral affections, being sometimes one of the earliest signs of deterioration, and in others a transient phenomenon. The essential feature for its occurrence appears to be some general, although slight, clouding of consciousness, but when there is in addition an appropriately placed focal cerebral lesion, the probability of its being present is increased.

BIBLIOGRAPHY

228 BRAIN, W. R. (1947). "Diseases of the Nervous System," p. 107. 3rd Edn. Oxford University Press, London.

229 WILSON, S. A. K. (1908). A contribution to the study of apraxia. *Brain*, 31, 164.

230 MAGOUN, H. W. (1954). In "Brain Mechanisms and Consciousness." Blackwell, Oxford.

231 BAY, E. (1953). Disturbances of visual perception and their examination. *Brain*, 76, 515.

232 ETTLINGER, G. (1956). Sensory defects in visual agnosia. *J. Neurol. Psychiat.*, 19, 297.

233 REINHOLD, M. (1950). A case of auditory agnosia. *Brain*, 73, 203.

234 WECHSLER, I. S. (1933). *Arch. Ophthal.*, 9, 957.

235 VON HAGEN, K. O. (1941). Two clinical cases of mind blindness (visual agnosia), one due to carbon monoxide intoxication, one due to a diffuse degenerative process. *Bull. Los Angeles neurol. Soc.*, 6, 191.

236 ADLER, A. (1944). Disintegration and restoration of optic recognition in visual agnosia. *Arch. Neurol. Psychiat.*, 81, 243.

237 FRANÇOIS, J. (1942). Hemianopsie homonyne par intoxication oxycarbonée aigue. *Ophthalmologica*, 103, 143.

238 NIELSEN, J. M. (1948). "Agnosia, Apraxia, Aphasia. Their Value in Cerebral Localization," p. 16. 2nd Edn. Paul B. Hoeber, New York.

239 HURWITZ, L. J. and Allison, R. S. (1955). Recurring mental confusion after portacaval anastomosis. *Brit. Med. J.*, 1, 388.

240 HÉCAEN, H. and AJURIAGUERRA, J. DE (1956). Agnosie visuelle pour les objets inanimés par lésion unilatérale gauche. *Rev. Neurol.*, **94**, 222.

241 LIEPMANN, H. (1905). Der weitere Krankheitsverlauf bei dem einseitig Apraktischen und der Gehirnbefund auf Grund von Serienschnitten. *Mschr. Psychiat. Neurol.*, **17**, 289.

242 KLEIST, K. (1934). " Gehirnpathologie." Barth, Leipzig.

243 BRUN, R. (1921-22). Klinische und anatomische Studien über Apraxie. *Schweiz. Arch. Neurol. Psychiat.*, **9** and **10**.

244 MAYER-GROSS, W. (1935). Some observations on apraxia. *Proc. Roy. Soc. Med.*, **28**, 63.

245 PIERCY, M., HÉCAEN, H. and Ajuriaguerra, J. DE (1960). Constructional apraxia associated with unilateral cerebral lesions—left and right sided cases compared. *Brain*, **83**, 225.

CHAPTER XI

The Differential Diagnosis of Organic Brain Disease in Later Life

Two chief problems arise in the differential diagnosis of organic brain disease: its recognition and its cause. The first presents little difficulty when mental symptoms are accompanied by unequivocal neurological signs, or when illness has been ushered in abruptly by fits, hemiplegia or aphasia. But when symptoms are unfolded gradually and have a vaguely neurotic or depressive quality, and no definite signs can be found on examination, the condition has to be distinguished from psychoneurosis or an affective disorder.

Differential diagnosis must also take into account the problem of apparently healthy persons taken ill with acute confusional mental symptoms. When the existence of organic brain disease has been established, there is the differentiation of focal from diffuse cerebral lesions and consideration of ways and means of determining their probable nature.

PSYCHONEUROSIS AND AFFECTIVE DISORDERS

In theory past history should supply the necessary clues to diagnosis of a *psychoneurosis* because this is a constitutional disorder affecting those of predisposed personality and temperament, the first appearance of symptoms seldom, if ever, being delayed until later life. Usually, in such cases, enquiry shows that there have been previous breakdowns and extended periods of ill-health, due to " overwork ", " rheumatism ", or other equally ill-defined causes. Many psychoneurotics take patent medicines or " tonics " regularly and their work record may reveal that there have been frequent changes of employment, although not always for the better, the reasons given for changing often being trivial, as for example, " the hours were too long ", or " the workroom was too hot ".

The second point in making a diagnosis of neurosis is to obtain evidence of recent psychological stress due to some hindrance encountered by the patient in his working or domestic life. This is not easy on account of the neurotic's tendency to turn a blind eye to such matters and protest that he has no worries, but a talk with relatives may bring it to light. In our experience, common exciting causes of breakdown in middle-aged men are industrial injuries and fear of permanent disablement—a fear, incidentally, which it is always difficult to disentangle from interest in securing compensation through successful litigation. Bereavement is also a common exciting influence, especially when the patient has been overdependant on the lost one. Other causes include: changes in management or conditions at the factory in which he works; demotion, promotion (with consequent need to undertake greater responsibilities), or retirement. The last-named often affects the neurotic adversely, on account of his never having developed any outside interests or hobbies. In women some of the chief exciting causes are: the menopause, bereavement, severance of ties with a favourite daughter through her marriage, worry over a husband's ill-health, his drunkenness or unfaithfulness.

It is well to reflect, however, that such psychogenic factors, although genuine enough, may be unrelated to the symptoms in question and one should always be wary of making too much of them in cases where careful history taking has revealed no evidence of previous neurotic behaviour. Psychoneurosis and organic disease often coexist and more convincing evidence must be obtained before the diagnosis can be made with confidence. Next to history, direct observation of the patient at the first interview is probably the best guide because both his symptoms and behaviour should be typical and the results of physical examination negative.

This statement, although axiomatic, requires definition. Increased emotional lability with tears, anxious and tense attitudes are common in psychoneurosis and often thought to be indicative, but in fact they are far from being so and, as has been seen, may occur in organic as well as in depressive states. Of more importance are the patient's attitude towards the examiner and the manner in which he details his symptoms. In organic brain disease the patient conveys the impression of doing his best to conceal his defects or, at least, of trying to make light of them. In some respects, indeed, his attitude resembles " la belle indifférence " of the hysteric; but the resemblance is only superficial; as examination proceeds and more questions are put, his apparent complacency explodes into catastrophic reactions, which effectively destroy any illusionary quality of indifference his previous behaviour may have given. Actually, apart from post-traumatic neurosis, in which florid symptoms of hysteria were often seen, gross hysteria was seldom encountered in this older age group and we had only one instance of hysterical memory loss. There was little evidence, too, of personal dissociation, a feature which may be more characteristic of hysteria in young adults, and no clear-cut distinction could be drawn between anxiety states and conversion hysterical reactions, in most cases ingredients of both kinds being intermixed.

Characteristic of the neurotic as opposed to the patient with organic disease was the impression he conveyed of trying to influence the examiner into believing that his symptoms were of great severity. When the first ones he mentioned failed to invoke any corresponding expression of concern, or he was reassured as to their insignificance, he would proceed without hesitation or embarrassment to describe other complaints which, he indicated, disturbed him no less greatly. When this happens it is difficult not to be carried away and lost in detail, but it is important to try and obtain answers to two questions in particular. First, are the symptoms of which the patient complains actually present at the time, and second, what effect do they have on him? The psychoneurotic usually answers the first question in the affirmative, which enables one to note the discrepancy between his account of their severity, e.g. a headache being " like a nail driven into my head " or " like a tight band pressing on my forehead ", and his appearance and talk, neither of which reveal any great disturbance of mind or bodily function. Other characteristics of the psychoneurotic are their excessive us of gesture in reinforcing statements, the frequency of palpitation, precordial discomfort, gastro-intestinal symptoms and panic reactions, the last-named being often associated with fear of crowds or shut-in places, e.g., churches, cinemas. On examination the hands may be cold and sweating, and tremor, sighing respiration or air swallowing may be observed. To the second question the patient will readily admit that his symptoms have made him excessively tired, miserable or depressed and that life has not been " worth living ", although he will firmly deny that he has ever had any suicidal intentions.

Faulty memory is often mentioned, but appropriate tests reveal no difficulty in registration or in reversing series. Orientation is perfect and no tendency to perseveration is seen. Clinical examination, electroencephalography and other tests are negative. The following is a fairly typical example of a post-traumatic neurosis. The patient was a man of 50 who had sustained a minor head injury at work some 9 months before and was at the time of examination involved in litigation to secure damages. His wife, who accompanied him, said that his chief complaint had been loss of memory.

He made no reply to the conventional greeting and after being helped to a chair sat there quietly with his gaze directed into space. His face was flushed and breathing audible at times and he wore a frowning resentful expression. When asked simple questions he turned to his wife who readily answered them, the patient himself remaining silent. When one approached him to examine the pupils and laid a hand on his head he gave a violent start and this type of response occurred repetitively throughout the greater part of the physical examination. He had a coarse shake of the right hand which became more pronounced when he attempted to do anything but it was more apparent at the beginning of the interview than at the end and lacked the characteristic qualities of either action, rest or static tremor. He undressed and dressed himself without difficulty. Systematic examination disclosed no evidence of abnormality in the nervous system or other organs.

A few days later, when he was examined again, he still claimed loss of memory but his behaviour had changed: the resentful tense attitude had gone, there were no startle reactions and he would now answer questions, although he made no attempt to offer information spontaneously. Organic mental tests revealed no evidence of clouding of consciousness or specific defects and although at times his answers were wrong, the ones he gave had the character of "near misses" i.e. Tuesday for Wednesday, 1957 for 1958, etc. and on performance tests with matches, drawing arrows and in the use of Kohs' blocks, there was no evidence of defective grasp or constructional difficulty. Despite his inability to recall any events since his accident, he was able to give the names of several cities, vegetables and birds and in doing so no trace of perseveration was observed.

Affective disorders in later life commonly take the form of depression and it is especially important to recognize this type of reaction because of its responsiveness to early and appropriate treatment. In many such cases, the interplay of three chief aetiological factors can be discerned: heredity, acquired disease, psychological stress and the extent to which each of these contributes to the individual case varies greatly. Consequently, depression may be seen in association with psychoneurotic features and with organic brain disease or it may be a symptom of schizophrenia.[246] At one time it was thought that the appearance of depressive symptoms in later life almost invariably indicated underlying cerebral deterioration, but it is now recognized, as Roth and Morrissey[247] and others have shown, that depressive disorders are not uncommon in later life and that they often occur without there being any co-existing brain disease. Thus, although the diagnosis of psychoneurosis in the elderly must be made with care and even reluctance, the possibility of symptoms being due to a potentially curable depression must always be considered, especially when the signs pointing to organic disease are equivocal or there are symptoms not readily explicable on that basis.

Affective disorders are so named because the disturbance is emotional, thought and behaviour not being primarily affected, although they often become so. Hereditary factors are pronounced in the recurring manic depressive form and the influence of constitution can be discerned in the involutional type. In the latter, although depressive symptoms may not have appeared until relatively late in life, the previous history usually bears the strong imprint of rigidity of outlook, overconscientiousness and mildly obsessive tendencies. The term " reactive depression ", which is passing into disuse, reflects the belief that in some cases hereditary and constitutional influences may play but little part and that depression is brought about by worry or personal physical suffering. However, such cases overlap too much with psychoneurosis on the one hand and with involutional depression on the other to make it often possible to recognize reactive depression as a distinct entity. Thus, there may be strong exciting extraneous causes in involutional cases, which appear to be responsible for precipitating breakdown and, not infrequently, " endogenous " features—self reproach, ideas of reference, delusional thinking—are seen in cases which otherwise would correspond to the concept of reactive depression.

In distinguishing depression from psychoneurotic anxiety, the following points were found to be helpful:

The previous work record of depressive patients is often exemplary. If there have been previous breakdowns, these have been fewer but more clear-cut and disabling in their effects. Depressed patients look ill and often show considerable loss of weight. The appearance of psychoneurotics belies their claims. Depression has a diurnal character, being usually most pronounced in the morning. Further, sleep loss is almost a constant feature in " endogenous " depression, the patient waking in the early hours of the morning and not obtaining more than 1–3 hours' sleep at night. By contrast the neurotic, although he may have difficulty in getting off to sleep, once asleep remains so until the usual hour of awakening. Unless agitated, when they became restless, weep and talk freely, depressed patients are usually silent or have little or nothing to say, answers to questions being delayed, given in low monotonous tones and as brief as possible. Their attitude alone, however, is sufficiently eloquent to proclaim their misery. Patients with post-traumatic neurosis, in whom it is difficult to decide how much behaviour is " unconsciously " motivated and how much related to malingering, often present the same appearance. But this lacks the genuine stamp of depression, resentment colouring it all too plainly, and it tends to disappear towards the close of the interview, when this has been conducted tactfully, the patient then exhibiting a friendly " relieved " attitude and a corresponding lightening of spirits, which contrasts oddly with his former sullen and resentful behaviour.

In psychoneurotics loss of interest is never global but attached to some activities more than others. So, whilst a patient may claim that life is not worth living, or that he has no interest in anything, these are clearly overstatements because, when the topic is pursued further, it becomes evident that there has been no loss of natural affection for relatives and friends, that he has never seriously contemplated suicide and that he hopes to get better. By contrast depressed patients are often convinced that there is no hope for them and mean what they say in declaring that life is not worth living.

An essential difference between psychoneurotic and depressed patients lies in their way of thinking. In depression not only is thought retarded but it often assumes an unworldly or unreal character. Psychoneurotics blame their illness on overwork, the shock of personal loss or physical ill-health. " If I could only get rid of this headache," they say, " I would feel better." Depressive illnesses often begin in the same way with morbid preoccupation over tinnitus, constipation, headache or other somatic complaint. But before long the patient tends to shift the blame to himself and finds what, to him, is some discreditable explanation in his past life to account for it. Alternatively, he may become paranoid and attach blame to the allegedly hostile intentions of other persons, these morbid ideas usually being followed by the appearance of organized delusions.

The distinction between true psychotic depression and organic mental disease is easy when the features are typical and physical examination, the results of electroencephalography and other tests are negative. In many cases the diagnosis was made on history, the results of physical examination and organic mental tests alone. But in others, where the two conditions co-existed, depression being severe and signs of organic mental deterioration slight, treatment directed to the former was most rewarding as the following case illustrates. The patient was a man aged 65 when first seen in 1952. His chief complaint was of difficulty in concentration at work and depression of spirits. He had had a previous bout of depression 5 years before, which had responded well to electric shock treatment, and had been wounded in the head during the First World War. However, the head injury had left no lasting effects and he had been moderately successful in building up a manufacturing business, of which he was owner.

His wife confirmed his statement and said that there had recently been a general loss of interest and that he had been unusually taciturn, inclined to "dither" over business decisions and the signing of forms. Although he went to sleep at night, he awoke early in the morning and would get up and pace his room. He had lost some weight.

General and neurological examination was negative except for an oval-shaped small bone defect in the left parietal region. He wore a sad worried expression and was restless and fidgety, disinclined to talk. He answered slowly but distinctly and seemed to have great difficulty in describing his symptoms, but although he said he was depressed he wanted to get better and had no suicidal thoughts. On organic mental testing there were no signs of general cerebral impairment or clouding of consciousness other than some impairment of memory for recent events. E.E.G. showed a dominant alpha rhythm at 10–13 c/s. but slower waves at 6–8 c/s. were noted, these being symmetrical and increased by overbreathing and photic stimulation. No epileptic features or signs of a focal lesion were found.

During the first ten days in hospital there was no change. He slept not more than 2–3 hours at night, although he made up for this to some extent by dozing during the day. His attitude, which suggested indifference or unconcern more than depression, the forgetfulness for recent events and the E.E.G. findings raised the possibility of some underlying organic condition, possibly connected with the old head injury but the cerebro-spinal fluid was normal and lumbar encephalography disclosed only some dilatation of the lateral ventricles, although there was practically no air over the vertex of the brain. Spontaneous improvement in his condition resulted and within two weeks he was discharged home in the best of spirits.

This man kept well for 4 years and then in 1956 was re-admitted with identical symptoms, relapse with recurrence of depression having been noted some three months previously. Again the findings on neurological examination and mental testing were normal, but it was discovered that he was refusing to drink because he believed attempts were being made to poison him. A psychiatric opinion was called and the opinion expressed that although there were some organic mental features, his condition was chiefly one of depression. Accordingly he was given 6 electric convulsion treatments at weekly intervals. All symptoms disappeared and 3 years later, at the time of writing, he has had no relapse and is in good health. Despite his age, 72, there are no obvious signs of mental deterioration. The case is described in some detail because it illustrates the importance of recognizing the depressive element when psychoneurotic, depressive and organic mental features are intermixed.

Acute Mental Symptoms in Elderly Patients

The term " acute toxic confusional psychosis " is sanctioned by long usage but it is important to understand that it does not imply the existence of some mental disease upon which acute symptoms are superimposed. This is not so. The condition, which occurs in previously healthy subjects as it does in the mentally afflicted, is characterized by the appearance of acute mental symptoms, due to some physical exciting cause, the prompt recognition and removal of which brings about their disappearance and the return of the patient to normality. These symptoms are the result of clouding of consciousness or general disturbance of brain function and differ in no essential respect from those already described in Chapter V. Post-traumatic and anoxic encephalopathy are, indeed, clinical varieties of the same syndrome. The form it takes, although coloured to some extent by previous personality and temperament, depends less on the nature of the offending cause than upon the duration and extent of exposure to it, age of the patient and the presence or absence of pre-existing organic brain disease. Defective capacity for registration and grasp give rise to disorientation and disturbance of mood which may be facile and euphoric, apprehensive, tearful, irritable or violently aggressive and corresponding behaviour disturbances occur which render management difficult. Perseveration is invariably seen as is defective memory for recent events, the latter usually being associated with confabulation, motor restlessness and other signs of delirium. Hallucinations are common in drug-induced cases and tend to have a distinctive character, depending on the toxin responsible, i.e. fearful visual hallucinations occurring in delirium tremens, Lilliputian hallucinations in belladonna poisoning.

Clouding of consciousness may be induced in one of two ways. First, by direct action of a nocious agent on the cerebral cortex so that the neurones undergo degenerative changes. Chromatolysis, in which there is breaking up of Nissl granules in cells, is not simply a proteolytic effect but due to the action of ribonuclease, Richter.[248] Swelling of neurones is due to changes in osmotic pressure within the cell caused by liberation of smaller nucleotide molecules and protein fragments. Provided the cause has not been too long operative and is promptly removed, these changes are slight and reversible, but otherwise permanent effects result from neuronal necrosis. The second way in which consciousness may be disturbed is through lesions affecting the diencephalon and brain stem. These may be caused either by toxic cellular damage or by mechanical pressure effects within the skull. Wernicke's encephalopathy, which is associated with bilaterally symmetrical lesions in the corpora mammillaria, periaqueductal grey matter and posterior colliculi,[249] is an example of toxic cellular damage. Trauma, rapidly expanding cerebral tumours and cerebral vascular accidents, all three of which may be associated with considerable intracerebral oedema and coning, are examples of the other.

So many aetiological factors may be responsible for precipitating an acute toxic encephalopathy that the problem of diagnosis cannot be said to be solved until the particular cause in a given case has been identified. Many of these have already been referred to in previous chapters, but a list of some of the most important, especially as they affect elderly patients, is given below:

Post-traumatic encephalopathy. In closed head injuries prolonged clouding of consciousness is related to oedema, disturbance of the cerebral circulation leading to secondary stagnant hypoxic effects and in some cases to actual brain stem injury, or the formation of an acute extradural or subdural haematoma. Haematoma formation is recognized by the patient recovering consciousness after the injury but becoming drowsy and relapsing into deepening unconsciousness some hours or a day or two later and presenting neurological signs confined to one side, e.g. hemiparesis with an extensor plantar response, inequality of pupils with dilatation of the pupil on the side of the lesion. Some years ago, a remarkable instance was seen in the case of a man of 50 who had fainted after coronary artery occlusion and in doing so bumped his head on a radiator. There was no bruise or other evidence of head injury, which at the time was not even suspected, and he was treated for the coronary occlusion by rest in bed and anticoagulant drugs.

Ten days later, by which time his cardiac state had improved, he suddenly complained of severe frontal headache and became truculent, abusive and quite unlike his usual self. After being given an analgesic and sleeping he felt better and when seen some hours later behaviour was entirely natural, there being no evidence of clouding of consciousness or focal neurological signs. The optic discs were flat and normal in appearance except that the edges on the nasal sides were blurred. The next day, however, the severe headache recurred, again with noisy behaviour but this time followed by signs of deepening unconsciousness. There were still no lateraling signs, but on making bifrontal burr holes a large subdural haematoma was found and evacuated. Owing to his drowsy stupor, only local anaesthesia of the skin had been used, but as soon as pressure within the skull was released, and whilst he was still on the table, consciousness began to return so that within an hour or so this had fully been regained and his subsequent recovery was entirely uneventful.

Another emergency associated with trauma is *fat embolism.* Sevitt,[250] in a series of 100 post-mortems performed on patients dying after injury, found evidence of systemic embolism in 24% and of pulmonary embolism in practically all (89%). He points out that although the latter is very common after fractures, it rarely gives rise to symptoms or clinical signs referred to the lungs. On the other hand, the effects of systemic and cerebral embolism are always apparent, although incomplete or partial syndromes occur more often than the classical variety. We have encountered two such cases in recent years. The first was a woman aged 68 who had sustained multiple fractures of the tibiae and fibulae. Although badly shocked on admission she was not unconscious, but after a lucid interval of 14 hours she passed into coma from which there was no recovery, death occurring on the fifteenth day after injury. Fat was present in the urine, but there was no skin rash. Fat emboli were found in the brain after death. The second patient survived. Drowsy stupor had suddenly appeared the day after multiple injuries with fractures had been sustained and had lasted 48–72 hours. Fat globules were recovered from the urine and there was a typical petechial rash on the anterior axillary folds and lateral aspects of the chest wall. Both plantar reflexes were extensor. In cases without rash, the difficulty in distinguishing the condition from extradural or subdural haemorrhage is often great, especially if there is hemiparesis or epileptiform convulsions occur. As a rule, however, the development of clouding of consciousness is more rapid in fat embolism and lateralising signs are less pronounced. As regards the time interval after injury, Sevitt states that the first symptoms of systemic embolism generally develop soon after injury (36 hours) and not after the third day as is commonly stated. Of his 75 cases, symptoms were noted in 23% within 12 hours of injury, in 60% within 24 hours, in 80% within 36 hours and in over 90% within 48 hours.

Acute mental symptoms in organic brain disease. Transient phases of clouding of consciousness causing mental confusion may be the first signs to draw attention to hitherto unrecognized organic disease. This generalization refers especially to such diseases as general paralysis, pernicious anaemia, cerebral arteriosclerosis and chronic subdural haematoma. Minor cerebral vascular accidents are readily detectable when there is transient hemiparesis, but when the lesion involves the temporo-parietal or parieto-occipital region the only physical sign may be a contralateral visual field defect, which is easily overlooked or difficult to demonstrate in such patients unless special techniques are employed (see p. 43). The occurrence of unrecognized minor epileptiform fits may also be responsible for causing transient disturbances of behaviour in slowly dementing patients.

Anoxic and hypoxic encephalopathy. The vitality of neurones depends on oxygen, glucose, glutamic acid and certain non-carbohydrates such as pyruvic and lactic acids and any interference with their supply or capacity to utilize these nutriments promptly results in signs and symptoms of clouding of consciousness. Although anoxia is no longer the hazard in industry it used to be owing to improvement in working conditions and ventilation in factories, *coal gas poisoning* is still one of the chief sources of anoxic admissions to hospital. But, even more important than these accidental and suicidal cases are patients already in hospital in whom unrecognized hypoxic effects may arise as side-effects of medical or surgical condition or, occasionally, of treatment being directed towards their relief. Actual oxygen lack in these cases is less responsible for producing hypoxic effects than is cerebral circulatory inadequacy or failure.   This may be brought about by deficiency in the pumping action of the heart, by diminution of the total blood volume or by pronounced lowering of systemic blood pressure.

In *chronic congestive heart failure* clouding of consciousness is usually more apparent at night than by day, although in severe cases it may be continuous. Epileptiform fits are liable to occur in heart block, but these may not be so obvious as the disturbances of mood and behaviour that follow them.

Hypoxic effects, consequent upon diminution in volume of the total circulating blood and of fall in blood pressure, are also seen after severe *gastric or intestinal haemorrhage*, but for every such case there are many more in which the mechanism of cerebral circulatory failure is less clear or in which more than one factor is concerned.   The effects of *dehydration* and of *alkalosis* have already been referred to in Chapter II. The reverse state to dehydration—*water intoxication*—although less likely to occur, is probably of equal importance. At one time individual susceptibility to epilepsy used to be tested in this way, that is by deliberately hydrating the patient.   Copious draughts of water and intramuscular injections of pitressin were given. In non-epileptics fits might not be induced but most subjects complained of severe headache and were drowsy, many becoming disorientated and a few developing delirium with noisy and violent behaviour.   It was for these reasons that the test was abandoned.

Body-water volume is regulated chiefly by the kidneys which increase or decrease the volume of urine and electrolytes excreted; changes in the latter may indeed be the primary mechanism involved in its control, Bull.[251]   In practice, water intoxication effects may occur in chronic alcoholics who drink more than usually large quantities of beer and in psychotics who are subject to delusions. In mentally-stable persons it has been brought about by too enthusiastic washing out of a colostomy, Clayton-Jones,[252] and in one of our patients it was precipitated by too much intravenous fluid replacement.   Other conditions that may predispose are: the drinking of large quantities of water after excessive sweating or being on a low salt intake, and the presence of chronic nephritis or anuria.   As the retained water is chiefly intracellular, it is rare to get oedema and the only physical signs may be extensor plantar reflexes with over-active tendon jerks.   The serum sodium is always low, Wynn.[253]

Modern treatment of systemic hypertension by the hexylmethonium group of drugs has been most successful in *lowering blood pressure*, but this can be dangerous in elderly patients and especially those in whom absent-mindedness and other early signs of organic cerebral disease are already apparent. Failure to bear this in mind, indeed, was responsible for the occurrence of mental confusion in one of our patients, whose condition, however, slowly improved after withdrawal of the hypotensive drug, so that three years later, despite his hypertension and advancing years, he is still comparatively well.

Clouding of consciousness due to altered content of the blood substrate. Second to oxygen the most important item required to maintain full consciousness is glucose, lack of which in the elderly is usually related to overdosage with insulin in diabetes. Kepler and Moersch[254] rightly stressed the fact that mental symptoms may dominate the clinical picture of *insulin hypoglycaemia* and this point was made even earlier by Wauchope,[255] although unfortunately it seems often to be lost sight of, the occurrence of undue fatigue, apprehension, faintness, unsteadiness, palpitation, warm perspiration and dimness of vision being more emphasized. Indeed, before giving instructions to middle-aged and elderly diabetics as to how to deal with hypoglycaemia, one should first test their capacity for registration, memory and constructional ability so as to ensure, if defects are found, that their relatives at least will be capable of taking avoiding action against hypoglycaemia, should the need arise. Relatives should be warned also to look out for any peculiarities in the patient's talk and behaviour which strike them as being unusual, uncalled for or inappropriate to the situation. These are often the first expressions of clouding of consciousness in hypoglycaemia and may be sufficiently pronounced as to impair insight, judgment or lead to perseveration. Thus, as Wauchope observed, a patient may dimly realize that something is amiss but feel compelled to continue what he is doing, e.g. driving a car, and in a negativistic way, although he may have some idea that he requires sugar, refuse to take it.

Vitamin deficiency. Utilization of glucose by the nerve cell is dependent on the enzymatic action of certain vitamins, notably vitamin B_1 (aneurine, thiamine). When this is deficient oxidization cannot occur and conditions analagous to those seen in hypoxia are created, which soon give rise to symptoms of clouding of consciousness. Pyruvic acid, which is an intermediate product of the oxidization of glucose, accumulates in the blood in the form of pyruvate. Deficiency may arise in old people, who are living alone, through their diet being inadequate, too much tea, bread and butter being consumed and too little vegetables and fresh meat. Vitamin deficiency also may be conditioned by overindulgence in alcohol or by heavy metallic intoxication—drugs like arsenic or mercury combining with the protein component of the vitamin and so interfering with the oxidation of pyruvic acid, Thompson.[256] Overdosage or long continued medication with barbiturates may have similar histotoxic effects.

Clouding of consciousness due to endocrine disorders. Apart from insulin hypoglycaemia, there was no instance in our series of primary or *idiopathic hypoglycaemia.* However, many such cases have been reported, one of the best accounts being that given by Romano and Coon.[257] Their patient had been subject to recurring attacks of mental confusion in which bizarre behaviour had been noted. These were at first thought to be hysterical, but later they were proved to be due to an islet-cell tumour of the pancreas. An admirable account is given both of the mental and physical state. In a small proportion of these cases, according to Whipple[258] there may be multiple tumours, in others the results of laparotomy are negative and the spontaneous hypoglycaemic attacks appear to be functional in origin. The diagnosis of idiopathic hypoglycaemia is suggested when symptoms indicative of clouding of consciousness recur either shortly after heavy meals or between meals and are accompanied by craving for food. The symptoms are relieved dramatically by eating a piece of chocolate or any other easily assimilable foodstuff and the electroencephalogram may be of value in demonstrating a correlation between disappearance of high amplitude slow waves during attacks and the taking of sugar. The finding of abnormally low blood sugars at these times and the response of the blood sugar level to insulin and to fasting are further aids towards confirmation of the diagnosis. However, individuals differ greatly as to the level to which the blood sugar must fall for symptoms to appear and in Addison's disease, for example, this may not be less than 60 mg.%.

In descriptions of *myxoedema*, as in hypoglycaemia somatic signs and symptoms tend to take pride of place over mental aspects, but the latter often predominate. Diagnosis is important because of the successful results attending treatment and because of the fatal consequences that may so easily ensue if the patient is allowed to become chilled or is treated with barbiturates (see p. 28).

Thyrotoxic crises are more common in young adults than in older age groups but must be borne in mind in thyrotoxic patients displaying a mounting pulse rate and temperature, restless delirium and other symptoms pointing to clouding of consciousness. Acute mental symptoms may also be precipitated in such cases by intercurrent throat infections, trauma, surgical operations, emotional shock and are intensified by the administration of bromides or barbiturates.

Idiopathic hypoparathyroidism is another occasional cause of acute

16

confusional mental symptoms, Robinson *et al.*[251] These authors describe a case in a woman of 61, whose symptoms had begun some years before with depression, following the death of her husband. Some time later, bilateral cataract operations had been performed. Mental confusion and loss of memory had heralded finally the development of epileptiform fits and on her admission to a mental hospital she was disorientated and unable to carry on a rational conversation. On physical examination the principal abnormalities noted were: slurring dysarthria, fine lateral nystagmus, depressed tendon jerks and doubtfully extensor plantar reflexes. Chvostek's sign was positive and skull X-rays showed calcification in the region of the basal ganglia. Serum calcium was 6·5 mg.%, inorganic phosphate 10·4 mg., and serum alkaline phosphatase 4·5 King-Armstrong units. Treatment by intravenous calcium gluconate and dihydrotachysterol (A.T.10) was successful in stopping the fits and improving her mental state.

Exogenous and endogenous toxaemias. Bromide psychosis is now rarely seen as the drug has largely passed into disuse, but barbiturate intoxication is fairly common and may occur unexpectedly in elderly arteriosclerotics, who are the subject of epileptiform fits and have been taking phenobarbitone for their control. In such cases, the dose should not be allowed to exceed 1 gr. daily or treatment must be changed, e.g. to soluble phenytoin sodium. It is also advisable to give supplementary doses of vitamins B and C. Apart from epileptics, the sudden withdrawal of *barbiturates* from persons accustomed to their habitual use is liable to precipitate fits and/or acute delirium with hallucinations. The incautious use of *morphine* or *opiates* often has similar effects in predisposed persons and there is especial risk in prescribing these drugs to patients with hypopituitarism, myxoedema or Addison's disease. In the treatment of Addisonian crises acute mental symptoms may be precipitated in the first day by overdosage with *cortisone*.

These are only a few instances of the toxic mental effects that may be traced to drugs and the possibility of such causes must always be taken into account in acute mental illness, especially when hallucinations are prominent and the unusual behaviour of the patient suggests the presence of some ideomotor apraxia, e.g. difficulty in dressing himself.

Mild or unsuspected infections such as influenza or bronchopneumonia, or even constipation may precipitate confusional symptoms in the elderly, especially those already showing evidence of organic brain disease. Recurring mental symptoms may also precede the appearance of more obvious signs of *liver failure* in patients with multilobular cirrhosis or after portacaval shunt operations, and in suspected cases the therapeutic test of giving a low protein diet for some days and combining this with Neomycin is worth a trial, rapid improvement in the mental state on such a regimen being in favour of an hepatic encephalopathy.

THE DIFFERENTIATION OF FOCAL FROM DIFFUSE CEREBRAL DISEASE

The differentiation of focal from multiple or diffuse lesions is important in later life on account of the frequency of cerebral vascular disease and because recent work has shown that in many apparently classical cases of apoplexy the lesions are not solitary and thrombotic but multiple and ischaemic in origin. In chronic brain disease, where mental symptoms may predominate over physical signs, differentiation is equally important because intracranial tumours and often solitary and circumscribed space-occupying lesions may, on occasion, readily be mistaken for global dementia.

Acute cerebral vascular accidents.

In cerebral vascular accidents the problem used to be to decide whether symptoms were due to thrombosis, haemorrhage or embolism; when hemiplegia resulted it was assumed that the most probable site of the lesion was in the lenticulostriate or one of the other perforating branches of the middle cerebral artery. The discovery that intracerebral haemorrhage could result from rupture of an aneurysm broadened this concept, but only in recent years has it been recognized that, whilst thrombotic, embolic and haemorrhagic lesions of intracerebral vessels still have to be reckoned with, the primary lesion is often situated on the proximal or cardiac side of the circle of Willis and involves the carotid or vertebral arteries, before their entry into the skull. As has already been mentioned, cerebral infarction is not invariably thrombotic but may be ischaemic in origin, tissue damage being due to hypoxia. Further, it is known that occlusion of one carotid or vertebral artery may occur without any serious consequences accruing, the remaining vessels being capable of maintaining an adequate circulation. But should intravascular clotting be extensive or a second main artery become occluded, cerebral circulatory failure usually results. This disaster can also be brought about in patients with carotico-vertebral atheroma by sudden falls in systemic blood pressure.

The actual vascular mishap that brings the patient under observation may thus be representative more of the epilogue than of the first act in the individual tragedy of cerebral vascular disease. But, fortunately, in most instances this is not so. The damage due to atheroma may be limited to a small area in the internal carotid artery just distal to the bifurcation, which means, if occlusion occurs and other things are equal, that some regression of symptoms is to be expected with opening up of the collateral circulation. In effect, these patients may remain free of further symptoms for many years.

Methods of investigation have been discussed on pp. 35–37 and will be dealt with further in the succeeding section, but as soon as the condition of the patient permits repeated examinations should be made for indications of any variation in the mental and physical state and to determine the extent to which the signs are suggestive of a single focal lesion or of multiple lesions. When obstruction of a large intracerebral vessel occurs abruptly there is swelling of the affected hemisphere, due to oedema, and usually coma, which is followed by clouding of consciousness for some days. Steady and progressive lessening of its depth, however, is to be expected as oedema subsides and the collateral circulation begins to function so that within 7–10 days there may be little or no sign of it, despite the fact that the residual hemiplegia may still be absolute. With focal intracerebral haemorrhage, contrary to the classical view, the reverse picture may be seen, hemiplegia appearing rapidly and being ushered in by severe headache without any clouding of consciousness. But this usually occurs later with expansion of the haematoma and mounting cerebral oedema.

In carotid stenosis or occlusion fleeting motor, sensory or visual disturbances may have been noted some days, weeks or months previous to the onset of hemiplegia, but, unlike obstructive intracerebral vascular lesions, consciousness is not lost abruptly although mental confusion is often seen, the patient showing perseveration, disorientation and impairment of memory. Thus, at first evidence of clouding is often slight but during the succeeding days it may become more pronounced, this sequence of events not being unlike that seen after asphyxia from coal gas, where the late appearance of secondary stagnant hypoxic effects creates the illusion that some complication of a more serious nature has arisen. However, we have not seen consciousness in such cases fall to the level of drowsy stupor, mental confusion usually resolving slowly with disappearnce of the hypoxic effects.

Occasionally it may be possible to distinguish a classical apoplexy, i.e. due to a capsular thrombosis, haemorrhage or embolism from carotico-vertebral atheroma (complicated by occlusion of one carotid) by the character of the physical signs. Thus, a capsular lesion, if sufficiently extensive, could cause contralateral hemiplegia, hemianaesthesia and hemianopia, but one would not expect it to cause hemiparesis and hemianopia. Such a finding without corresponding sensory impairment, and especially if there were a discrepancy between the extent of paralysis and the visual field defects, would be more in keeping with the presence of at least two separate lesions, one situated anteriorly and the other posteriorly in the substance of the hemisphere.

Other signs which would favour the diagnosis of carotico-vertebral atheroma, complicated by cerebral circulatory failure and the formation of multiple ischaemic infarcts in the cerebral hemispheres, would be persistence of an extensor plantar response on the side opposite to the hemiplegia, the repeated demonstration of an exaggerated jaw jerk or of a bilateral snout reflex. Post-ictal oedema from occlusion of or haemorrhage from an intracerebral vessel may also give rise to bilateral neurological signs through swelling of one hemisphere causing displacement and coning downwards of the brain stem through the tentorium. But at this stage the patient is likely to be in drowsy stupor, the level of consciousness being more acutely and severely depressed than it is in circulatory inadequacy and there may be other distinguishing features such as inequality of the pupils and neck stiffness.

Chronic organic mental states.

Examples have been given earlier of intracranial tumours and other space-occupying lesions simulating dementia, and someone has remarked cynically that, in attempting to differentiate such focal lesions from diffuse cerebral cortical atrophy, 10 c.c. of air are of more value than the most painstaking clinical examination! This may be so in patients who have reached the stage of becoming surgical emergencies before their true nature has been suspected. But lumbar encephalography and angiography, however indispensable as preliminaries to surgical intervention, are far from being reliable in the early stages of organic brain disease and may sometimes prove actually misleading. For example, if lumbar encephalography is performed in elderly subjects at a time when their physical signs are still equivocal and symptoms indicative chiefly of loss of initiative and memory impairment, the finding of symmetrical dilatation of the ventricles may be accepted as confirmatory evidence of an early dementia when, in effect, the appearances are physiological, Heinrich,[260] and symptoms are due to some other cause, e.g. a slow-growing infiltrating tumour not yet causing ventricular deformity. Further, neither air encephalography nor angiography can be used indiscriminately because they carry a certain risk. We have had experience of unfortunate consequences such as acute clouding of consciousness, transient hemiplegia and aphasia, and other authors, Rowbotham,[261] Perese[262] have reported similar happenings. Robinson[263] has also described a case in which lumbar encephalography led to the formation of a subdural haematoma.

When an organic mental state is suspected, therefore, it is safer and usually more rewarding to watch for physical signs, the appearance of which may enable one to decide whether there is a focal circumscribed lesion or diffuse brain disease. The comparative infrequency of headache and papilloedema in elderly patients with tumours has already been noted. Epileptiform fits may occur both with focal and diffuse lesions, although it was our impression that major seizures with convulsions were less common in dementia than were minor attacks, the only indications of which might be some transient disturbance of behaviour. In a few cases of tumour the site of the lesion was indicated either by the aura or the unilateral character of the fits.

As regards *physical signs*, these are to be expected at some stage of the illness in both types of case, but in dementia their distribution is almost invariably bilateral and symmetrical. No matter how suggestive symptoms may be of a primary dementia one should always hesitate to make this diagnosis when signs are strictly unilateral or disproportionately greater on one side than on the other. This, of course, is axiomatic but real difficulty can be experienced in appraising the significance of slight differences in tendon reflexes or of decrease or increase of muscle tone on making passive movements. Motor deficit in patients with anteriorally-placed tumours in the contralateral hemisphere may be so slight as to cause only slight weakness of the hand grip, weakness of dorsiflexion at the wrist, or a tendency for the limb to fall away slightly when the arms are extended. Early signs of unilateral sensory impairment may be even more difficult to appraise and can only be detected by repeated observation of the patient's behaviour in showing neglect of the affected limb and by application of the tests described in Chapter III. The same may be said of visual field defects.

Character of intellectual defects.

Study of the intellectual defects shown by patients with organic mental disease is also of value in helping to differentiate between focal and diffuse cerebral lesions. Some years ago we tried to do this on a statistical basis by selecting two groups of patients, one with focal cerebral lesions and the other with diffuse cortical atrophy and giving them tests to determine their capacity for registration, memory and orientation. Observations were also made for changes in mood and behaviour, insight, language and dyspraxic difficulties. It was anticipated that with focal lesions there would be no defects or that certain functions only would be impaired, depending on the site of the lesion, and that with diffuse lesions there would be thinly, but more or less evenly, spread defects in all aspects of mental activity. This was true on the whole but the numbers were too small and performances too variable to enable any valid conclusions to be drawn. Another source of error was that, at the time of examination, many patients with focal lesions were already showing evidence of intracranial complications, due to increase in size of the lesion and cerebral oedema causing brain displacement. This had the effect of inducing symptoms of clouding of consciousness which were, of course, very similar to those seen in diffuse cortical atrophy, although the mechanism of their production was different. So, although it is possible with psychometric tests to correlate intellectual defects with the sites of uncomplicated focal lesions, a qualitative approach is more rewarding when the object is to differentiate between focal and diffuse lesions. When this is done many distinguishing points emerge and these may now be considered.

Alterations in mood and behaviour.

Mood and behaviour are related and disturbances of both are common in organic mental disease. They depend on the interplay of several factors, chief among which are:

Premorbid Personality and Temperament. These serve to "colour" affective changes and may partly determine the reasons why some patients show anxiety, tension or depression and others hostility or suspicion.

Clouding of consciousness. This interferes with the patient's awareness of himself. Moods of unconcern, indifference, expansive good humour and denial of illness are usually accompanied by impairment of insight. But this is not always so for one of our patients, an intelligent woman who showed neither clouding of consciousness nor lack of insight, when questioned about the good-humoured and jocular attitude she adopted towards her afflictions, replied that it was like being poor, i.e. " You can do nothing about poverty, so why not make a joke of it!" Clouding of consciousness also plays a big part in determining abnormalities of behaviour, e.g. perseveration leading to senseless repetition of acts, disorientation and defective grasp to the patient being found wandering and ideomotor apraxia to difficulties in dressing, shaving, etc.

Nature of Underlying Pathology. The most pronounced mood changes are seen with rapidly developing lesions, whether focal or diffuse, and this is especially true of cerebral vascular accidents, subdural haematomas, actively infiltrating or expanding tumours, secondary deposits, general paralysis and the toxaemic and hypoxic encephalopathies. Mood changes are often pronounced at an early stage of Pick's disease, but in the presenile dementias due to diffuse cortical atrophy, although invariable and often the first symptoms to draw attention to the patient, their development may be so insidious as to make it impossible to fix even the approximate year of onset. The same may be said of diffuse cerebral atherosclerosis in which insight may be retained until relatively late. But in chronic vascular disease the inconspicuous mood changes are apt to be livened from time to time by unaccountable mood swings with corresponding alterations in behaviour, these being related probably to fluctuations in the cerebral circulation, the efficiency of which has been impaired owing to atheroma of main arterial trunks.

Anatomical site of the Lesion. The transient disturbances of affect that accompany fits in temporal lobe disease and the buoyant or over-confident mood and uninhibited behaviour displayed by some patients with frontal lobe tumours suggest that lesions in these situations may have special significance in determining the kind of affect seen. But in many of our frontal tumour cases such changes did not occur and Bleuler[15] believes that the so-called " frontal syndrome " may be found with lesions in other sites. Analysis of our own material indicated that neither the site of the tumour nor its position in the dominant or subordinate hemisphere made much difference. The factor in tumour cases most often responsible for promoting mood changes was clouding of consciousness, due to intracranial complications having arisen and affecting midbrain and diencephalic structures. Thus, of our 38 cases in which observations were made, complications were present in 27 and among these mood changes were found in 85%. By contrast, of the remaining 11 patients without complications mood changes were found in only 37%.

As regards the type of change seen, moods of unconcern and fatuous euphoria were more common in diffuse than in purely focal lesions, but as a differential diagnostic point this cannot be relied upon; similar moods were encountered in chronic subdural haematoma and in some of our patients who were found to have meningiomas. Rowdy aggressive behaviour was also seen twice with haematomas although it was more distinctive of the toxic and hypoxic encephalopathies. Anxious, tense or depressed moods were seen fairly often with focal lesions, less commonly with diffuse and then usually only in the early stages of a dementia. In 7 of our tumour cases persistent moods of anxiety were early and pronounced features, their appearance antedating other symptoms and signs, and in 3 of these patients the chief anxiety was that they might have a tumour!

This brings one to some more reliable points of distinction between focal and diffuse lesions. Insight is more likely to be retained in the former so that patients' anxiety tends to centre around their symptoms or disabilities, e.g. hemiplegia, altered sensation. Dementing patients with diffuse cortical atrophy are less aware of themselves and, if they show anxiety or depression, it is more related to fragmentary and poorly systematized delusional thinking in relation to their environment, e.g. that the man in the next bed has stolen their money, that they have no home. Further, the extent to which abnormalities of behaviour may develop differs. Patients with focal lesions may become noisy and difficult to control; they may get up and pass water in the corner of the ward, but rarely is their behaviour so bizarre or truly antisocial that it lands them in trouble with authority.

Before leaving the subject some mention must be made of the possible diagnostic value of *increased emotional lability* and *catastrophic reactions*. Increased emotional lability is common in atherosclerosis and is seen especially in cases where there is relative cerebral circulatory inadequacy and in which focal thrombotic or ischaemic infarcts have occurred. Some of these deeply situated lesions may involve the centres or tracts concerned with emotional expression. In such cases there is " emotional incontinence ", outbursts of tears or laughter, or of both, occurring on the slightest provocation and often being incongruous to the situation. Insight, however, may be preserved so that the patient is embarrassed and as a result may be rendered more anxious and tense. We have had no personal experience of patients with tumours or others with global dementing features exhibiting these symptoms to the same extent, although minor degrees of emotional instability are not uncommon in all forms of organic mental disease.

Catastrophic reactions differ from increased emotional lability in that they usually have a definite precipitating cause. That is, the patient has been doing his best to conceal his defects and is suddenly confronted with a situation which is beyond his powers. Such reactions are easily provoked in some patients but not in others and premorbid temperament probably has some influence in determining their occurrence in individual cases. Their occurrence denotes some retention of insight, but that this is often defective was shown by their frequency in our general paralytics, in most of whom pronounced reactions were readily evoked. In post-anoxic and traumatic states and in diffuse cerebral atherosclerosis and Alzehimer's disease they were also seen on occasion. But with the exception of general paralysis they were perhaps most common in focal lesions and especially those involving the dominant hemisphere and causing expressive dysphasia. When catastrophic reactions take the form of tears difficulty may be experienced in distinguishing them from increased emotional lability, but the circumstances in which they occur usually provide the clue.

Impairment of factual memory for past events.

Amnesic defects, although present in most organic mental states, are often concealed by the patient and in those who lack insight may not be brought to light until some obvious blunder due to "absent-mindedness" occurs and draws attention to them. Three chief differences could be discerned in the pattern of memory impairment shown by our patients with focal and diffuse lesions respectively.

First, there was the duration of memory impairment and its order of appearance among other symptoms. In patients with tumours the duration was rarely longer than a few weeks or months at the most, an observation which suggests that in these cases its appearance (like changes in mood and behaviour) may be correlated with the development of intracranial complications. Enquiry among relatives usually brought out this point very clearly: " Oh, no! . . . he used to have a good memory . . . that's the strange thing about it . . . it is only in the past 6 months that we have noticed anything wrong with it." In dementing patients, on the other hand, it was usually impossible to fix the time of onset and memory defects had been apparent for a much longer time.

The second point is a corollary of the first. In dementing patients disintegration of intellect is often slow and for long periods at a stretch may remain more or less stationary. Until their decline has reached an advanced stage, patients can rearrange their lives to some extent to compensate for faulty memory. Forthcoming events are noted in a dairy, arrangements for the next day are recorded on scraps of paper. Personal belongings are always put in the same place. The point is that, although not all dementing patients avail themselves of these stratagems, they have the opportunity to do so, whereas this is denied to the patient with a tumour or other focal lesion by reason of the rapidity with which his memory impairment develops.

The third point of distinction relates to the extent and character of memory impairment seen in these two classes of patient. Although both may display temporal or spatial defects, naming difficulties or simply amnesic indifference, temporal and spatial defects are rarely as extensive in focal lesions as they may become in dementia. Eccentricities of behaviour such as getting up in the middle of the night to go to the office or making a journey to the city on a Sunday to transact business are typical of slowly dementing states, although, as noted on p. 126, they may occasionally be caused by a meningioma, but we have not seen topographic memory loss in patients with focal lesions develop to the extent that they lose themselves out of doors or have difficulty in finding their way about their homes.

Disorders of speech and language.

Most accounts of the speech and language disorders seen in dementia have centred around Pick's and Alzheimer's diseases, the expressive character of the dysphasia in the former conditon having been correlated with its predilection for the frontal and temporal lobes and the mixed expressive and receptive forms seen in the latter with early involvement of the parietal and occipital lobes.

Anteriorially-placed lesions in the dominant hemisphere tend to disturb expression more than comprehension but as noted earlier, the great majority of our patients showed both kinds of impairment. Many features, also, which have been described as typical of Pick's or Alzheimer's disease were noted in post-anoxic and cerebral vascular cases and, on occasion, in patients with tumours. It is not proposed, therefore, to compare individual diseases but to consider only what points of distinction can be drawn between the speech defects shown by patients with focal and diffuse or multiple lesions respectively. These may be summarized as follows:

(1) Pronounced disturbances of speech and language with only slight or no symptoms of clouding of consciousness are suggestive of focal lesions involving the speech area and the reverse is true of global cerebral affections. Occasionally, however, in dementia isolated speech defects were among the first symptoms observed, e.g. difficulties in naming, word blindness, but, as a rule, although some specific defects could always be demonstrated these were much less obvious than changes in mood and behaviour, absent-mindedness, difficulty in registration etc. With focal neoplastic lesions there was often little evidence of dysphasia until intracranial complications supervened, after which they invariably became pronounced. Apparently abrupt onsets might raise the suspicion of cerebral thrombosis but with tumours there was often a previous history of fits, accompanied by transient dysphasia, which had been more numerous, more fleeting and more selective in their character than would have been expected had a large vessel been undergoing gradual occlusion.

(2) Insight is retained to a greater extent with purely focal lesions than diffuse ones and this may account for the anxious, tense and depressed moods shown by many of our dysphasic patients, and for the frequent occurrence of catastrophic reactions which were often apparent at an early stage before the development of clouding of consciousness.

In the global dementias, by contrast, unless speech defects occurred early, the patient was usually either oblivious or unconcerned about them.

(3) Perseveration is of no special diagnostic value in organic brain disease, but when there are no other signs of clouding of consciousness and it is observed to occur solely in connection with speech, this is an indication of the presence of a focal lesion involving the speech area. It was rarely found to be so marked in patients with tumours as it was in those with focal vascular lesions and in doubtful cases the pronounced character of the sign may be helpful in distinguishing between the two.

(4) Spontaneous speech. Some patients in the early stages of global dementia manage to preserve a façade of normality by indulging freely in "small talk" but gradually their repertoire becomes more limited and stereotyped, more laced with clichés or set phrases, until they reach the stage when they do not speak unless spoken to. Their habitual silence is related to general intellectual decline and paucity of ideas; they show no embarrassment or concern and make no pretence of taking part in conversation, remaining aloof and indifferent to what is going on around them. Patients with focal vascular or neoplastic lesions on the other hand often show " push of talk " in their efforts to express themselves and become greatly embarrassed when others fail to understand. If possessed of sufficient insight to recognize their defects they may keep silent, but they attend to people talking and make signs to indicate they are interested in listening.

(5) As regards the character of their expressive defects, dementing patients in replying to questions often break off in the middle of sentences, leaving the rest unfinished. They use periphrasis but to a lesser extent than do patients with purely focal lesions causing expressive rather than receptive difficulties. Dements, instead of trying to bypass their difficulty in word finding by circumlocution may resort to such phrases as " that thing " or " the what you may call it ". Paraphasia, which was less common than periphrasis was not observed in any of our patients with purely focal lesions, and when it occurred in dementing states was frequently associated with disorientation and moods of euphoria or unconcern.

(6) Gesture and pantomime. It is our impression that although patients with diffuse cortical atrophy may be capable of reproducing gestures or of miming acts they seldom make use of either as a means of communication. Their attitude in this respect is very similar to that seen in amnesic indifference. Patients with focal lesions causing dysphasia are willing to employ them and sometimes do so most effec-

tively, that is provided comprehension is relatively intact, but in many cases their gestures have an inept, clumsy quality due to associated apraxic defects.

(7) Naming from sight and naming from memory. This is a useful point of distinction. Patients with focal lesions have as much difficulty in trying to name objects which they are allowed to see and handle as they have in trying to recall names from memory. Dementing patients have special difficulty in recalling names from memory; their performance with sighted objects is often surprisingly good.

(8) Responses to simple concrete questions and abstract propositions. Patients with both types of lesion have greater difficulty in responding to abstract questions but, no matter how simple the questions, the patient with a focal lesion will betray in his answers some defect in word finding or sentence construction, whereas in the early stages of a global dementia the patient may be capable of coping with simple questions without difficulty. It is only when he is given abstract propositions that his speech defects become apparent.

(9) Gross receptive difficulties in dementing patients are always accompanied by general symptoms and signs of clouding of consciousness. In the absence of any such signs, difficulties in comprehension of spoken or written speech are usually indicative of the presence of a focal lesion. Further indications in favour of such are afforded by the behaviour of many patients with dyslexia who may find they can read slowly provided they trace the letters with their fingers or repeat the alphabet over to themselves until they come to the required letter.

Disorientation.

Although disorientation was a fairly common symptom both in focal and diffuse lesions the combination of total lack of orientation in time, place and for persons was never seen in patients with strictly focal or circumscribed lesions. It was only occasionally seen in cerebral vascular lesions resulting in hemiplegia and prolonged clouding of consciousness and its occurrence, to all practical purposes, was more or less confined to advanced cases of dementia, due to diffuse cerebral cortical atrophy or multiplicity of lesions in both hemispheres. Such patients usually had no idea of the time of day or night or the place they were in and they mistook relatives and friends for other persons or persons deceased, or regarded them as strangers. In patients with tumours disorientation was relatively late in its occurrence, and it was rare to find it before intracranial complications had supervened. In early cases of global dementia, on the other hand, disorientation could usually be traced back for a much longer period, and it was possible to show that it had grown up, as it were, alongside their amnesia, temporal aspects being first disturbed and later spatial orientation becoming affected. Some considerable time then usually elapsed before the patient became disoriented to persons, but the slow unfolding of disorientation in this order was very typical of diffuse lesions, whereas in patients with tumours, disorientation invariably made its appearance late—over a period of a few days—and it never developed the full-blown picture seen in advanced dementia.

Because of this late appearance of disorientation it was usually not possible to demonstrate by means of house drawing and map tests evidence of abstract disorientation in patients with rapildy developing focal lesions. But, the routine use of such tests was of assistance in the recognition of abstract disorientation in diffuse cortical atrophy and its presence was invariably observed at some stage in the course of such maladies.

As regards fragmentary aspects of disorientation: prosopagnosia, right-left bodily disorientation, finger agnosia, all these could at times be demonstrated in patients with diffuse cerebral lesions and little focal significance may be attached to them unless it can be shown that other aspects of orientation are unaffected.

Agnosias and apraxias.

In slowly dementing patients whose chief symptoms are related to impairment of factual memory and changes in behaviour, picture agnosia and constructional apraxia were often found at an early stage in their decline, and in doubtful cases were helpful in distinguishing a dementia from a purely affective disorder. But visual object agnosia and ideomotor apraxia were seldom encountered as isolated early symptoms. Indeed, the sudden appearance of these symptoms was so frequently associated with toxic encephalopathy, that when mental confusion is of short duration and these are prominent features the suspicion of drug intoxication, liver disease, anoxia or hypoglycaemia should be aroused.

As regards the significance of agnosic and apraxic defects in focal brain disease, unilateral tactile agnosia or astereognosis was sometimes of great value in helping to distinguish a focal parietal lesion from a global dementia and in a few cases the transient occurrence of ideo-motor apraxia following minor epileptiform seizures was the first indication to give a lead to the diagnosis. In one right-handed man who was later found to have a right parieto-occipital tumour, the earliest demonstrable signs were contralateral hemianopia and some cortical sensory impairment. His only mental defect was constructional apraxia and this was marked and constantly present from day to day. However, having regard to the great frequency with which agnosic and apraxic defects are found in association with clouding of consciousness, one would hesitate to attach any focal significance to them unless they were accompanied by other suggestive signs and it could convincingly be demonstrated that consciousness in general was little affected.

ANCILLARY METHODS IN DIAGNOSIS OF FOCAL AND DIFFUSE CEREBRAL LESIONS

1. *Electroencephalography.*

Electroencephalography was performed routinely in all our cases, recordings being repeated at intervals, when required, in order to detect signs of deterioration when none was at first apparent or to note changes in the constancy and extent of previously noted abnormalities. Criteria of abnormality were the same as those recommended by Grey Walter, Cobb *et al.*[264] and a 6-channel machine was used. The E.E.G. was of considerable help in differentiating focal from diffuse cerebral lesions, but reliance was placed more on correlation of clinical and other data with the results than upon these findings alone.

Diffuse cerebral cortical atrophy. Records are available from 28 cases in which the absence of focal neurological signs, the chronic amnesic character of the symptoms and results of investigation were all indicative of diffuse cortical atrophy, due to a variety of causes. Represented among these were diffuse cerebral atherosclerosis, post-traumatic and anoxic cases and patients with Alzheimer's disease, general paralysis and Huntington's chorea. The characteristics noted in the E.E.G. may be summarized as follows:

(1) In 5 instances (case No. 39 cerebral atherosclerosis; case Nos. 49, 95, chronic amnesic syndromes of unknown origin; case Nos. 69, 73, post-anoxic dementia) the records were normal or equivocal. There was an α rhythm of good amplitude and symmetry: diffuse slower activities at 4–7 c/s. were sometimes seen, but these were of lesser amplitude than the alpha. The same applied to faster activities, which were occasionally picked up from the frontal regions. Both types of rhythm could often be induced by overbreathing or photic stimulation and were accentuated by these procedures.

(2) Abnormalities were found in the other 23 cases, these being of three chief types:

(*a*) α rhythm, although symmetrical was infrequent, poorly developed or absent, the records being dominated by slow frequencies at

4–7 c/s. These were symmetrically distributed and of greater amplitude than the α rhythm (case Nos. 13, 16, 20, 22, 23, 24, 26, 27, 29, 31, 47, 60, 98, 104, 144).

(*b*) Low amplitude or flat records, there being little activity on either side of the brain (case Nos. 13, 29, 34, 60, 74, 83, 93, 98, 104, 121). Three of these were patients with Huntington's chorea.

(*c*) Records showing focal activity or asymmetry. These were only seen occasionally. In case No. 77 (chronic atherosclerotic dementia) rhythms occurred at 1–2 c/s. which became focal in the left frontal region, and in case No. 191 (general paralysis) a focus was found at 3–4 c/s. in the left temporo-occipital region. In another case (No. 16), a patient with a chronic amnesic syndrome and fits of unknown causation, slow activity was observed at 1–2 c/s. in both frontal regions. In 2 other instances (case Nos. 28 and 60), although an actual focus could not be demonstrated, activity was asymmetrical, α rhythm being less affected on one side and slower rhythms being more prominent on the other.

Cerebral tumours. Results are available in 29 cases of cerebral tumour, the site and pathology of which was determined at operation or autopsy. As in the dementias, a proportion of the records—about one fifth— were normal or equivocal. In one case (No. 181) this was probably explained by the tumour (an ependymal astrocytoma of the fourth ventricle) being too deeply seated to disturb cortical rhythm. There was a good α rhythm at 8–9 c/s., which was perfectly symmetrical and apart from some low amplitude fast activities in the frontal region there was nothing ususual. In another case (No. 117), in which an astrocytoma was found in the left parietal cortex, E.E.G.'s were per- sistently normal. This gave rise for a time to the suspicion that the symptoms might be hysterical, as physical signs were equivocal and only the patient's mental state was abnormal. In the other 3 cases in which there were negative E.E.G. findings, meningiomas were found —case No. 133, left temporal (sphenoidal electrodes were also nega- tive), case No. 167, right temporal and case No. 86, right parietal.

In the remaining 24 cases, the E.E.G. was consistently abnormal and was often of value in suggesting either the position of the tumour or the side upon which it was placed. Three chief types of abnormality were seen:

(*a*) There was a normal α rhythm, but this was interrupted by frequent, symmetrical slow wave activity at frequencies ranging from 4–7 c/s. to 2 c/s. These were of high voltage and present in all areas. In the only case (No. 97) in which this type of record was seen, the findings were interpreted as being indicative of a deep-seated midline tumour and this proved to be correct for at operation a pinealoma was found, which was causing some dilatation of the third and lateral ventricles.

(*b*) In 10 cases there was more or less normal α rhythm, which, at times, was interrupted by slow frequencies on one side. These were of greater amplitude than the α and were constantly present, being quite unaffected by overbreathing or photic stimulation. In three patients in which the slow activity became focal, a tumour was found at or near the site designated.

Case No. 88. Normal α rhythm with slow activity at 1–2 c/s. focal in left temporal region (left fronto-temporal astrocytoma).

Case No. 36. Normal α rhythm with slow activity at 2 c/s. focal in R-frontal region (right frontal meningioma).

Case No. 106. Normal α rhythm with slow activities at 6–7 c/s. becoming focal in left posterior parietal region (left temporo-parietal glioblastoma).

In the other 7 cases, no focus could be demonstrated, but in most instances the unilateral character of the high amplitude slow activity indicated the side upon which the tumour was situated. Unfortunately, in one case (No. 85), a glioblastoma in the parieto-temporal region was invading both hemispheres by way of the corpus callosum so that the right-sided abnormality was misleading, and in another (No. 45) with a meningioma growing from the falx cerebri, abnormal activity was most pronounced at a site some distance from the tumour.

Case No. 99. Normal α rhythm present at 8 c/s. with slow 1 c/s. activity in left parietal region, the α rhythm being less well developed on this side than on the right; no focus (left temporal meningioma).

Case No. 51. Low amplitude α rhythm seen at 9–10 c/s. with slow activities of higher voltage on the left side most marked in the parieto-occipital region. No focus (left temporo-parietal astrocytoma).

Case No. 140. Normal α rhythm present but constant slow activities seen in the right fronto-temporal region (right parasaggital meningioma extending over the right parietal lobe).

Case No. 48. Normal α rhythm with some slower activities at 5–7 c/s. Diffuse activity at 2–3 c/s. recorded from right frontal area. No focus (right frontal meningioma).

Case No. 139. An irregular but fairly symmetrical α rhythm present at 8 c/s. However, there was excess 6–7 c/s. activity which was frequently of greater amplitude. Slow waves of higher amplitude at 2–3 c/s. recorded on both sides but chiefly over left hemisphere. No focus (left parietal astrocytoma).

Case No. 85. α rhythm at 8–10 c/s. of fair amplitude and symmetry with slower activities at 7 c/s. Diffuse slow ½–2 c/s. waves of greater amplitude over the left hemisphere. No focus (temporo-parietal glioblastoma in both hemispheres, spreading across through corpus callosum).

17

Case No. 45. α rhythm of good amplitude and symmetry at 11–12 c/s. Slower rhythms at 8–9 c/s. and 4–6 c/s. present on the left side, which were increased by overbreathing. On repeated examination some weeks later these appearances were unaltered but some slow 1–4 c/s. activity was observed in the right occipital region. No focus (meningioma of falx cerebri).

(c) In 13 cases there was little or no α rhythm, or it was present on one side only. Dominant slow rhythms were recorded from both sides, which were asymmetrical and sometimes focal on the side upon which they were most pronounced. In 4 cases, in which a focus was demonstrated, a tumour was found at or near the site indicated, in a fifth case the tumour was on the same side but in the posterior fossa.

Case No. 46. Little or no α rhythm, the record being dominated by low amplitude slow waves at 4–7 c/s. and these were focal and of greater amplitude in the right temporo-occipital region (right occipital oligodendroglioma).

Case No. 148. α rhythm at 10–11 c/s. only seen on left side, high amplitude slow activities at 1–2 c/s. being prominent on the right and focal in the right temporo-occipital region (right occipital oligodendroglioma).

Case No. 87. α rhythm normal on right side but absent on left, where it was replaced by slow waves at 3–6 c/s. These became focal at two points in the left frontal and left fronto-temporal regions respectively (left frontal astrocytoma—tumour confined to frontal lobe).

Case No. 89. Fairly normal α rhythm on left side but absent on right, where it was replaced by slow waves of greater amplitude at 4–7 c/s. These occurred at the rate of 1–2 c/s. in the parietal region, where they became focal (right parietal meningioma).

Case No. 163. Only a little α rhythm at 8 c/s. seen, slower activities at 4–7 c/s. being dominant and bilateral and of greater amplitude on the left side, where they became slower at 2–3 c/s. and focal in the parieto-temporal region (left acoustic neuroma, large cystic tumour).

In 2 other cases showing foci, metastatic tumours were present. These were secondary to primary intrathoracic carcinomata.

Case No. 143. Only a little diffuse α rhythm at 8 c/s., which was irregular and asymmetric, being less on the right side than the left. Slower activities at 2–6 c/s. recorded over the right hemisphere which became focal at times in the right temporal region (right frontal secondary tumour—squamous-celled carcinoma of the bronchus).

Case No. 134. No α rhythm seen. Bilateral 4–6 c/s. activity, of higher amplitude on left side and becoming slower at 1–2 c/s. in the left temporal region, where it was focal at times (multiple secondaries in frontal regions and left temporal lobe).

In the remaining 6 cases no focus could be demonstrated. In 2 instances a midline tumour was found and in the other 4 the side upon which the tumour was situated was indicated by slower wave forms of higher amplitude.

Case No. 72. Irregular and asymmetrical rhythm of low amplitude, the record being dominated by slow activity at 1–3 c/s., which was symmetrical and of high voltage. Fast activities at 14–20 c/s. were also recorded. No focus (epidermoid suprasellar cyst).

Case No. 151. Scanty α rhythm at 8 c/s., slow 6 c/s. rhythm being dominant. On the left side these were at 3–4 c/s. and on repeated examination fell to 1–3 c/s. No focus (mid-brain glioma).

Case No. 94. Only occasional α rhythm with slow frequencies predominating and of greater amplitude. These were asymmetric and most pronounced in the right frontal region. No focus (right frontal oligodendroglioma).

Case No. 59. No α rhythm seen. Bilateral asymmetric activity at 5–6 c/s. becoming slower and of greater amplitude in left temporal area. No focus (left frontal astrocytoma).

Case No. 70. No α rhythm seen. Both fast and slow activities recorded with frequencies ranging between 8–18 c/s. On left side high amplitude 1–3 c/s. waves and occasional theta activity at 4–7 mc/s. No focus (left parieto-temporal anaplastic astrocytoma).

Case No. 174. α rhythm was seen only on the right side, slower activities at $1\frac{1}{2}$–2 c/s. being recorded from the left and these were of greater amplitude. Some theta activity was also found but no focus (left fronto-temporal astrocytoma).

In cortical affections, it is recognized that abnormality in the E.E.G. is dependent on the acuteness and severity of the lesion. Unilateral vascular lesions give rise to transient abnormalities on the side affected, but later the rhythms tend to revert to normal. The same is true of the presenile atrophies; during acute phases there is often much abnormality, which may be focal, but later as the patient's condition becomes more static rhythms may again become normal, Hill.[265] This author, incidentally, was the first to describe the peculiar absence of cortical rhythmical activity which is seen in Huntington's chorea, although it is not pathognomonic of that disease. Delay *et al.*[266] noted a normal rhythm at 10 c/s. in the frontal region of a case of Pick's disease in which ventriculography had shown both frontal lobes to be atrophic. Cerebral tumours are electrically inert and the high amplitude slow activity, which may be focal at the site or more pronounced or confined to the side of the tumour, is due to the partially damaged or oedematous tissue surrounding it. Slow-growing, infiltrative, supratentorial tumours may create so little disturbance of cellular metabolism that this slow activity does not result, but fast-growing tumours and actively expanding and compressing tumours may excite marked abnormality, Millar.[267] Analysing results in a series of 87 confirmed cases of primary supratentorial neoplasms, this author found that the

E.E.G. correctly foretold the side affected in 79 cases, localized the tumour in 52 and was normal in only 5 cases. By contrast a normal record or evidence of generalized abnormality was the usual finding in posterior fossa tumours. Comparing the value of the E.E.G. with clinical methods, however, Renfrew *et al.*[268] conclude that in lateralizing and localizing a tumour the E.E.G. most often serves to confirm clinical opinion, in only a few cases the information provided by it being distinctly additive in character.

The principal differences in the E.E.G. between our cases of tumour and diffuse cortical atrophy are summarized in Table 17. Normal records were found in about the same proportion in both groups, but it is of interest that in the 5 tumour cases with normal records 3 were

TABLE 17.—*Diffuse Cerebral Cortical Atrophy v Cerebral Tumour: Comparison of E.E.G. Results*

E.E.G.	Diffuse atrophy (26 cases)	Tumour (30 cases
Normal	5 (20%)	5 (17%)
Asymmetry of record (amplitude and/or frequency)	6 (23%)	26 (86%)
α rhythm present on one side only	0	4 (13%)
α rhythm scanty or absent	17 (65%)	13 (43%)
Focal activity (unilateral)	3 (11%)	10 (33%)
Bilateral foci	1 (4%)	0

slow-growing meningiomas and amenable to surgery. The frequency with which this particular tumour may simulate a presenile dementia has already been remarked in Chapter I. It may be concluded, therefore, that a consistently normal E.E.G. does not rule out the possibility of an organic mental state, but that when records are abnormal the E.E.G. is of value in distinguishing between focal and diffuse lesions. In diffuse cerebral cortical atrophy it is unusual to find any pronounced asymmetry in the amplitude or frequency of prevailing activities, whereas such occurs in a high proportion of patients with tumour. By contrast, slowing of α rhythm and its replacement by bilateral, more or less symmetrical slow frequencies, behaving as an α rhythm, is more typical of diffuse atrophy, in which group of cases no instance of unilateral normal α rhythm being preserved was found. Foci of abnormal activity were seen at or near the site of the lesion in about one-third of the cases of tumour. The occurrence of more than one focus indicated usually the presence of multiple metastases or of diffuse cortical atrophy.

The really difficult records to interpret were those in which the α rhythm was scanty and replaced by bilateral slow activities, which were so pronounced on both sides as to make one doubt they could be associated with a solitary focal lesion in one hemisphere. It was in these that serial records were of especial value in enabling the consistency of any asymmetric features to be assessed. The accidental occurrence of dehydration, heavy sedation by barbiturates, fall of blood pressure or vitamin deficiency may produce such features in the records of patients suffering from early presenile dementia and it is advisable to correct any such defects as may exist and repeat the test 7–10 days later, before attributing any focal significance to them.

The E.E.G. in chronic subdural haematoma. In the chronic variety of subdural haematoma, E.E.G. changes may be slight or absent. When the record is normal, the mental state is correspondingly so. When a haematoma is suspected on clinical grounds, then an asymmetry of α rhythm should be accepted as the surest guide to its correct lateralization, but when there is no such asymmetry the presence of unilateral slow and/or focal activity may point to the side of the lesion, Millar.[269] In 2 of the 7 cases in this series, the records were normal. In the other 5, the appearances corresponded to one or other of the three types of abnormality known to occur in this condition, Grey Walter *et al.*[264]

(*a*) A localized focus of activity at delta frequency in an otherwise normal record, Short and Dunster (1940).

(*b*) Diminished amplitude of wave forms over the site of the haematoma, Jasper *et al.* (1940).

(*c*) High voltage fast and slow activities on the side of the lesion, Sjaardema and Glaser (1942).

Other uses of E.E.G. in organic mental states. Although in chronic dementing states or arrested cases of dementia the E.E.G. may be normal, it is, as already mentioned, extremely sensitive to acute or subacute biochemical or pathological changes occurring in the brain. Weinstein and Kahn *et al.*[270] used amobarbital to bring-up abnormalities and claimed that testing patients with organic mental states by this means enabled focal activity or pronounced asymmetry to be demonstrated, which was of assistance in differential diagnosis. Some years ago we carried out similar experiments on a mixed group, half of whom were normal persons aged between 40–60 and the other half patients in whom the signs pointed to the presence of a tumour, the results of E.E.G. and mental tests being compared before and after pentothal administered intravenously.

As drowsiness supervened too rapidly to enable them to be studied closely, pentothal was discontinued and 1 oz. absolute alcohol substituted, this being given orally. In a series of 10 cases with an equal number of controls, no appreciable differences were noted in the extent of falling-off in the performance of mental tests or in the E.E.G. Of great value, however, was the E.E.G. control of patients suffering from hepatic encephalopathy, as changes in the character of the record preceded the actual appearance of clinical symptoms, so that one could test the effects of diets of differing protein constitution without harmful effects, protein being reduced on the first appearance of such changes.

Another use of the E.E.G. was in patients recovering from acute cerebral vascular accidents, in which one expected to see in serial records, repeated at intervals of 2–3 weeks, as oedema subsided and a good collateral circulation was established gradual improvement and disappearance of abnormal focal activity, which was at first pronounced. Persistence of marked unilateral abnormalities were sometimes indicative of clot formation or of a tumour, and persistent bilateral abnormalities were suggestive of cerebral circulatory inadequacy with multiple areas of anoxic softening and lack of establishment of a satisfactory collateral circulation.

2. *Cerebrospinal fluid.*

Examination of the cerebrospinal fluid, whilst essential to the diagnosis of general paralysis and in the differentiation of spontaneous subarachnoid haemorrhage from meningitis, gives little information of diagnostic value in other organic mental states. The procedure is indeed risky in cases of cerebral tumour or subdural haematoma and in any case there is little in the way of information to be gained from it. We agree with Bull[271] that raised intracranial pressure is more safely estimated by clinical, opthalmoscopic and radiological methods and that lessened density of the clinoid processes in a plain X-ray of the skull may be an even earlier sign of increased pressure than papilloedema. As a rule, therefore, lumbar puncture was delayed until it was reasonably certain that a space-occupying lesion could be excluded, or, in cases in which there was strong suspicion, air pictures could be made simultaneously.

As regards abnormalities found in the fluid, in all our cases of general paralysis, the Wassermann reaction was strongly positive and the cellular content typical. Total protein and globulin were increased and the colloidal gold test was of paretic type. In about half of the tumour cases and in slightly more of the cases of diffuse cerebral cortical atrophy the fluid was normal in all respects. A rise of total protein above 50 mg.%

was observed in 15% of proved cases of tumour and in about 19% of the cortical atrophies, the proportions being about the same for globulin. Raised protein levels were also often found in cerebrovascular disease. In 3 patients with tumour—case No. 163 (acoustic neuroma), No. 143 (metastatic frontal lobe tumour), No. 72 (suprasellar epidermoid cyst) —the colloidal gold curve was meningitic in type, but in no instance were tumour cells found.

3. *Radiography.*

Plain radiograms of the skull were taken in all cases, occasionally information of great value being obtained from them. In presenile dementing patients the appearances were normal although occasionally frontal hyperostosis was seen. This, however, was not peculiar to these cases being seen sometimes in patients with focal lesions.

In about three-quarters of patients with tumour, plain X-rays of the skull were normal. Calcification of the pineal gland occurs normally in over 50% of skulls of persons aged 40 and over and is more common in men than women, Vastine and Kinney.[272] According to these authors, Schüller (1918) and Naffziger (1925) were the first to note the value of displacement of the pineal shadow in the diagnosis of intra-cranial lesions. In our cases, pineal shift was observed in about one-third, but in only two instances was there a significant shift (more than 3 mm.) to one side. In the remainder, measurements showed that the opacity was in the midline, although a tumour, which was later shown to be causing displacement, was present in one or other hemisphere. Useful information was obtained by plain radiography of the skull alone in about 13% of cases later found to have a tumour. In No. 19, the site of the meningioma, later removed at operation, was easily identified by extensive calcification in the right frontal region, and in No. 163 (left acoustic neuroma), there was erosion of the left petrous temporal bone. In the few other cases in which abnormalities were present, although suggestive of the presence of a space-occupying lesion, these were insufficient in themselves to indicate its site. They included: prominent vascular markings in one particular region of the vault of the skull; opening up or ballooning of the sella turcica, due to pressure from a distended third ventricle; asymmetric erosion and decalcification of the clinoid processes, and displacement to one side of a calcified pineal gland.

Radiograms were also taken of the chest in cases where the possibility of an intrathoracic tumour arose, and in cerebral vascular cases to find out if there was any evidence of aortic atheroma or cardiac hypertrophy.

Angiography. We have only adopted this procedure in recent years as a means of investigating organic mental cases. Serious consequences in the form of hemiplegia and aphasia may follow its indiscriminate use, especially in chronic cerebral vascular disease, but it has proved valuable in certain instances where the clinical features have suggested the likelihood of intracerebral haemorrhage with clot formation or occlusion of one common carotid or internal carotid artery. There was usually no difficulty in deciding the side to inject, but when signs were equivocal it was sometimes necessary to do both sides in turn. Needless to say, this was never considered without good reason and was only undertaken after attempts to localize the lesion by other means had failed. Some of the methods that may be used to do this have already been referred to in Chapter II, i.e. palpation of the vessels in the neck, ophthalmodynamometry. For a time, when no pulsation could be felt in the neck, we tried to feel the pharyngeal pulse, but few patients would tolerate the gloved finger inserted, as it has to be, through the mouth to behind the tonsil. Local anaesthetic applications were of little help and further, when pulsation was felt in this situation one could never be sure that it was not being transmitted from the external carotid or due to clonic-like contractions of the stylopharyngeus muscle.

Another method sometimes advocated is to test the effect of temporary carotid compression upon the character of the E.E.G., but we have always felt anxious about the propriety of this procedure, which at the best of times does not provide as valuable information as can be obtained through angiography. In one-quarter of their 6o patients, Skillicorn and Aird[273] noted E.E.G. abnormalities, which appeared within 10–20 seconds of unilateral carotid compression below the sinus. Admittedly, these invariably precede clinical signs of clouding of consciousness, but a check on the latter can, be kept equally well by the simple expedient of getting the patient to count whilst his carotid is being compressed. The theory underlying the test is that compression of an already occluded vessel will have no effect on the E.E.G., whereas in cases where collateral circulation has not been established, compression of the healthy vessel on the other side will render the brain hypoxic. In practice, results are often difficult to interpret although, occasionally, they may be of considerable assistance in enabling one to predict the chances of successful operative interference.

Vertebral angiography (although the only means of visualizing the basilar system of arteries) was rarely undertaken in patients in later life because of the danger of causing the artery to go into spasm. This may happen when the needle point fails to enter it at the first attempt. Such an event might have little effect if the vessel were already occluded, but if patent and the opposite vertebral artery were not, the effect of spasm through wounding of the unaffected vessel could have serious consequences. This hazard may be overcome by brachial arterial catheterization, which is now coming into use. However, by comparison, carotid angiography is a relatively simple procedure, provided cases are carefully selected and only dilute solutions of contrast medium used.

Angiography was used as a confirmatory aid to the diagnosis of intracranial tumours, especially in patients whose physical signs and E.E.G. had already indicated the probable side upon which the tumour was situated. It was also of value in helping to distinguish intracranial clots from neoplastic lesions, and in cases in which the history was of comparatively short duration and the signs indicative of mounting intracranial pressure, it was preferred to air encephalography because it caused less dangerous reactions. In such cases, too, there was often doubt as to the presence of a chronic subdural haematoma and, as lumbar encephalography could not be considered it saved the necessity for making ventriculograms.

Of the 30 cases of cerebral tumour, angiography was performed in 16, but in 7 of these air pictures had to be made in addition to provide the necessary pre-operative knowledge as to its site and probable character. In the remaining 9 cases, the information obtained from angiography alone was sufficient to enable the surgeon to proceed. This information was derived from study of the angiograms in relation to displacement of the anterior, middle or posterior cerebral vessels upwards, downwards or in the case of the anterior cerebral across the midline. In 4 cases the typical appearances of a tumour circulation with sacculation of blood vessels were seen.

Air encephalography. Ventriculography was sometimes done as a preliminary to craniotomy when an angiogram or lumbar encephalogram had not provided sufficient information to enable the surgeon accurately to determine the site and extent of a tumour. In most cases, however, lumbar encephalography is to be preferred, being a simple procedure, requiring no special preparation, and in selected cases the appearances it may reveal are as reliable as those obtained from the more complex undertaking, Norton and Wickbom.[274] In some ways, however, this is perhaps unfortunate for it encourages too free use of the test and possibly also its substitution for more detailed examination. Thus, in one patient seen recently, a diagnosis of early Alzheimer's disease had been made because there was symmetrical ventricular dilatation. But organic mental tests showed no evidence of intellectual deterioration and repeated neurological examination brought out some brain-stem signs in the form of paresis of conjugate gaze upwards and defective convergence, these signs being associated with difficulty in reading and cerebellar ataxia.

Also, although simple to perform, lumbar encephalography is not without risk. Subdural haematoma, as already noted, may result and in some of our patients, who were already showing signs of clouding of consciousness, deepening of the level was observed for some days and accompanied by such undesirable consequences as incontinence of urine; this is especially liable to occur in chronic amnesic patients although it tends to disappear as soon as consciousness has returned to its previous level and regular habits are reinstituted.

So, lumbar encephalography was used sparingly and principally as a confirmatory test in patients with amnesia to distinguish between the possibility of a tumour or other space-occupying lesion and diffuse cerebral cortical atrophy. Usually the history was of shorter duration than is found in dementia, neurological examination and electro-encephalography were equivocal, but under clinical observation odd features about the patient had been noted, e.g. the occurrence of fits, unexpected incontinence, frequent headaches. For the test 10–30 c.c. of air were injected into the lumbar subarachnoid space and, after time had been allowed for the air to ascend into the skull, radiograms were taken. In diffuse cerebral cortical atrophy these showed the typical appearances of symmetrical dilatation of the lateral ventricles, absence of any filling defect or displacement, a normally outlined third ventricle and air in the subarachnoid space beneath the vertex and over the lateral surfaces of the hemispheres.

Lumbar encephalography was also of value in suspected cases of aqueduct or third ventricle obstruction, when combined with a contrast medium, so that the basal cisterns and fourth ventricle could be accurately outlined. With suspected tumours of the fourth ventricle, however, it was usually necessary to make burr-holes to demonstrate with air, and possibly a small amount of an opaque medium, the outline of the third ventricle.

The question sometimes arises as to what one should do in the event of failure with lumbar encephalography, that is to say when radiograms show no evidence of filling of the ventricles or of air over the vertex. Such a result could be due to a technical fault, e.g. the air being injected extradurally, but when patients have been selected with care and lack of experience can be discounted, failure to demonstrate air in the ventricular system is almost pathognomonic of obstruction to its free flow by a deep-seated tumour blocking the aqueduct, third or fourth ventricle. This happened in case No. 81, a man aged 62, who presented with " functional " features (although these had some unmistakable organic mental characteristics) and ataxia. Lumbar encephalography showed air in the cisterna magna and cisterna ambiens, but none in the ventricles or over the hemispheres. At first it was thought this was due to mischance but, later, by means of ventriculography a tumour was found blocking the fourth ventricle and invading both cerebellar hemispheres. In such instances, repetition of previous failure will only result from further attempts at lumbar encephalography, and if it is felt there is a reasonable chance of helping the patient, a ventriculogram should be done. In the case referred to, the tumour was an ependymal astrocytoma and Torkildsen's operation was performed successfully.

BIBLIOGRAPHY

246 Behind the Depressive Symptom (1959). Annot. *Brit. Med. J.*, **2**, 102.

247 ROTH, M. and MORRISSEY, J. D. (1952). Problems in the diagnosis and classification of mental disorder in old age. *Jnl. Ment. Sc.*, **98**, 66.

248 RICHTER, D. (1959). Protein metabolism of the brain. *Brit. Med. J.*, **1**, 5132.

249 CAMPBELL, J. and BIGGART, J. H. D. (1939). Wernicke's encephalopathy. *J. Path. Bact.*

250 SEVITT, S. (1960). The significance and classification of fat embolism. *Lancet*, **2**, 825.

251 BULL, G. M. (1953-54). " Body Water Control." Lectures on the Scientific Basis of medicine. Vol. 3, XIII, p. 219.

252 CLAYTON-JONES, E. (1959). Water intoxication. *Brit. Med. J.*, **2**, 306.

253 WYNN, V. (1956). Water and electrolytes: water intoxication and serum hypotonicity. *Metabolism*, **5**, 490. Quoted in Annot. *Brit. Med. J.* (1959), **2**, 556.

254 KEPLER, E. J. and MOERSCH, F. P. (1937). The psychiatric manifestations of hypoglycaemia. *Amer. J. Psychiat.*, **91**, 89.

255 WAUCHOPE, G. M. (1933). Hypoglycaemia: critical review. *Quart. J. Med.*, **2**, 117.

256 THOMPSON, R. H. S. (1952). Discussion on recent work on peripheral neuropathies. *Proc. Roy. Soc. Med.*, **45**, 661.

257 ROMANO, J. and COON, G. P. (1942). Physiologic and psychologic studies in spontaneous hypoglycaemia. *Psychosom. Med.*, **4**, 283.

258 WHIPPLE, A. O. (1944). Hyperinsulinism in relation to pancreatic tumours. *Surgery*, **16**, 289.

259 ROBINSON, K. C., KALLBERG, M. H. and CROWLEY, M. F. (1954). Idiopathic hypoparathyroidism presenting as dementia. *Brit. Med. J.*, **2**, 1203.

260 HEINRICH, A (1939). Das normale Enzephalogramm in seiner Abhängichkeit von Lebensalter. *Z. Alterforsch.*, **1**, 345.

261 ROWBOTHAM, G. F., HAY, R. K., KIRBY, A. R., TOMLINSON, B. E. and BOUSFIELD, M. E. (1953). Technique and the dangers of cerebral angiography. *J. Neurosurg.*, **10**, 602.

262 PERESE, D. M., KITE, W. C., BEDILL, A. J. and CAMPBELL, E. (1954). Complications following cerebral angiography. *Arch. Neurol. Psychiat.*, **71**, 105.

263 ROBINSON, R. O. (1957). Subdural haematoma in an adult after air encephalography. *J. Neurol. Psychiat.*, **20**, 131.

264 WALTER, W. GREY, COBB, W. A., WHITTERIDGE, D., GREVILLE, G. D. and HEPPENSTALL, M. E. (1950). " Electroencephalography." Macdonald, London.

265 HILL, D. (1947). Discussion on the electro-encephalogram in organic cerebral disease. *Proc. Roy. Soc. Med.*, **41**, 242.

266 DELAY, J., NEVEU, P. and DESCHAUX, F. (1944). Les dissolutions du langage dans la maladie de Pick—diagnostic de l'atrophie cérébrale par l'encéphalographie et la ventriculographie. *Rev. Neurol.*, **76**, 37.

267 MILLAR, J. H. D. (1955). Some observations on the electroencephalogram in cerebral tumours. *J. Neurol. Psychiat.*, **18**, 68.

268 RENFREW, S., CAMERON, J. H. and HAGGER, I. C. (1953). The value of the electroencephalogram in the diagnosis of intracranial tumours. *Brain*, **76**, 92.

269 MILLAR, J. H. D. (1960). The electroencephalogram in subdural Haematoma. *Scot. med. J.*, **5**, 123.

270 WEINSTEIN, E. A., KAHN, R. L., SUGARMAN, L. A. and LINN, L. I. (1953). Diagnostic use of amobarbital sodium in organic brain disease. *Amer. J. Psychiat.*, **109**, 889.

271 BULL, J. W. D. (1959). Lumbar puncture. *Brit. Med. J.*, **1**, 48.

272 VASTINE, J. H. and KINNEY, K. K. (1927). The pineal shadow as an aid in the localization of brain tumours. *Amer. J. Roentgenol.*, **1**, 320.

273 SKILLICORN, S. A. and AIRD, R. B. (1954). Electroencephalographic changes resulting from carotid artery compression. *Arch. Neurol. Psychiat.*, **71**, 367.

274 NORTEN, G. and WICKBOM, I. (1958). The relative value of encephalography and ventriculography for the investigation of intracranial tumours. *J. Neurol. Psychiat.*, **21**, 1.

CHAPTER XII

Treatment

SPACE precludes detailed discussion of the treatment of organic mental states for information relating to which reference should be made to other sources. But the fact that these conditons occur so often in elderly subjects does not mean that, on occasion, they cannot be treated as successfully as in younger persons. At present the chief causes of failure are: uncertainty as to their etiology; the absence of adequate preventive measures, and delay in their recognition, because often by the time appropriate treatment is undertaken it is too late to be effective. The knowledge gained in the past 50 years, however, encourages one to believe that further advances in this field will be made before the end of the century so that, to paraphrase Rolleston's words[3] the Psalmists' threescore years and ten and its sorrowful extension to four-score may be so often exceeded by human beings, who appear normal, that the possibility of a far longer existence is raised.

TREATMENT OF THE CAUSE

Space-occupying lesions.

In this particular series expanding or infiltrative focal lesions of traumatic or neoplastic origin were found in approximately one-quarter of the patients—a high proportion—but probably more a reflection of the close association in which we worked with our neurosurgical colleagues than of the true incidence of these causes in organic mental disease in general. There were 8 cases of *chronic subdural haematoma*. All but three of these recovering fully after evacuation of the clot through appropriately-placed burr-holes. Of the three failures, in two the condition was not recognized in life and in the third, although the clot was successfully localized and evacuated so that the patient was able to resume routine work, signs of a chronic amnesic syndrome persisted until his death two years later as the result of an accident. In this case the dementing process, which was probably arteriosclerotic in origin, had been evident for some years and had clearly preceded the signs and symptoms relating to the haematoma. In the other cases in which operation was curative, mental and neurological symptoms had been of short duration and of periods ranging from 6 months to 2 weeks. The rapidity with which deterioration had occurred was often very striking. Thus one man, a farmer, aged 65, admitted on account of left-sided neurological signs, presented the picture of an advanced dementia, being doubly incontinent, aggressive and resistant, disorientated in time and place and totally unable to register or to recall past events. A large right parietal haematoma was evacuated and within 3 weeks recovery was sufficient to enable him to return home. Subsequently he resumed work and when last seen 3 years later had fully recovered.

Another patient (details of whose case are given elsewhere (see p. 120), had a large right frontal aerocele, which was successfully dealt with surgically by repair of the tear which had led to air gaining access to the skull through the right frontal air sinus. His recovery was also uneventful.

There were 39 *intracranial tumours*. Of these 6 were metastatic and secondary to bronchial or mammary carcinomata. In 5 no operative treatment was feasible but in the sixth, a man of 64, in whose case ventriculography had demonstrated the presence of a space-occupying lesion in the right frontal area a solitary metastatic growth was successfully removed. The features of this case were so unusual that they may briefly be recorded:

Case No. 143, male, aged 64 (1956). In the autumn of 1955 he had complained of cough, pain in the chest and haemoptysis. A bronchial carcinoma invading the upper zone of the left lung was found and successfully excised, partial pneumonectomy being performed. Recovery was uneventful. Some four months later, in February 1956 he complained of headaches and was noticed to be absent-minded, lacking in initiative and having no clear recollection of recent events. His mood was irritable, tense and depressed. He was partly disorientated, incontinent of urine, incapable of registration or of recalling past events and when pressed for answers would burst into tears and wring his hands in a despairing gesture. There were no neurological or chest signs. Electroencephalography showed slow activity at 2–3 c/s. over the right hemisphere and a focus in the right frontal area. Ventriculography confirmed the presence of a space-occupying lesion which at craniotomy was found to be circumscribed and easy to remove. On section this proved to be metastatic and identical histologically with the bronchial tumour (a squamous-celled carcinoma). Recovery was uneventful and there has been no recurrence of symptoms. When seen three years later he appeared to be normal both physically and mentally and had resumed his former occupation.

In 16 cases an *intracerebral astrocytoma or glioblastoma* was found, the situation and infiltrative character of which limited the surgical approach either to confirmation by biopsy of the histological nature of the growth or to its partial removal, this being followed by deep irradiation when the histological appearances were considered favourable to such treatment. One elderly woman, despite a rapidly-growing and diffusely infiltrating glioblastoma in the temporal region of the dominant hemisphere, which had been irradiated, showed remarkably little disturbance of intellect and speech for some 6 months afterwards until increasing frequency of fits finally led to her death in status epilepticus. A man with a type III astrocytoma in the same situation continued a vegetable-like existence for 3 months before his death. But a clergyman, with a cystic astrocytoma in the right cerebellar hemisphere, made a good recovery after partial excision of the tumour, evacuation of the cyst and deep irradiation, and was able to resume his parish duties for 4 years before symptoms from extension of the growth led to his death in coma. Two other cases also made good initial recoveries and lived for a year after operation but 11 survived for only a few days or weeks after operation.

Of the remaining 17 cases of tumour there was one *acoustic neuroma*. This was partially excised and the patient is still alive 6 years later but the chronic amnesic syndrome, which had been apparent for a year or so before her tumour was recognized, has persisted and the result is disappointing. The same applies to 2 other cases with *deep-seated tumours involving the third ventricle* (pinealoma) and fourth ventricle (ependymoma) respectively. For these Torkildsen's operation was performed. By contrast, a woman of 46 with a large suprasellar epidermoid cyst, who had been amnesic and disorientated for a year or so before operation, recovered dramatically after the cyst was exposed and emptied in 1952. Further aspiration was necessary within a year but until 1956, when contact with her was lost, there had been no recurrence of symptoms. In 2 other cases *oligodendrogliomata* were found at operation, occupying the right frontal and right posterior parieto-occipital regions respectively. In both instances it was possible to excise the growths in their entirety by either frontal or posterior parieto-occipital lobectomy and the patients made good recoveries. Even more favourable results were obtained in 8 of the 11 cases of *meningioma*. Many of these were large and judging by the duration of symptoms, had been present for some years before their existence was suspected. In one case, that of a man aged 65, with amnesia of a few months' duration, and paresis of the left arm and lower face, the tumour was small, circumscribed and situated just beneath the right frontal pole. Its removal would have presented no technical difficulty but unfortunately ventriculograms were misleading in suggesting that the tumour was situated on the lateral convexity of the lobe, and at operation it could not be located. In a second case a large meningioma was successfully removed but as in the preceding case the patient died within 2 days of operation. The third fatality, which followed the successful removal of a large left temporal meningioma, was unexpected because the patient was showing promising signs of recovery when he died suddenly a week later from pulmonary embolism. In the remaining 8 cases in which meningiomata were successfully removed the subsequent course was uneventful, symptoms and signs of mental impairment disappearing within a month or two of operation, except in one case in which some expressive dysphasia persisted.

Post-anoxic and traumatic encephalopathy.

In more severe cases with persistent coma or drowsy stupor, the patient was barrier-nursed, recumbent in the lateral decubitus, the foot of the bed being slightly raised and air passages kept clear. Penicillin was ordered when there was any possibility of intracranial infection. To prevent pressure sores the skin was frequently cleansed and changes in posture were made every few hours, exposed parts such as the heels being protected by cotton wool dressings. Higgins, Lewin et al.[275] have shown in closed head injury that although about 10% of the cases develop no metabolic disturbance, about one-quarter show either hyperchloraemia and hypochloruria or hypochloraemia and hyperchloruria, or water deficiency, and that over 60% have transient metabolic disturbances with proteinuria, elevated blood urea, blood sugar and glycosuria. Therefore, one of the first considerations is to assess electrolyte balance, samples of blood being taken for estimation of the blood urea, plasma chloride, bicarbonate, sodium and potassium levels, both in the serum and urine. Fluid intake, urinary output, specific gravity and pH should also be estimated. Blood transfusion may be required in the first 24 hours, but after that feeding should be begun by a naso-oesophageeal tube passed into the stomach. Lewin and his colleagues fed their patients with 2 oz. of water or diluted milk hourly or two-hourly for 4–8 hours, before each feed the stomach being aspirated. A milk-glucose-water regimé was then begun so that the patient received 3 pints of milk, 1–3 pints of water and 300 g. of glucose in the 24 hours (225 calories; 50 g. protein and 0·85 g. sodium). After 24–48 hours, unless there was hyperchloraemia a pint of Ringer-Fischer solution was substituted for the same amount of water and the sodium intake increased gradually to 2 g. daily. If the blood urea were normal and the patient still in coma the protein intake was increased to 100 g. daily by the addition of eggs, soya flour and full-cream dried milk to the feeds. Vitamin supplements were also provided (riboflavine 2 mg., aneurin hydrochloride 5 mg., nicotinamide 20 mg., pyridoxine 2 mg. with vitamin A, 4,500 I. U., and vitamin D, 1,000 I. U. daily).

Hyperpyrexia was treated by removing bedclothes and tepid sponging, but if persistent a wet sheet was placed over the patient and an electric fan turned on to induce hypothermia, ice bags being placed in the axillae and groins and chlorpromazine being given to abolish shivering and reduce the temperature. This was maintained at $84 \cdot 2°$ F ($29°C$); any further reduction is inadvisable on account of the danger of ventricular fibrillation.

When unconsciousness is prolonged, however, the chief danger is cerebral hypoxia, due to insufficient pulmonary aeration or obstruction of the air passages. Continued hypoxia leads to damage of the endothelium of the cerebral capillaries and dilatation of the capillary bed so that engorgement and diapedesis of blood elements occurs into the surrounding tissues (delayed cerebral oedema). In such cases the intravenous injection of hypertonic glucose or urea in fructose solutions may be advisable.[276] But even more important is it to ensure a free airway from the commencement of treatment. When there is much secretion blocking the upper air passages a catheter should be passed into the trachea and mechanical suction used, a cuffed endotracheal tube being inserted. Respiration can then be maintained either with an anaesthetic bag and valve attached to an oxygen cylinder or by means of a mechanically-driven positive pressure machine. When these measures prove inadequate because of continued hypersecretion or bulbar weakness a tracheotomy should be done, positive pressure respiration thereafter being maintained by means of a suitable apparatus. Assisted respiration may be given in this way for periods up to 12 weeks, but frequent assays of electrolytes and of blood gases are necessary, Dreifuss *et al.*[277]

General paralysis of the insane.

General paralysis accounted for 12 cases or about 6% of the total clinical material. Except for one man, whose condition was too far advanced to benefit, all were treated by penicillin on the lines recommended by Purdon Martin[278] some years ago.* Most of our cases were seen between 1946–1955 and a few of the earlier ones had fever therapy, followed by penicillin and repeated courses of arsphenamine. But in latter years we have abandoned these other methods, being convinced that the disappearance of cells in the cerebrospinal fluid and the return of the protein content and colloidal gold curve to normal may as effectively be secured by bismuth and penicillin alone.

---

* In a later paper[279] this author remarks: " Some of my patients treated with pencillin alone in 1945 have now been under observation for ten years, and nearly forty have been followed up for more than five years. . . . I have seen no relapses, either clinical or as evidenced by the C.S.F."

Hahn *et al.*,[280] who recently conducted a survey of 1086 cases treated
in the United States, came to similar conclusions and affirm that
if syphilis is energetically treated by penicillin general paralysis can
be prevented. Whether this is true or not in the long term remains
to be seen but fresh cases have certainly been infrequent in recent
years, Kidd.[281] In the initial course of treatment penicillin was
given in its crystalline form intramuscularly in divided doses every
three hours throughout the day. Those treated between 1946–1950
received initial courses of 10–15 mega units but later cases had 30 mega
units. Before commencing treatment patients had a careful organic
mental and physical examination, attention being paid especially to
their behaviour in hospital, the state of the cardioaortic system, renal
function, vitamin intake, water and electrolyte balance. During this
preliminary stage they received every fifth day intramuscular injections
of 1 grain (65 mg.) bismuth. The treatment was sometimes combined
with potassium iodide in doses of 15 grains (1 g.) daily. Barbiturates
and other potentially toxic sedative drugs were avoided.

After 3 weeks, when it was apparent that there was no untoward reaction, penicillin was cautiously introduced in doses of 10,000 units
three hourly. Patients were kept in bed at first and on the first two days
hourly records were made of the pulse and temperature. Any sustained
changes or alteration in the level of consciousness led to the dose of
penicillin being halved or the treatment temporarily suspended in favour
of further bismuth therapy alone. In the absence of reactions the dose of
penicillin was steadily increased so that within a week the patient was
receiving 1 mega unit in each 24 hours. Following completion of the
initial course bismuth was resumed, injections being given at weekly
intervals until the limits of tolerance had been reached. Re-examination
of the cerebro-spinal fluid immediately after treatment usually gave
disappointing results, the character of the fluid being little changed, but
after three months cells had usually disappeared, total protein and
globulin been reduced and the colloidal gold curve altered, although
the Wassermann reaction often continued to be positive. Persistently
positive Wassermann reactions in the absence of any other changes in
the cerebrospinal fluid, however, were not considered to be indications
for further treatment.

Further courses of penicillin (15 mega units) and bismuth were given
after the lapse of 6 months to a year and repeated tests of the cerebrospinal fluid made for the succeeding 2 years, persistent changes in the
protein content and in the colloidal gold curve being regarded as
indications for further treatment on the same lines. But in many of the
cases the serological results were so good as to make this unnecessary,

all signs of activity (with the possible exception of a persistently positive Wassermann reaction) having disappeared—although, unfortunately, these welcome changes were seldom accompanied by corresponding degrees of improvement in the patient's mental state. However, the inadvisability of pursuing treatment with powerful spirochaetocides in such patients is illustrated by the case of a man of 50 in whom preliminary examination had revealed no signs or symptoms of cardiac disease. Some 5 weeks after the commencement of penicillin treatment he developed congestive failure with auricular fibrillation and died following cerebral embolism, post-mortem examination revealing that this had been brought about by recent degenerative changes in the heart muscle and aorta, which was the seat of chronic syphilitic aortitis.

This was the only fatality related to the setting-off of a Herxheimer reaction through treatment. Of the 10 other cases, a business director and a professional man were enabled to resume their former lives and activities, the former treated in 1951 and now aged 71, being retired but in good health and the latter, a younger man, being only 49 in 1946 when treated, having been enabled to continue since then in routine clerical duties and maintain his family. Three of the others have since died, one is under treatment at the time of writing, 3 have a chronic amnesic syndrome which precludes employment, but are well adjusted so that they can live at home, and the remaining 2 cases are severely demented and in mental hospitals. These results, disappointing as they are, suggest not that treatment was ineffective but that it was undertaken too late and only after irreversible and major brain damage had occurred.

Cerebral vascular disease.

Diffuse cerebral atherosclerosis is not amenable to any present day method of treatment. In these patients, the clinical picture can be that of advanced dementia but in others, although the cerebral circulation is barely adequate there may be when first seen few symptoms beyond absentmindedness and loss of initiative. Epileptiform fits may occur and a history of multiple and transient strokes is common. A high mortality is associated with diffuse cerebrovascular disease, more especially in males.[282] *Transient clouding of consciousness with mental confusion,* however, may readily be precipitated by sudden falls in systemic blood pressure, disturbances in electrolyte or water balance or inadequate vitamin intake. Potentially histotoxic drugs such as the barbiturates may also have the same effect. *Elderly diabetics* under treatment by insulin run the risk of hypoglycaemia, the effect of which is increased by the existence of cerebral circulatory insufficiency and it is unwise to pay too strict attention to maintaining " normal " blood sugar levels. Chlorpropamide (Diabinese), an oral antidiabetic drug, is especially suitable for the treatment of diabetes of late onset. Hypoglycaemic symptoms were not observed in any of the cases treated by Grant and Boyd.[283] In one of our cases, as mentioned earlier, a hypertensive man aged 68, there had been no symptoms apart from failing memory and occasional fits until a ganglion-blocking drug was incautiously prescribed with the object of reducing his blood pressure. The desired effect was obtained but within a week the patient had become restless, confused and disorientated and 6 months elapsed after the drug was withdrawn before he reverted to his previous self. Supplementary doses of vitamins B and C were often helpful during these transient episodes of clouding of consciousness in accelerating recovery and, at times when there was great mental confusion, we have given, as recommended by Gould,[284] as much as 1,000 mg. aneurine hydrochloride, 640 mg. nicotinamide, 16 mg. riboflavine, 200 mg. pyridoxine, 20 mg. calcium pantothenate and 300 mg. sodium ascorbate with 4 g. of dextrose intravenously. The ascorbate and dextrose are stored in separate ampoules and mixed with the other preparations just before injection. In less severe confusional reactions following influenza, pneumonia, acute bladder infections or pyelitis one-quarter of the above initial doses may be given intramuscularly and thereafter twice daily for 2 or more days, Dawson.[285]

The possible adverse effects of *anaesthetics* and *surgical* operations in patients with cerebral atherosclerosis should never be allowed to deter one from recommending what may prove to be a life-saving procedure, but the choice of anaesthesia must be carefully made, each case being judged on its own particular merits or demerits and steps taken to ensure during actual anaesthesia that both a free airway and control of blood pressure are secured. Apparatus for inflating the lungs with oxygen must be at hand and pre- and post-operative medication restricted to the minimum requirements. Pre-operatively, chlorpromazine may be given for its sedating effects and is safer than barbiturates, but thiopentone may be required for induction as a preliminary to gas and oxygen. It is quickly eliminated through the lungs under such conditions but should not be used in cases of respiratory obstruction, gross dyspnoea due to disease of the heart or lungs, or in severe renal and hepatic disease or myxoedema.[286] Bedford suggests that during operation elderly patients should be placed in the Trendelenberg position, whenever practicable, and that they should be kept recumbent until the blood pressure is stable at its pre-operative level.

Post-operative prolonged clouding of consciousness, however, may still occur in these patients if attention is not given to their water and electrolyte requirements. Thus, mental disturbances occur in some

2–3% of all cases of *cataract* following operation, Greenwood,[287] Clark,[288] and cases have been reported where delirious patients have so injured the operated eye that it had subsequently to be enucleated. Preventive measures consist of: (1) admission of the patient to hospital 2 or 3 days before operation so that fluid intake and output can be measured if necessary and any tendency to dehydration corrected. (2) Care in the use of barbiturates; these are often given for sedation but in effect their overprescription contributes to the development of delirium, Allison.[181] If a sedative effect is desired chlorpromazine should be used and a safe and effective hypnotic is chloral hydrate, 20 gr. in syrup and water. Other useful sedatives in old people with atheroma, in whom it is desirable to avoid barbiturates, are glutethimide (Doriden), 250–500 mg. at bedtime or methylpentynol (Oblivon) 250–750 mg.[289] (3) Operation should if possible be conducted under local anaesthesia. (4) Post-operatively, a nurse should be in attendance to reassure the patient and make sure that a sufficient intake of fluid is maintained. It may be desirable to bandage both eyes for a few days after operation so that the eyeballs may be kept at rest and the pupils shielded from light. But a confused patient who still retains sight in his unoperated eye may become agitated and assume, because he cannot see, that the operation has been a failure. In such circumstances it is probably best to uncover the unoperated eye and waive the risks of leaving it unbandaged. (5) As soon as possible the patient should be got out of bed and encouraged to take assisted gentle exercise.

Intracerebral haemorrhage with haematoma formation usually occurs from rupture of an aneurysm, bleeding from a localized angiomatous formation or an atherosclerotic vessel. The sudden onset of hemiplegia and severe headache may be preceded by one or more epileptiform fits, but as a rule consciousness is not lost, although clouding or deepening unconsciousness may supervene later, should the haematoma expand. Surgical treatment by exposure and evacuation of the clot is usually called for and in experienced hands has yielded excellent results, McKissock.[290] There were 2 such cases in this series, in one the source of haemorrhage being obscure and in the other a ruptured aneurysm. Both made a good recovery.

Anticoagulant therapy* is of value in cerebral embolism and within

* Commencing with heparin, 10,000 units intramuscularly every 6 hours for about 36-48 hours. Also on the first day the patient was given Warfarin ("Marevan", Evans) 9 mg. orally. Subsequent daily maintenance doses of Warfarin, usually 3-6 mg. were determined by prothrombin estimations. Patients remained in hospital until prothrombin levels were adjusted to 20–25%. On discharge they attended once a week for blood tests, the interval being increased to once every ten days or a fortnight, if satisfactory control had been maintained. Any tendency for prothrombin levels to fall below 15-20% was met by omitting the drug for a few days and by subsequently reducing the dosage.

the last 2 years we have adopted it for certain patients in whom there have been *transient symptoms pointing to atheroma of the carotid or vertebral systems* and in whom it was feared vascular occlusion might occur. Such symptoms included transient dimness of vision, hemiparesis, hemiparaesthesiae, vertigo, diplopia, ataxia, dysarthria. In all treated cases the diagnosis had been confirmed so far as possible by the results of angiography, ophthalmodynanometry or carotid compression. Patients with symptoms or signs of gastro-duodenal ulceration, liver disease or papilloma of the bladder were excluded. Time will show whether the results of this treatment are as good as they appear to be in coronary disease. Caution is necessary in interpreting short term results for, as is well known, the occlusion of one internal carotid artery may not be followed by other similar vascular accidents for many years. Further, as Carter and others[291] have shown, the suspension of anticoagulant treatment, once begun, may not be without risk owing to increased coagulability of the blood resulting from its abrupt withdrawal. It is estimated that the " rebound " effect may last 6 weeks and this may explain the unfortunate experience of one of our patients who had been taking Warfarin, following a coronary occlusion. After some months, as he appeared to have fully recovered, the drug was omitted but within 2 weeks he had developed a right hemiplegia and aphasia. At the time this was thought to be a coincidence. It may have been but other similar cases have been reported and it is advisable, therefore, when such a step is contemplated that frequent estimates of blood prothrombin levels should be made and that the dose of anticoagulant should gradually be reduced before being omitted. Another difficulty that arises over this treatment is that of getting patients to attend regularly and of ensuring that the drug is having the desired effect. We agree with Foley and Wright[292] that only intelligent and co-operative patients are suitable for long-term therapy. Haemorrhage is another potential danger. Groch *et al.*[293] who report favourably on the treatment, state that although some 20% of their 108 cases had haemorrhagic complications this only led to its discontinuance in 1 out of 18 patients, who had been followed-up for more than a year. They point out, however, that despite weekly or bi-weekly blood tests " it is impossible to maintain any large group of patients within therapeutic range for a prolonged period of time ", and that this observation is especially true of patients in the older age groups of 60–70.

Immediate operation on the affected vessel is the logical step when the carotid artery has become stenosed or blocked by thrombus formation. Operation was successfully performed by Strully[294] more than 7 years ago and in Great Britain Rob and his colleagues[295] have had most experience of it. Time, however, has a determining influence because in cases of thrombosis, if the clot has spread from the cervical to the intracranial portion of the internal carotid, it is too late to hope for success in removing it. Rob and Wheeler recommend thrombo-endarterectomy as the operation of choice and, failing this, localized resection of the diseased portion (often the part just distal to the bifurcation), and end-to-end anastomosis. To reduce the risk of anoxia consequent upon temporary clamping of the carotid artery, operation is done under hypothermia, body temperature being kept at 28–30° C. In cases where there is stenosis and clotting has occurred distal to the bifurcation, re-establishment of blood flow may take place naturally through opening up of the terminal twigs of the external carotid and ophthalmic arteries, blood passing via the external carotid and ophthalmic artery (in which the direction of flow is reversed) to enter the carotid syphon above the seat of obstruction. This fact often has been demonstrated by arteriography and may account for some of the remarkable recoveries that now and then follow the appearance of apparently disastrous hemiplegic and aphasic signs. As regards the situation of those parts of the cerebrum which have been deprived of their normal blood supply through blocking of a main vessel, here again the chances of their survival depend to a great extent upon establishment of a collateral circulation. The functional validity of meningeal arterial anastomoses in establishing collateral circulation has been demonstrated in 3 cases of middle cerebral arterial occlusion by Rosegay and Welch.[296] By means of angiography they were able to show in their first 2 cases that filling of an occluded middle cerebral artery could occur from branches of the anterior cerebral artery. In their third case they demonstrated a flow of blood in the opposite direction, i.e. from the middle to the anterior cerebral, and for this to occur, of course, the proximal connection of the anterior cerebral with the circle of Willis has to be completely interrupted. By way of such anastomotic channels blood supply may be restored to part of the cortex normally dependent on the middle cerebral artery, and the same may occur when in turn the anterior cerebral or posterior cerebral arteries are the seat of occlusion. In the opening up of the collateral circulation the maintenance of an adequate systemic blood pressure plays an important part. This is important in treatment, and in cases of internal carotid or basilar artery atheroma, in which occlusion of a main vessel has occurred and the possibility of clot formation is suspected, a mixture of 5% carbon dioxide in oxygen may be inhaled by the patient through a B.L.B. mask for some 5–15 minutes each hour in the hope that its vasodilating effect may hasten establishment of collateral circulation. Stellate ganglion block has been abandoned as being both ineffective and unphysiological.

Although self-limiting in many of its effects, *cranial or temporal arteritis* may cause blindness. Prompt treatment is often effective, however, and when vision becomes impaired, Parsons-Smith[73] recommends 15 mg. prednisoline orally as an emergency measure, followed by 5 mg. thrice daily. As soon as possible this treatment should be switched to adrenocorticotropic hormone (ACTH), the drug being given in doses of 25 units intravenously on the first 2 days and thereafter, for 21–28 days, 20 units intravenously twice daily. In his experience prognosis depends on early treatment, i.e. commenced within a few hours of the onset of blindness and in none of his cases, so treated, did visual impairment progress to total blindness.

There were 3 patients with *hepatic encephalopathy*. One of these is capable of light work 4 years after the condition was first recognized, by which time he had had two severe episodes of coma. The second patient, after the lapse of 6 years is partly demented and requires continuous hospital care. The third died in coma. In the presence of threatened coma we have relied on a protein-free dietary; fluids, glucose and electrolytes being given intravenously, when necessary. Oxytetracycline is administered in doses of 0·5 g. 6-hourly. This treatment is usually effective and as soon as full consciousness is regained the antibiotic is omitted and the patient allowed small and increasing amounts of protein up to 10–60 g. daily. For maintenance treatment we have allowed 60 g. protein daily, but once every 10 days advised a low-protein diet. Oedema of the ankles from restriction of protein is treated by bandaging the limbs below the knee and resting the patient in the recumbent position at intervals, but ascites presents a more difficult problem as its treatment and that of the encephalopathy are to some extent mutually antagonistic. In such cases " a balance must be struck between the mental status and the ascites, and an endeavour made to control the ascites while keeping the patient sensible. If this cannot be achieved, then the mental state must take priority ", Montgomery.[297]

REHABILITATION OF THE BRAIN-INJURED

Patients with hemiplegia or other physical disabilities resulting from brain disease or injury need help to enable them to walk again, an accomplishment which can usually be achieved in uncomplicated cerebral vascular accidents in some 10 to 12 weeks. Passive movements of the affected limbs are first made, then with the first signs of recovering voluntary power, slings are arranged to support the leg and encourage the development of active movements, Adams.[298] By the end of the second or third week the patient is sitting out of bed and exercises in standing are introduced. From then on he passes through successive stages with the use of mechanical appliances until finally he can walk unaided. The extent of recovery depends largely on the severity and permanence of the brain lesion, but two other factors are of equal importance, namely the strength of the patient's resolve to walk again and absence of any further signs of activity in the lesion responsible for causing the disability.

The same principles apply to those whose brain injury has left residual defects in the sphere of intellect and in disturbances of mood and behaviour. Examples are patients recovering from severe cerebral anoxia or trauma, treated cases of general paralysis and others who have had an intracranial tumour successfully removed. Mental disabilities, however, are often less obvious than their physical counterparts and one of the difficulties in management is that relatives and friends, impressed by the apparent recovery of the patient, decide to take him home at a stage when he is still unfit. Harm may result from acceding to such requests, especially in cases where there has been severe brain damage. Thus, one post-anoxic patient shortly after his return home was found wandering and in great distress so that he had to be admitted to a mental hospital. A second, who had been allowed to return prematurely to work, caused a disturbance by accusing other workers of stealing his tools, which, of course, he was constantly mislaying. Another man, a fitter, tried to cover up his mistakes by alleging that his neighbours at the work bench were deliberately " spoiling the job " when his back was turned. These patients, by dint of careful rehabilitation, were eventually enabled to adjust themselves to their altered mental capabilities and the same was true of many others in whom no permanent mental disablement resulted, but whose premature return to domestic or working life was liable to precipitate similar reactions, due to their being faced with problems with which their intellectual capacity at the time was unable to cope.

Exercises in registration and in the performances of simple repetitive tasks.

In the case of post-anoxic and traumatic patients mental rehabilitation should begin as soon as the level of consciousness has risen sufficiently to make this possible: that is during emergence from the stage of disorientation and at a time when there is still defective capacity for registration and recall and inability to undertake simple constructional tasks. By then the patient can usually dress himself, attend to his physical needs and take his food unaided. But if not, he must be assisted by the nurse until he can accomplish these elementary activities on his own account. Ambulant patients in whom the residual disability is more mental than physical should be encouraged to assist in other activities not directly related to themselves, such as carrying trays, helping to lay the table, clearing up after meals and rolling bandages. At their daily visits the doctor and nursing sister in charge should make a point of stopping to talk to them, even though conversation may be almost entirely one-sided or entail no more than the exchange of a few banalities. On each occasion the name of the hospital should be mentioned and the patient encouraged to repeat it, a simple enough matter, although a few minutes later he will probably have forgotten what he has just been told. But this failure must be passed off lightly because it is essential that the patient should not become emotionally upset. When he finally succeeds in retaining the information, the next step will be to get him to give the names of other patients in adjoining beds or wards whom he should visit, afterwards finding his way back to his own bed unaided. Later, when he has become orientated in place, the same procedure may be adopted to encourage return of orientation in time, the day, month and year being noted in that order.

Simultaneously with the above, for a quarter of an hour or so each morning and afternoon, and thereafter for increasing periods up to an hour, he should be given some easy repetitive task such as sorting objects, the occupational therapist or nurse staying with him until he is capable of carrying on unaided. Provided there is no gross receptive speech defect, visual object or colour agnosia, wooden bricks or beads, painted in two colours, may be used, these being sorted by the patient into separate piles, one for red and the other for white. If this proves too easy he may thread them on to a piece of string with the colours arranged alternately. Or, differently shaped pieces of cardboard can be used, the object being to separate the circles from the triangles and squares, the test being later further complicated by cutting the centre out of half of the cards and leaving the other half whole, thus providing other ways of sorting. Somewhat similar is the Form Board, to use which the patient must insert objects of different shapes in the appropriate slots provided for them. A plain baize-covered table or tray covered by a plain dark cloth should be provided as patients with disturbances of figure-background relationships readily become confused when working against a multi-coloured or variegated background. It is also essential, of course, that spectacles are worn by those that require them. Left to themselves few patients remember to use them.

When such simple tasks have been mastered more difficult ones should be selected, for example, sorting peas and beans, nuts and bolts or pieces of string of differing lengths and colours. Old illustrated magazines may also be provided from which the patient has to cut out with scissors pictures of men or women, motor cars, children, animals, etc. These are then pasted in a large size scrap-book.

Occupational therapy.

More organized and extended occupational therapy is required for two chief types of patient: those in whom amnesic indifference and lack of motive are pronounced and others with residual signs of specific intellectual defects either in speech, orientation or constructional ability. The successful planning and carrying out of such treatment depends on observance of three chief principles:

(1) The work selected must provide incentive. That is to say not only must it have interest, but it should enable the patient to derive some satisfaction from its completion. So, previous occupation, interests and hobbies have to be taken into account in deciding upon suitable tasks. For women there is a wide choice ranging from rug making, weaving, embroidery, to making mats or doing leather work; and for men carpentry, bookbinding or making wooden toys. The latter may be assembled from lengths of wood already cut and shaped to represent, for example, the hull of a ship, its superstructure, masts, funnels and boats. These are then nailed or glued together by the patient and the completed model painted. Persons formerly interested in spare-time drawing or painting may be invited to make a start by copying simple coloured figures or designs or applying colours to objects in a picture, which have previously been outlined in pencil. An interesting example of the use of drawing in rehabilitation was given by the late Forster Kennedy[205] in his account of the different stages through which a professional artist passed in recovering her natural drawing ability. Two pictures were painted by one of our patients, a working man of 64, who although only an amateur and self-taught, had indulged in his hobby for many years before a head injury. Hemiplegia and severe dysphasia were the immediate sequelae to the injury and it was a year before he had recovered sufficiently to leave hospital, but he continued to attend for occupational therapy and 2 years after his injury completed the second picture. The first, done before his accident, showed good composition and perspective with plenty of warmth and colour. The second, although remarkably good considering his state in the preceding 2 years, lacked these qualities, the colours in particular being drab and conveying a sombre effect. Alajouanine's[299] interesting account of the effect of brain damage on artistic ability as it affected a writer, musician and painter should be read.

(2) The work must neither be too difficult nor too easy but graded according to the patient's previous intellectual status and residual defects. The presence of physical handicaps such as hemiplegia, hemianopia and sensory loss must be taken into account as also the question of fatigue. Instead of providing suitable materials and leaving the patient to work on his own, arrangements must be made for him to attend the occupational therapy department for gradually increasing periods, beginning with half an hour and extending this to 2 or 3 hours at each session. Not only does this provide contrast in the daily hospital routine but it fosters the idea of work being an essential part of daily life.

(3) The work should be of increasing complexity. Once a start has been made and it is obvious that the patient can manage unaided and is deriving satisfaction from what he is doing, modifications should be introduced so as to make it more difficult. The length of time spent at work is also increased. These advances must be made in easy stages and not before sufficient rapport has been established between therapist and patient as otherwise catastrophic reactions will occur, the patient becoming angry and resentful at interference, refusing to continue or becoming agitated and bursting into tears. One must be at pains to avoid these reactions except possibly in the later stages of rehabilitation. It is permissible then to create situations likely to precipitate them with the object of finding out whether the patient has reached the stage when occupational therapy may be discontinued and actual work considered. Patients with residual constructional difficulties should be given simple jig-saw puzzles consisting of some half a dozen large sections which, when fitted together, form an easily recognised figure. Later they may be encouraged to copy in 2 or 3 dimensions designs made with blocks. The assembly of wooden toys from pre-prepared parts is another way of assisting recovery but before apraxic patients may be considered fit to resume work, it is essential that they should have demonstrated their ability to understand simplified blue-prints and be able to construct models from them. The rôle of the trained occupational therapist at this stage is chiefly to determine and advise whether failure to progress is due to lack of motivation* or to severe residual brain damage. In the latter case the goal of ultimate return to work can never be achieved and it is best to concentrate

* Lack of motivation is a common feature in the elderly. The popular belief that " you cannot teach an old dog new tricks " may act as a deterrent to aspiration and display itself in an unwillingness to submit to tests and activities in which they fear they may fail. Such remarks as: " You don't really want me to do it?" " After all, I'm nearly sixty," " So this is where you make a fool of me, is it?" illustrate this tendency as does the visible relief and pleasure they may show when told they have done very well.[300]

before his return home on those activities of which the patient is still capable. But instances of this kind are in the minority, lack of motivation being usually more important in delaying progress and this in turn being often dependent on persistent mood changes—the patient remaining anxious or depressed, unduly obsessional or adopting a negativistic attitude. In such cases it is always worth while persevering with treatment, although breaks in its continuity are beneficial. The relatives should be told that the patient has done well in reaching his present level of performance and that he may return home, but that after a month or two he should come back for further treatment. In this way, by allowing " holidays " and setting reasonable goals to be achieved at each readmission, many patients within 1 to 2 years ultimately succeed either in returning to work or becoming adjusted to the routine of ordinary domestic life and activities. In 2 patients in whom depressive features became so pronounced as to interfere with progress in rehabilitation, the serious step was taken of ordering electric convulsion therapy. One was a man of 65 with a left-sided hemiplegia, the result of ischaemic infarction from carotico-vertebral atheroma. Although he was able to walk unaided after 3 months and had recovered some useful power in the arm, his mood remained persistently tense and enbittered so that he refused to admit any progress, dwelt continually on his past achievements and expressed the wish that he were dead. At home he was peremptory in his manners and subject to frequent catastrophic reactions. It was in this setting, when his admission to a mental hospital was under consideration, that 3 electric shock treatments were given at intervals of a week. There was no untoward reaction and he became more composed and amenable. This was $3\frac{1}{2}$ years ago and (although he died early this year) he had continued in reasonably good health and been enabled to resume part of his work as a business agent. The other case was a man of 55 with parkinsonism and a chronic amnesic syndrome, but the depressive features were very similar and the response equally good.

Speech therapy.

As already mentioned disturbances of speech and language were found in a number of our patients with organic mental states, 21 being attributable to cerebral vascular accidents, 17 to tumours and 26 to diffuse cerebral cortical atrophy. When a tumour had been successfully removed recovery of speech usually took place rapidly under therapy, but in the diffuse cerebral cortical atrophies the tendency to continuous slow deterioration usually annulled any benefits. The patients considered most suitable for speech therapy were those with cerebral vascular accidents in whom there had been little or no evidence of preceding intellectual deterioration and in whom neurological examination indicated a focal rather than diffuse or scattered lesions. However, it was not always possible to anticipate results, and some who were thought to be poor prospects, on account of signs pointing to disease of both hemispheres, responded better than it had been thought they would. In retrospect it seems probable that in these the cerebral circulation, despite blockage of a main vessel, had been restored to adequacy through opening up of collateral communications in undamaged vessels. Unfortunately in 2 such patients who had regained much of their powers of expression within 2 years of commencing speech therapy, the good results were swept aside in an instant by the recurrence of further cerebral vascular catastrophies, which led to their deaths.

In the first few days or weeks following a stroke, whilst there is still some residual clouding of consciousness, active speech therapy is uncalled for. Perseveration is usually very pronounced so that attempts at communication break down within a minute or less of their inception, and if persisted in only lead to the patient becoming distressed or showing other signs of a catastrophic reaction. However, as Joyce Mitchell points out,[187] once a patient has become aware of his speech and language loss, support is vital and later the therapist can help by interpreting and creating opportunities for communications at some level at which he is still capable. Visiting relatives and staff should be advised to limit their conversation to simple remarks which can be answered by a nod or shake of the head. Even when there is marked perseveration patients can often repeat series, and this exercise is of value in demonstrating to them that their speech has not been wholly lost. After spending a few minutes examining the patient and reassuring him generally one may invite him to join in counting, not bothering about pronunciation but just trying to follow on after the examiner. When this has been explained one should count quickly from 1 to 10 and then begin again more slowly saying: " one ", to which the patient will usually respond " one ", " two ", to which he will usually perseverate, repeating " one ", " three ", to which he may again repeat " one "; " four ", to which he may respond correctly: " five ", again correctly " six ". Once having succeeded in getting him to follow 2 or more sequences correctly in this way the exercise should be stopped before he becomes tired or perseveration again asserts itself. This method does not succeed in all patients and should be discarded if its effect is only to induce distress, but when successful one can then move on to getting the patient to repeat days of the week and months of the year. Repetition of material that may have possible affective significance, such as " The Lord's Prayer ", however, is best avoided.

The inimical effects which disturbances of affect have on performance make it essential that good rapport be established between the therapist and the patient, as otherwise little headway in re-education can be made. In most aphasics, and especially those with purely focal lesions affecting the dominant hemisphere, one expects moods of tension, anxiety, frustration, increased emotional lability or actual catastrophic reactions, it being difficult for such patients, whose insight is largely preserved to submit philosophically to this most disabling of symptoms. Increased emotional lability due to frustration usually disappears in time as rapport is established and means of communication found, but when persistent, occurring spontaneously and unrelated to failure in performance it is usually of bad prognostic significance and indicative of more general cerebral damage than the physical signs would actually suggest.

Only a few examples need be given of the methods employed in treating expressive and receptive speech disorders. The former were most often due either to oral apraxia or amnesic defects. When oral apraxia is pronounced it is useless to expect the patient to learn words by simple repetition or imitation. He must first be taught by the aid of touch, sight and hearing to place his lips, tongue and soft palate in the required positions to reproduce the component sounds. When this has been mastered the sounds are then incorporated into words and later into sentences. Thus, one patient, who had been originally speechless, was able after a year to repeat words sounded in his hearing and could make up some sentences, although these were uttered hesitatingly. Affective influences were still playing a big part in retarding progress for when he was alone, or in the company of people he knew well, he did much better than with strangers or others in whom he sensed some criticism of his efforts. When the difficulty in speaking is primarily amnesic one should determine whether the defect is chiefly aural or visual, or a combination of both. For example, a patient may be able to reproduce a word better by hearing it spoken than by being presented with the object that it represents. In all classes it is essential to arrange for frequent practice in identifying pictorial representations of objects with their written and spoken symbols, because only in this way can memory patterns of speech be re-established. A few patients with right-sided hemiplegia and especially those who have been exclusively right-handed, resist all efforts to get them to use the left hand in writing, but in most patients this is possible and recovery of writing proceeds simultaneously with that of spoken speech, the acquisition of one skill reinforcing that of the other. Two chief defects in writing ability were seen: those related to constructional apraxia, where there is difficulty in shaping letters, and amnesic disturbances where spelling, syntactical and punctuation defects are most apparent. Patients with constructional apraxia were kept under the care of the occupational therapist until this defect had in some measure been overcome when they were then instructed in the copying of letters, words and sentences.

On the receptive side, reading difficulties were fairly common and each case had to be treated individually. The woman with right-sided hemiplegia, hemianopia and dysphasia, whose case has already been referred to, see p. 161, had to be persuaded to look to her right and the only way she could read at first was by fixing her gaze on a word and then moving the head and eyes to bring the next word into view. Affective disturbances were very pronounced and she repeatedly declared that it was useless for her to try to read. But despite numerous setbacks, within 2 years she was able to read headlines and captions under pictures in illustrated newspapers and even to attempt novel reading, although most of this had still to be read aloud to her.

Another patient, also with a right half-field defect had no defect of eye movements. But, although able to speak without much difficulty and to write fluently, she could not understand what she had written. Her dyslexia was literal, only a few letters of the alphabet being recognizable by sight and this was associated at first with marked constructional apraxia. When she ran her finger over a letter so as to trace its shape she knew it at once, but the difficulty lay in persuading her that it was worth while to do this and to prevent her from guessing at a word, when she was less than halfway through with her tracing of its component letters. This tendency to guess seemed to be related chiefly to fatigue and lowered motivation and was common especially in patients with isolated speech defects. The same sort of behaviour was occasionally seen in oral apraxics whose capacity for gesture was intact; they might be so competent at expressing themselves by this means as to make them disinclined to undertake the much harder task of reacquiring speech through imitation of lip and tongue movements.

Social rehabilitation.

Unsatisfactory home conditions may undo much of the good accomplished in hospital and when the time approaches for the patient's discharge the services of the almoner or psychiatric social worker are required to look into these matters and make adjustments, whenever possible. In practice it was often necessary to arrange for the provision of temporary home helps, and with many there was the problem of their resettlement with relatives who were willing to have them. Further, when the patient had recovered sufficiently as to enable him to resume his former employment it was advisable to get in touch with the firm's industrial medical officer or to arrange for the social worker to visit the factory or office so as to ensure that on his return consideration would be shown to him and allowance made for any possible shortcomings. Ideally, such patients should have a preliminary spell of light work, with no great responsibilities attached so that later, if their rehabilitation has been successful, they may be reinstated in full work. For those whose residual disabilities have rendered them incapable of resuming their previous work the problem is more difficult. Suitable alternative employment may not be at once available but whilst efforts are being made to find such, the patient can be tided over the period of waiting by arranging for him to join an industrial rehabilitation course or, failing that, to continue attending the occupational therapy department as an out-patient once or twice a week. Full use was made of the services of the Disablement Resettlement Officer attached to the Ministry of Labour who, under the terms of the Disabled Persons Employment Act and subsequent legislation, administers the " designated employment " scheme by which certain suitable occupations must be reserved for registered disabled persons. The Disablement Resettlement Officer also ensures that all firms employ their statutory quota (3%) of disabled persons and, where re-training is necessary, he arranges this through training schemes coming under the auspices of the Ministry of Labour or of voluntary training bodies.

BIBLIOGRAPHY

275   HIGGINS, G., LEWIN, W., O'BRIEN, J. R. P. and TAYLOR, W. H. (1954). Metabolic disorders in head injury. *Lancet,* **1**, 61.

276   Cardiac arrest and the central nervous system. (1960). Annot. *Brit. Med. J.,* **1**, 558.

277   Dreifuss, F. E., Hurwitz, L. J. and John, C. (1957). Polyneuritis requiring artificial respiration. *Lancet,* **2**, 59.

278   MARTIN, J. P. (1948). The treatment of neurosyphilis with penicillin. *Brit. Med. J.,* **1**, 922.

279   MARTIN, J. P. (1956). The modern treatment of neurosyphilis. *Practitioner,* **176**, 142.

280   HAHN, R. D., WEBSTER, B., WEICHARDT, G., THOMAS, E., TIMBERLAKE, W., SOLOMON, H., STOKES, J. H., MOORE, J. E., HEYMAN, A., GAMMON, G., GLEESON, G. A., CURTIS, A. C., CUTLER, J. C. (1959). Penicillin treatment of general paralysis (dementia paralytica). *Arch. Neurol. Psychiat.,* **81**, 39/557.

281 KIDD., C. B. (1959). Changing trends in general paralysis. *Ulster med. J.*, **28**, 197.

282 MARSHALL, J. (1959). The natural history of cerebrovascular disease. *Brit. Med. J.*, **1**, 1612.

283 GRANT, A. P. and BOYD, M. W. J. (1960). Experience of chlorpropamide in 100 cases of diabetes mellitus. *Irish J. med. Sci.*, **417**, 408.

284 GOULD, J. (1953). Treatment of delirium, psychosis and coma due to drugs. *Lancet*, **1**, 570.

285 DAWSON, D. J. C. (1957). Acute toxic confusional psychosis. In " Whitla's Dictionary of Medical Treatment ", 9th Edn., ed. Allison R. S., and Crozier, T. H, Baillière, Tindall and Cox, London.

286 Contra-indications to thiopentone therapy (1955). Annot. *Brit. Med. J.*, **2**, 836.

287 GREENWOOD, A. (1928). Mental disturbances following operation for cataract. *J. Amer. med. Ass.*, **91**, 1713.

288 CLARK, W. B. (1949). The important complications of cataract surgery. *New Orl. Med. Surg. J.*, **102**, 248.

289 HOWELL, T. H. (1960). Sedation and analgesia in old age. *Practitioner*, **184**, 45.

290 McKISSOCK, W. (1959). Primary intracerebral haemorrhage. Results of surgical treatment in 244 consecutive cases. *Lancet*, **2**, 31, 683.

291 CARTER, S. A., McDEVITT, E., GATJE, B. W. and WRIGHT, I. S. (1958). Analysis of factors affecting the recurrence of thromboembolism off and on anticoagulant therapy. *Amer. J. Med.*, **25**, 43. Quoted by Groch *et al.* (293).

292 FOLEY, W. T. and WRIGHT, I. S. (1956). The use of anticoagulants. *Med. Clin. N. Amer.*, **40**, 1939.

293 GROCH, S. N., HURWITZ, L. T., McDEVITT, E. and WRIGHT, I. S. (1959). Problems of anticoagulant therapy in cerebrovascular disease. *Neurology*, **9**, 786.

294 STRULLY, J. K., HURWITT, E. S. and BLANKENBERG, H. W. (1953). Thrombo-endarterectomy for thrombosis of the internal carotid artery in the neck. *J. Neurosurg.*, **10**, 474.

295 ROB, C. G. and WHEELER, E. B. (1957). Thrombosis of internal carotid artery treated by arterial surgery. *Brit. Med. J.*, **2**, 264.

296 ROSEGAY, H. and WELCH, K. (1954). Peripheral collateral circulation between cerebral arteries. *J. Neurosurg.*, **2**, 363.

297 MONTGOMERY, D. A. D. (1957). Diseases of the liver. In " Whitla's Dictionary of Medical Treatment ", 9th Edn., Baillière, Tindall and Cox, London.

298 ADAMS, G. F. (1960). Progress in the management of cerebral vascular disorders. *Brit. J. Clin. Pract.*, **14**, 361.

299 ALAJOUANINE, T. (1948). Aphasia and artistic realization. *Brain*, **71**, 229.

300 WELFORD, A. T. (1958). " Ageing and Human Skill." Oxford University Press, London.

INDEX

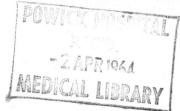

Acalculia, 84, 85, 189
Acoustic Neurinoma, 47, 255
Aerocele, post-traumatic, 120
Affect, influence of in: disorientation, 105; forgetting, 114; dysphasia, 164; bodily orientation, 184; visual agnosia, 208
Affective disorders, 224–7
— E.C.T. in, 227
— in focal and diffuse cerebral lesions, 240
— insomnia in, 225
— and psychoneurosis, 225
— reactive and endogenous depression, 225
— thought content in, 226
Agnosia, 202–10
— auditory, 47, 86, 202, 204
— colour, 44, 86
— in differentiating focal and diffuse lesions, 246
— finger, 185
— picture, 86, 87, 246
— tactile, 59, 202, 204, 246
— visual, 86, 127, 202
Agraphia, 79, 80, 148, 153, 154, 188
Akinetic mutism, 94
Alkalaemia, 25, 38, 98
Alzheimer's disease, 2, 240, 243, 247
Ambidexterity, 167
Amnesia: character of in differential diagnosis, 242–3; and consciousness, 97; dyscalculia due to, 85; with visual agnosia, 209; retrograde, 105; in men and women, 116; hysterical, 222, 224
Anaemia, 32
Anaesthetics in the elderly, 268
Aneurysm, intracranial. Olfactory hallucinations with, 42
Angiography, 256–7
— complications of, 237
— disorientation after, 174
Anosodiaphoria, 194
Anosognosia, 39, 196, 208
Anoxia, cerebral: encephalopathy due to 103–4; amnesic indifference after, 114; causing: Gerstmann's syndrome, 191, visual agnosia, 204; treatment of, 280

Anticoagulants, 269–70
Anxiety, 221, 224
Aphasia, 132–72
— aetiology of, 132
— anatomical factors in, 75
— Head's classification of, 76
— in differentiating focal from diffuse lesions, 243
— tests for, 77
Apperception, 202, 209
Apraxia, 210–19
— in differential diagnosis, 246
— of gait, 20, 21, 53
— pseudoapraxia, 101
— of tongue, lips, face, 48, 78, 137
Argyll Robertson pupils, 47
Arteriosclerosis, cerebral: 5, 34, 35; mood changes in, 240; insight retained in, 240; E.E.G. in, 247; treatment of, 267
Arteritis, cranial, 45, 272
Astereognosis, 56, 63
Auditory agnosia, 47, 86, 202, 204
Ataxia of gait, 53, 54

Barbiturates and the E.E.G., 253
Behaviour, disorders of: 9–13, 23–4, 69
— in aphasia, 78, 139, 143
— in disorientation, 104
— in focal and diffuse lesions, 239–42
Blindness: cortical, 46, 205; due to cranial arteritis, 45, internal carotid artery occlusion, 52
Body scheme or image, 182
Bronchoscopy, 37

Calcification, intracranial, 234, 255
Calculation, 84–5
— dyscalculia and hemianopia, 85
— — in Gerstmann's syndrome, 189
— — due to amnesia, 85
Caloric tests, 46
Carbon monoxide, 2, 98,230
Carcinoma: bronchial, 29; liver, 29; of meninges, 38; vagina, 28
Cardiac arrest, temporary, 98
Cardiac failure, 25, 33, 231

Carotico-vertebral atheroma, 35
— cerebral circulatory insufficiency and, 33
— clinical tests for, 35–6
— diagnosis of, 236, 237
— 'drop' attacks in, 21
— ischaemic infarction due to, 35, 235
Case-taking in organic mental states, 7–26
Cataract, post-operative treatment of, 269
Catastrophic reactions, 11
— in aphasia, 138, 141; rare in paraphasia, 139
— significance in diagnosis, 222, 241
Centrencephalic system, 96, 108, 115
Cerebral arteriosclerosis, atherosclerosis, 5, 34–5
Cerebral circulatory failure, 35, 231, 235, 254, 271
Cerebral damage, extent of, 15, 174
Cerebral vascular accidents, 235
— acute mental confusion with, 230
— disorientation after, 174
— due to cerebral circulatory failure, 237
— E.E.G. in, 254
— treatment of, 267
Cerebrospinal fluid, 254
Cerveau, isolé, 95
Chorea, Huntington's, 22, 53, 251
Chvostek's sign in hypoparathyroidism, 234
Cingulectomy, 94, 95
Colour blindness, 44
Coma, 94, 98
Confabulation, 106, 128, 196
Consciousness, impairment of, 93–6
— constructional apraxia in, 219
— delirium, 100
— in denial syndromes, 197
— disorientation, 102
— in dysphasia, 157, 158
— full consciousness, 107
— in Gerstmann's syndrome, 184
— ideomotor apraxia in, 211
— mood changes in cerebral tumour and, 240
Constructional apraxia, 212; in amnesic subjects 125–6; as early sign of brain disease 213, 214, 246; in Gerstmann's syndrome, 184; in literal dyslexia, 162; in non-aphasic with lesion of subordinate hemisphere, 168; and spatial disorientation, 176; tests for, 87–91

Corneal reflex, depressed in acoustic neurinoma, 47
Corporeal awareness, 182
Cortical blindness, 205, 206, 207
Cortical sensory loss, 56–63

Dehydration, 38, 98, 231, 253
Delirium, 100
Delusions, 23
Dementia, presenile, 1
— and disorientation, 174
— ideomotor apraxia in, 211
— simulated by space-occupying lesions, 7, 18
— speech disorders in, 134, 136, 243–5
— visual agnosia an early sign of, 207
Denial syndromes, 191–9
Depression, 224–7
— associated with brain disease, 9, 10 197, 198
Diagnosis in elderly organic mental cases, 221–59
— acute confusional states, 227
— affective disorders, 224
— air encephalography in, 257
— angiography in, 256
— cerebrospinal fluid in, 254
— electroencephalography in, 247
— focal from diffuse cerebral lesions, 235
— psychoneurosis, 221
— radiography of the skull in, 255
Diarrhoea and opiates, effect of, 24
Diplopia due to cranial arteritis, 35
Disorientation, 102–7
— bodily, 182
— extent of and cerebral deterioration, 174
— in focal and diffuse lesions, 245–6
— spatial, 175
Dominance, cerebral, 166–9; and Gerstmann's syndrome, 190; and auditory and visual perception, 202; and constructional apraxia, 215
Drawing tests, 91, 175–82
Drop attacks, 21
Drugs precipitating mental symptoms, 234; Antabuse, 28; barbiturates, 234; bromides, 234; hypotensive drugs, 232; insulin, 232; opiates, 24
Dysarthria, 48, 136
Dyscalculia, 189; tests for, 84–5
Dysgraphia, 148–54; incoherence and jargon, 153; mirror reversals in,

154; tests for, 79–80; with
dyscalculia and bodily disorientation, 185
Dyslexia, 160–5; associated with
defective eye moves., 161; due
to visual inattention, 160; literal, 162; losing the place in
reading, 165; tests for, 81–4;
verbal, 164
Dysphasia, 132–71
— aetiololgy of, 132–4
— catastrophic reactions in, 241
— defective comprehension and level
of consciousness, 158
— dysarthria, 136
— expressive aphasia, 156
— in focal and diffuse cerebral lesions,
243–5
— jargon and incoherence, 142
— nominal defects, 137
— paraphasia and periphrasis, 138
— perseveration, 141
— reading defects, 160
— recurring, due to carotid occlusion, 52
— speechlessness, 135
— syntactical defects, 139
— tests for, 77–84
— writing defects, 148
Dyspraxia, 210–19

Electric shock treatment, 277
Electroencephalography, 247–54; and
carotid compression, 256; effect
of peripheral stimuli on, 95;
in cerebral tumour, 248; in
diffuse cortical atrophy, 247; in
Huntington's chorea, 251; in
subdural haematoma, 253; in
vascular lesions, 251
Emotional lability, increased, 222, 241
Encephalography, air, 237–8; 257–9
Encephalopathy, acute and subacute;
due to dehydration and alkalaemia, 38; hypotensive surgery,
34; porphyria, 39; vitamin
deficiency, 232; hepatic disease,
31; Wernicke's disease, 38, 228
Epilepsy; due to hypoparathyroidism,
234; infrequent with meningiomata in elderly, 23, and in
carotid occlusion, 52; Jacksonian fits with focal lesions, 133;
major seizures and global dementia, 19, 118; minor fits and
expressive speech defects, 140

Erosion, cranial, 47, 255
Euphoria, 70, 139
Eyeballs, defective conjugate moves.
of, 161

Fat embolism, 229
Finger Agnosia, 185; with visual
agnosia, 209
Figure-background relations, 202, 208,
209
Flapping tremor, 31
Focal and diffuse cerebral lesions,
differentiation of, 235
Frontal lobe syndrome, 240

Gait, disturbances of, 20–2; 'drop'
attacks, 21; due to apraxia 53;
in dementia, 119; in Hunting-
ton's chorea, 53
General paralysis of the insane:
E.E.G. in, 247, treatment of, 265
Gerstmann's syndrome, 183–91
Gestalt, 102, 162, 163, 202
Gesture and pantomime, 84, 136, 137,
223
Grasp reflex, 64

Haematemesis causing acute confusional symptoms, 37
Haematoma, chronic subdural: behaviour in, 7; with mental
confusion, 229; sensory inattention in, 58
Haemorrhage, intracerebral, 235-6, 256
Hallucinations, 228
— due to drugs and metabolic disorders, 102
— olfactory, 42
— proprioceptive, 24
— stereognostic, 23
— visual, 17
— visual after-images and, 24
Handedness, 48–9
— and cerebral dominance, 166
— left-handedness, 167
Headache, 17
— often absent in elderly, 18
— in intracerebral haemorrhage, 236
Heart block and acute confusional
symptoms, 231
Hemianopia, 43–4
— in Gerstmann's syndrome, 184
— and parieto-occipital vascular
accidents, 230
— and spatial disorientation, 175
— and visual inattention, 45

Hemiplegia, 49–50
— and agraphia, 148
— and disturbances of body awareness, 195
— due to intracerebral haemorrhage,
236
— sudden onset of with coma, 51
Hepatic failure, 31
— E.E.G. in recognition of, 254
— and ideomotor apraxia, 212
— mental symptoms early sign of, 32,
234
— treatment of, 272
Hepatic foetor, 32
Huntington's chorea, 53, 248
Hypertension, systemic, 34
— and carotico-vertebral atheroma,
34, 235
— effect of reducing blood pressure,
34, 232
Hypoglycaemia: from overdosage with
insulin, 25, 232
— idiopathic, 233
Hypoparathyroidism, idiopathic, 233–
234
Hypothyroidism, 28
Hysteria, 222–3

Ideatory apraxia, 211
Ideomotor apraxia, 87, 127, 139, 208,
211
— in recent toxic and global affections, 212, 246
— transient after fits, 246
— with visual agnosia, 208
Incoherence, 142, 153
Incontinence of urine, 64, 258
Insight, 69
— and catastrophic reactions, 241
— and constructional apraxia, 218
— defective in paraphasics, 79
— retained in cerebral arteriosclerosis,
240
Insomnia in the elderly, 269
Intellectual deterioration, 66–8
— and aphasia, 76
— and disorientation, 174
— and mind blindness, 203

Jâmais vue effects in chronic amnesia,
126
Jargon aphasia, 78, 142, 153

Korsakoff's syndrome, 104, 113
— with 3rd ventricle tumour, 94, 121

Learning ability, 67, 71, 72
Liver disease, 29, 31, 32

Memory impairment, 111–30
— anatomical regions concerned in,
113, 114
— due to indifference, 128
— duration of and aetiology, 121
— in focal and diffuse lesions, 242
— hysterical, 222, 224
— for names, 127
— for recent events, 124
— retrograde, 105
— tests for, 72
— for temporal sequences, 125
— for topographic detail, 126, 175
— in visual agnosia, 209
— in women and men, 116
Meningiomas: simulating dementia,
120
— in elderly with absence of headache
and papilloedema, 18
— parietal and wasting of hand, 50
Migraine simulated by carotid occlusion, 52
Mind blindness, 46, 127, 202, 203
Misoplegia, 197, 199
Mood, changes in, 10, 69, 104, 218,
239–42
Motor neglect in parietal disease, 50
Motor weakness:
— in arms, tests for, 49
— ipsilateral in leg with frontal
meningioma, 50
— pronator sign, 50
— recurring, due to carotid occlusion,
52
Muscular wasting in parietal disease,
50
Myxoedema, 28
— as cause of acute confusional
symptoms, 233

Nystagmus, optokinetic in hemianopia, 43, 184

Occupational therapy, 275–7
Ocular movements, 48
— in cortical blindness, 207
— deranged in visual inattention, 161
Ophthalmodynamometry, 36, 256
Organic mental states in later life,
237–47
— aetiology of, 2
— age and sex distribution, 2
— agnosia and apraxia in, 204

Orientation, 173

Papilloedema, 43
— absent in elderly subjects, 238
— in cranial arteritis, 46
Paraphasia, 79, 138–9
— of expression, 144
Parietal acalculia, 218
Parkinsonism, 30
Performances, variability of in inorganic mental states, 11, 239
Periphrasis, 79, 138
Perseveration, 100–1
— in aphasia, 79, 80, 141, 160
— in drawing, 87
— and paraphasia, 138
— in speech alone, 142, 244
— in topographic memory loss, 127
Personality and temperament, 25, 239
— in affective disorders, 225
— perfectionist drives and denial syndromes, 197
— in psychoneurosis, 221
Personification of hemiplegic limb, 199
Pick's disease, 2, 119, 240, 251
Picture agnosia, 107, 126, 209
— tests for, 86–7
Pineal shift, 255
Prosopagnosia, 174, 246
Protein low diet in hepatic failure, 32
Pseudo-athetosis, 55
Psychogenetic factors, 231–2
— false, 222
— in organic brain disease, 24
Psychoneurosis, 221–4
— behaviour in, 222, 223
— differentiation from affective disorders, 225, 226
— exciting causes of, 222
— post-traumatic neurosis, 223, 224
Psychosis, acute, 227–35
— anoxic, 230
— due to carotid stenosis, 236
— and endocrine disorders, 233
— and fat embolism, 229
— hallucinations in, 228
— due to hypoglycaemia, 232
— due to intercurrent infection, 234
— post-traumatic, 229
— due to vitamin deficiency, 232
Ptosis, 48

Radiography of skull, 255–9
— air encephalography, 257
— angiography, 256

Radiography of skull, (*Contd.*)
— frontal hyperostosis in dementia, 255
— intracranial calcification, 234
— pineal calcification, 255
Reflexes, tendon: absent in old age, 63; bilateral extensor plantar responses, 237; forced grasping and groping, 64; increased jaw jerk, 63; sucking reflex, 63.
Registration, 71
— in disorientation, 105
— in dysphasia, 72, 141
— in visual agnosia, 209
Rehabilitation of brain-injured, 272, 280
— in early stages, 273
— occupational therapy in, 275
— speech therapy in, 277
Reticular formation, 95, 96, 203

Sensation, 54–63
— cortical sensory impairment, 58
— inattention or extinction, 56
— motor neglect in sensory loss, 50
Series test, 70
Sleep, disturbances of, 21, 94
Spatial orientation, 175–82
— in constructional apraxia, 219
— in patients with naming difficulties, 124
— recovery of in post-anoxic cases, 106
Speech and language disorders, 132–171
— abstract topics, 140
— anatomical factors and, 75
— with antesiosly placed lesions, 243
— apraxia, oral, 137
— in differentiation of focal and diffuse lesions, 243
— dysarthria and, 136
— dysgraphia, 148
— dyslexia, an early sign of in dementia, 22
— dyslexia, literal, 162; verbal, 164
— expressive defects in, 156
— gesture and pantomime in, 244
— literary style, falling off in, 22
— names, early difficulty in recall of, 22
— naming sighted objects and from memory, 146
— paraphasia, 138, 244
— periphrasis, 138, 244
— 'push of talk', 142, 144, 244

Speech and language disorders (*Contd.*)
— receptive defects in, 157, 245
— sentences left unfinished, 244
— 'small talk', capacity for in, 244
— speechlessness in, 135, 136
— talk, spontaneous, 14
— tests for, 77
— word finding difficulties, 137
Speech therapy, 277–80
Stick tests, 88
Stratagems and evasions, 12, 122, 242
Stupor, 99
Subacute combined degeneration, 32
Surgical operations in elderly, 25, 268
Symptoms of intellectual deterioration, duration of, 16

Tactile agnosia, 204
Tactile inattention, 56
Thalamus, lesions of: and constructional apraxia, 218; literal dyslexia and expressive aphasia, 164
Thought content, 14
Time, telling the, 218
Tiredness, due to loss of initiative, 21
Tone of muscle increased in dementia, 119
Trauma, cerebral, 25, 120, 124, 174, 280

Treatment, 261–81
— cerebral vascular disease, 267
— general paralysis of the insane, 265
— hepatic encephalopathy, 272
— post-anoxic and traumatic encephalopathy, 264
— rehabilitation of brain-injured, 272
— space-occupying lesions, 261
Tremor, 48, 52
Tumour, cerebral, 5, 17, 18, 29, 43, 49, 64, 118
— aphasia often late in appearance with, 133
— disorientation in, 174, 245
— results of operation in, 261

Urine, incontinence of, 21

Ventricle, 3rd, tumours of, 94
— simulating dementia, 121
Vertigo, recurring in temporal lobe tumour, 47
Visual agnosia, 46, 127, 202
Visual inattention, 43, 45
Vitamin deficiency, 232–3, 253
Vomiting, persistent, 38

Water intoxication, 231
Wernicke's encephalopathy, 38, 228
Writing, 148–55
— apraxia of, 154
— tests for dysgraphia, 79